Management of Bone Metastases

Vincenzo Denaro • Alberto Di Martino
Andrea Piccioli
Editors

Management of Bone Metastases

A Multidisciplinary Guide

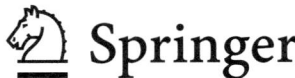

Springer

Editors
Vincenzo Denaro
Department of Orthopaedics and
Trauma Surgery
University Campus Bio-Medico of Rome
Rome
Italy

Alberto Di Martino
Department of Orthopaedics and
Trauma Surgery
University Campus Bio-Medico of Rome
Rome
Italy

Andrea Piccioli
General Direction of Health Program
National Ministry of Health of Italy
Rome
Italy

ISBN 978-3-030-08797-5   ISBN 978-3-319-73485-9   (eBook)
https://doi.org/10.1007/978-3-319-73485-9

Printed on acid-free paper

This Springer imprint is published by the registered company Springer International Publishing AG part of Springer Nature
The registered company address is: Gewerbestrasse 11, 6330 Cham, Switzerland

Foreword

Improving the success of anticancer therapies in recent decades has led to a marked prolongation of survival in patients suffering from cancer even in advanced disease. In this extended survival, many patients face persistent lesions or recurrences at the original or distant sites, and the skeleton as a whole is the third most frequent organ affected by distal metastases after the lungs and liver. Bone involvement frequently and seriously affects the life of the patients since it can cause severe pain and functional impairments; in addition, cancer therapy itself can alter bone composition. There is a need of therapies aimed at least at managing these aspects even when an effect on survival is not expected. It is also a public health matter since the burden of disease associated with bone metastases affects a wide population of cancer patients and consumes a relevant amount of health system resources; therefore, the selection of alternative therapeutic options should be based on solid knowledge. This manual provides an updated overview on the management of bone metastases, which is also clear and comprehensive, proposing an integrated multidisciplinary approach which is being more and more deemed as the most appropriate in many neoplastic diseases. The book covers several aspects of what is known about bone metastasis including basic science, *e.g.*, bone physiology and mechanisms determining homing and growth of tumor cells. Chapters address the different types of therapies, drugs, surgery, and physical agents, and also rehabilitation and possible complications are not neglected. Considerable attention is paid to the process of therapeutic decision, which is particularly important and complex in this field where most of the cases are not treated with curative intent but rather to limit the symptoms of the evolving disease and to ensure a better quality of the residual life. This book provides a description of evidence available, decisional algorithms, and software to assist in the complex path of clinical decision which has to be taken at an individualized level, considering clinical status and expected survival to balance the impact of therapies and benefits expected. Much attention is dedicated to orthopedic surgery, which has a key role in the management of bone metastases with several possible solutions and materials extensively described in the book. As it would be expected, several authors from well-known centers contributed to write a manual dealing with such a broad range of topics.

In conclusion, the editors make available to oncologists in general and to those specialized in the treatment of cancer bone metastases a valuable tool to assist them in the clinical management of such conditions.

Walter Ricciardi
President of the
Italian National Institute of Health
Rome, Italy

Preface

It has been estimated by AIRTUM (Italian Association of Cancer Registries) that there have been about 369,000 new diagnoses of cancer in Italy in 2017, approximately 192,000 males and 177,000 females. Overall, there are 1000 new diagnoses of cancer every day. These data are in line with those of the American Cancer Society (ACS), which estimates an incidence of 1.7 million new cases of cancer, half of which are prone to develop bone metastases. Despite the increased incidence, an increase in the survival of these patients has been observed in the last few years. According to the ACS, the 5-year overall survival of cancer patients has improved from 49% in the years 1975–1977 to 69% in the period 2006–2012. This outstanding result is due to the improvement in the integrated approach to the cancer patient.

Bone is the most common site for metastasis, mainly because of the contribution of breast and prostate cancers, which in postmortem examinations have showed a 70% prevalence of metastatic bone disease. However, bone metastases may occur in a wide variety of bone malignancies, with considerable morbidity and complex demands on healthcare resources. On the basis of the data of the Medical Expenditure Panel Survey (MEPS), the agency for healthcare research and quality estimated that the direct medical costs for cancer in the USA in 2014 were 87.8 billion dollars. Fifty-eight percent of those costs were for hospital outpatient or office-based visits and 27% were for inpatient hospital stays.

In fact, even though most cases of bone metastases are asymptomatic, these can cause pain and are complicated by the so-called skeletal-related events (SRE), which include pathologic fractures and impending fractures, spinal cord compression, and hypercalcemia. Therefore, the occurrence of a skeletal metastasis represents a severe event which negatively affects the prognosis of the cancer patient, above all if the lesion requires surgery. On average, a patient with metastatic disease will experience SREs once every 3 to 6 months, usually clustering around periods of progression of the disease, and becoming more frequent as the disease becomes more extensive. Moreover, occurrence of SREs is associated with an increase in the frequency of invasive procedures and in the number of outpatient and daycare visits of the oncologic patient.

This book aims to develop awareness of the need for an integrated approach to patients affected by bone metastases, by presenting major advances in medical, surgical, and radiological interventions for patients with metastatic cancer to the bone. Moreover, the approach to the cancer patient in terms of characterization of the patient's disease is fully discussed. The book consists of five parts, different in terms of contents and perspective with respect to the management of the bone cancer patient.

Part I is entitled "biology of bone metastases" and is devoted to the characterization of the pathology of bone metastasis, and to the medical treatments available today for patients with bone metastases, including bone modifying agents and anticancer agents with bone effects, and the bone-targeted therapies used in the adjuvant setting.

Part II is devoted to the "approach to the patients" affected by bone metastases, by giving guidelines to the clinician on how to characterize the single patient affected by bone metastases. In particular, some of the most difficult challenges for clinicians, like the determination of the patient's survival and the risk of fractures of bone lesions (the so-called impending fractures), are presented in a complete fashion. These issues influence most of the current work of oncologists, clinicians, and surgeons and represent the main issues in the care of the oncologic patient with metastatic disease to the bone. Current standards of radiation therapy to the long bones, pelvis, and spine are presented here indicating how this kind of treatment is currently crucial to the management of bone cancer patients. Finally, the guidelines of treatment of patients with metastases to the different bone segment (namely spine, long bone, and pelvis) are provided in separate chapters. We are extremely proud of this work, since it reflects the efforts of the Italian Orthopaedic Society (SIOT) Bone Metastases Study Group that in the last few years has drawn simple and reproducible criteria for decision-making in the clinical setting of the bone metastatic patient.

Part III deals with the surgical management of patients with bone metastases. In the last few years the development of newer instrumentation systems and biomaterials, together with less aggressive anesthesiological care, is reflected in more targeted surgery, and when possible with more aggressive surgery, even in the metastatic patient. This makes sense thinking of the increased survival time after surgery of the patients with metastases to the bone; therefore the implants and surgical techniques should be targeted to anatomical location, type of tumors, sensitivity to radiation, and adjuvant therapies, and above all to patients' survival. Many chapters are dedicated to the complications more commonly associated with these surgical interventions. In particular, infections, fractures, and failures around tumor implants are among the most feared complications that can occur in these patients. Two outstanding contributions are devoted to the correct staging and preoperative planning of patients before surgery—"Think, stage, then act" is a simple but quintessential rule!—and to the common pitfalls occurring in the management of patients affected by skeletal metastases, which most often determine the final surgical results. A full chapter is dedicated to the rehabilitation of patients operated on for metastatic disease to the bone, since after the management of pain and disability, the return to function is our main aim for these patients.

Dealing with immunocompromised patients, or when the expected survival is not enough to accept the risks associated with surgical interventions, surgery is sometimes not an option for patients affected by metastases to the bone. In this context, clinicians and interventional radiologists have developed newer minimally invasive techniques to manage these patients. This is the main topic of Part IV. In this context, other techniques like electrochemotherapy have been introduced into clinical practice in controlled studies and are now available to clinicians for the management of selected patients with bone metastases.

We end this book with a look to the contemporary directions in the management of bone metastases—what's new—and to the potential future directions of this discipline. We particularly thank Prof. Capanna for his visionary contribution to this book with his chapter entitled "Future Directions," which represents a leap into the next generation of treatments for patients affected by bone metastases.

We wish to thank our contributors for the outstanding work expressed in their respective chapters. They are well-known leading specialists worldwide in the topic of metastases to the bone and osteoncology, and we trust that this textbook will represent an international reference in the field of bone metastases. We do recognize that, given the rate of advancement of the knowledge in this field, some topics will need constant revision and update. However, today this textbook represents a collection of the most current knowledge on this subject and definitely reflects the tremendous advancements in the standard care of these patients worldwide.

Rome, Italy   Vincenzo Denaro
                                                                                                              Alberto Di Martino
                                                                                                              Andrea Piccioli

Contents

About the Editors

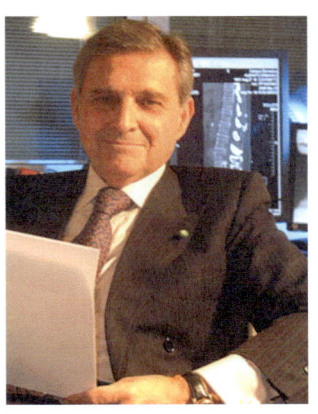

Vincenzo Denaro has been Full Professor in orthopaedic surgery and Dean at the University Campus Bio-Medico of Rome, and is one of the leading spine surgeons in Italy. His training included Professor Boni in Pavia, Professor Roy-Camille at the Hopital Pitie Salpetriere in Paris, and Prof. Macnab in Toronto. Being one of the founder members of the Cervical Spine Research Society of Europe, he has been President of the Italian Spine Society. His main fields of interest include the management of patients affected by spinal and tumour diseases. He is co-author of the National Guidelines on the management of bone metastases of the Italian Orthopaedic Society (S.I.O.T.), and of the Italian Association of Medical Oncology (A.I.O.M). He is author of more than 300 papers and book chapters, and has edited two books.

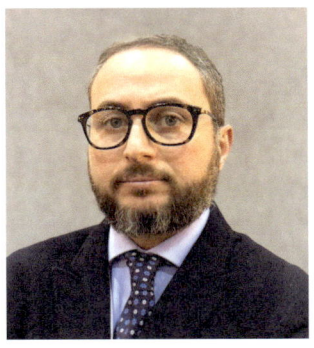

Alberto Di Martino is Assistant Professor in orthopaedics and trauma surgery at University Campus Bio-Medico of Rome. His main fields of interests include spine and tumour surgery, and basic research. He has a PhD in tissue regeneration in Orthopaedics, and is currently involved in the osteoncology unit at the University Campus Bio-Medico of Rome. His training included a Spine research fellowship at Thomas Jefferson University and the Rothman Institute of Philadelphia (USA), and is currently involved in the Spine and Oncology programs with Prof. Vincenzo Denaro at the University Campus Bio-Medico of Rome. He is the Editorial Coordinator of the Italian Orthopaedic Society Bone Metastasis Study Group of the Italian Orthopaedic Society (S.I.O.T.). He has authored more than 80 manuscripts, and is co-author of the National Guidelines on the management of bone metastases of the S.I.O.T., and of the Italian Association of Medical Oncology (A.I.O.M). He currently is board member of several leading journals in the fields of spine and orthopaedics.

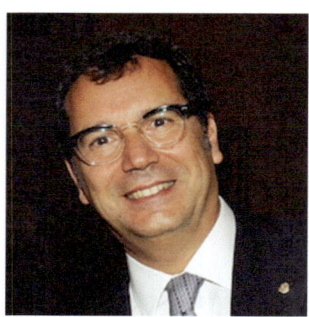

Andrea Piccioli is an orthopaedic surgeon skilled in musculoskeletal oncology, trained at the Memorial Sloan Kettering Cancer Center of New York. He is the Secretary of Italian Society of Orthopedic and Traumatology (S.I.O.T.) and the Coordinator of the Working Group on Bone Metastasis of the Italian Society. He has been Orthopaedic Oncologist Consultant in "Palazzo Baleani" of Policlinico Umberto I in Rome, and is currently member of the Scientific Committee of the "Istituto Superiore di Sanità". He is the Director of the 3rd Office for Quality, Clinical Risk and Hospital Program, General Direction of Health Program, National Ministry of Health. He is the author of several scientific papers in the field of orthopaedic oncology and traumatology, and he is also responsible for the S.I.O.T. National Guidelines on Orthopaedic oncology. His main interests are on musculoskeletal oncology, and public health.

Part I

Biology of Bone Metastases

Pathology of Bone Metastasis

Carlo Della Rocca and Claudio Di Cristofano

Abstract

Bone metastases are a frequent complication of advanced cancer. Interactions between cancer cells and marrow stromal cells and bone turnover mechanisms are crucial in metastases growth and the pathogenesis of bone damage. Metastatic tumour cells stimulate the bone remodelling and indirectly induce the osteocytes to release several growth factors that promote the proliferation of stromal, haematopoietic and neoplastic cells in a sort of vicious circle. Histological examination of bone metastasis of known origin is performed usually to define prognostic and/or predictive markers for target cancer therapy; in the 10–30% of patients in which the primary tumour is not identified, the histologic findings derived from bone biopsy could be diagnostic by morphological or immunohistochemical assessment of the neoplastic tissue.

1.1 Introduction

Bone metastases are a frequent complication occurring in patients with advanced cancer, and these are a significant problem in the management of cancer patients. Patients with bone metastases often have a poor prognosis, and it results from the systemic spread of tumour. The skeleton is the third most frequent site for metastatic carcinoma dissemination after the lung and liver, and its colonization causes significant morbidity in patients with solid tumours. The breast and prostate cancer are responsible for more than 80% of cases of bone metastases, but also haematopoietic malignancies, such as multiple myeloma, or sarcomas may develop bone metastases.

Bone metastases are often characterized as osteolytic, as in breast cancer, or osteoblastic, as in prostate cancer. Although each bone segment may be involved, the thoracic spine is the most frequently involved site, followed by the cervical and lumbosacral spine.

Pain is the most common symptom of bone metastases related to pathological fractures, microfractures or interruption of the cortical bone; more rarely it is secondary to mechanical disturbances due to deformities.

C. D. Rocca, M.D. (✉)
Department of Medical-Surgical Sciences and Biotechnologies, Sapienza University of Rome, Azienda Ospedaliera Universitaria Policlinico Umberto I, Rome, Italy
e-mail: carlo.dellarocca@uniroma1.it

C. Di Cristofano, M.D.
Pathology Unit, Department of Medical-Surgical Sciences and Biotechnologies, Sapienza University of Rome - Polo Pontino, Latina, Italy

© Springer International Publishing AG, part of Springer Nature 2019
V. Denaro et al. (eds.), *Management of Bone Metastases*, https://doi.org/10.1007/978-3-319-73485-9_1

Pathological fracture occurs in the absence of a mechanical stress sufficient to interrupt the continuity of the bone segment, but it is caused by pre-existing bone structural modifications, such as the presence of metastases.

The interest in the study of bone metastases is not only due to the high prevalence of these lesions in cancer patients but also because it is a model to study the interaction of tumour cells and the associate marrow stromal cells. Indeed, bone metastases represent the first good example of the importance of the microenvironment in metastatic spread.

The biological affinity of cancer cells for the bone is due to the high vascularization of the bone marrow; moreover the bone microenvironment produces factors that promote the survival and the proliferation of cells.

The metastatic cancer cells migrate to the bone marrow across the sinusoidal wall and proliferate and stimulate bone turnover with the development of osteolytic or osteoblastic lesions. These two radiological aspects of metastases represent the two extremes of the abnormal regulation of physiological processes involved in bone remodelling.

Under physiological conditions, the bone homeostasis requires a continuous bone remodelling to adjust its resistance according to the load to which it is subjected and to remodel its form according to mechanical stress, depositing new organic matrix and removing the worn part.

This balance between bone regeneration and degradation is guaranteed by the coupled action of osteoblasts and osteoclasts. Osteoblasts are involved directly in remodelling, secreting organic matrix components and adjusting the deposition of minerals. When the osteoblasts become trapped in the matrix and transform in osteocytes unable to proliferate, the bone formation is interrupted.

Osteoclasts are the major actors in bone resorption; they form an extracellular bone compartment where pouring hydrochloric acid, proteolytic enzymes and other proteins is required for the acidic digestion of the organic and inorganic bone matrix. Osteoblasts secrete lysosomal enzymes that degrade the calcium ions, collagen fibres, glycoproteins and proteoglycans. The action of the osteoblasts and osteoclasts depends on the systemic factors including hormones and cytokines that promote their proliferation and modulate their actions.

All types of bone metastases, characterized as osteolytic, osteoblastic or mixed, are due to osteoclast activation, and this is associated with increased serum biochemical markers of bone remodelling, such as pyridinoline (PYD) that reflects the degradation of mature collagens or bone-specific alkaline phosphatase (BALP) that is associated to bone formation.

Several studies have been performed to assess the utility of markers of bone turnover to evaluate bone metastases [1, 2] or to monitor anticancer treatment response [1, 3, 4], as well as to predict bone complications. However, the clinical practice guidelines do not recommend the use of bone turnover markers to understand the clinical data and the treatment response in metastatic patients [5–7].

1.2 Bone Turnover and Metastasis

The bone remodelling is the process whereby microscopic mature bone tissue is reabsorbed and equivalent new bone tissue is formed. The process takes place at the BMU (bone multicellular units) level. The BMU are temporary microanatomic structures with resorption of old bone by osteoclasts and by a reconstruction phase, with osteoblasts activity. The two phases are in equilibrium, and the more bone is reabsorbed, the more it will be formed. For a long time it has been believed that osteocytes were only viewer of this important process, but now it's well known that they play an important role in bone turnover control and regulation. Dendritic shape is a characteristic of osteocytes, and the dendrites are longer and more abundant in mineralized matrix close to the bone surface; moreover the number of osteocyte dendrites is inversely proportional to the cell size and activity. In the transformation of the active osteoblast in the corresponding osteocyte, dendrite proliferation is directly related to osteocyte maturation.

The network formed by osteocytes with their dendritic extensions allows to control, through chemical mediators, bone formation and resorption and haematopoiesis [8]. In this model, osteocytes "feel" the load variations in the bone and, for a sort of piezoelectric stimulus, begin to produce some factors, such as the sclerostin, that stimulate osteoblasts and osteoclasts to adapt bone microarchitecture to mechanical variations [9, 10].

Sclerostin is a protein expressed mainly by mature osteocytes (Fig. 1.1), but is not expressed in osteoblasts, and it has an inhibitory activity on Wnt-β-catenin pathway [11]. The β-catenin is involved in many processes; it plays a key role in cytoskeleton and intercellular junction stabilization. Moreover, when Wnt ligand interacts with the cell surface Frizzled receptor, the β-catenin is not degraded by proteasome, but it enters into the nucleus and acts as a nuclear transcription factor, leading to activation of genes involved in Wnt pathway. In the bone the Wnt-β-catenin signalling promotes the maturation of osteoblasts and the survival of osteocytes and indirectly inhibits osteoclastogenesis by inducing the expression of OPG by osteocytes.

In osteoclast precursors, osteoclastogenesis is a process linked to the activation of the nuclear receptor NF-kB (RANK, receptor activator of nuclear factor-kB) induced by interaction with its ligand, the RANK-L protein (ligand of receptor activator of nuclear factor-kB), produced by osteocytes [12]. However, the osteocytes also produce the osteoprotegerin (OPG) protein (Fig. 1.1) that by binding to RANK-L inhibits the interaction with RANK and consequently osteoclast differentiation. In bone tissue microenvironment, the RANK-L and OPG ratio is a key factor in the differentiation of osteoclasts and so in bone resorption [13, 14].

All these actions are summarized in Fig. 1.2.

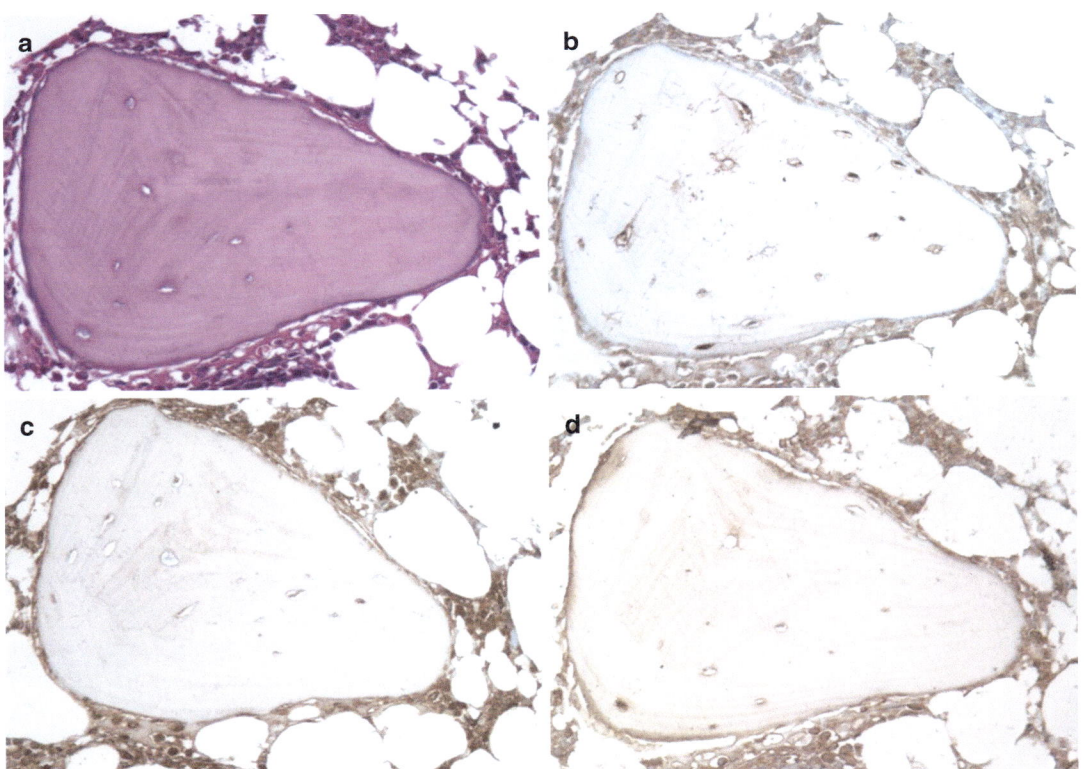

Fig. 1.1 (**a** HE 20X; **b** SOST 20X; **c** OPG 20X; **d** RANKL 20X) Sclerostin (**b**) and OPG (**c**) are clearly expressed in mature osteocytes, while RANKL (**d**) is only occasionally seen in the same cells

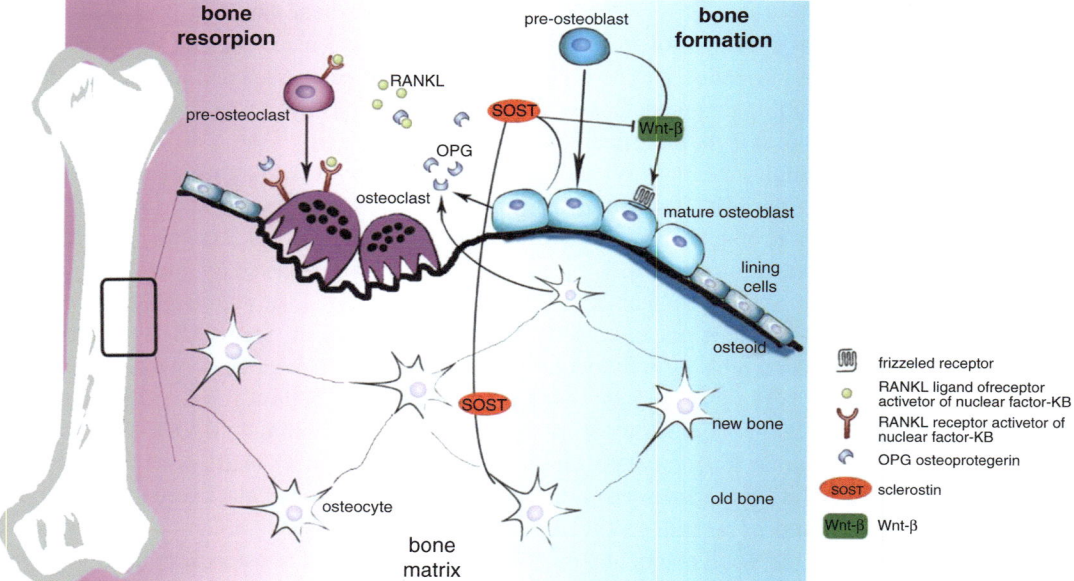

Fig. 1.2

During the development of metastasis, the malignant cells undergo genetic and epigenetic alterations that allow it to move away from the primary tumour site in order to enter into the bloodstream and eventually develop a secondary tumour at the other site. The molecular mechanisms related to the development of metastases and to the spread of circulating tumour cells (CTC) are not yet completely understood.

Through the vessels, the CTC arrive in highly vascularized bone marrow, and through the interaction with the haematopoietic cells and stromal microenvironment, they contribute to their survival. Metastatic tumour cells stimulate the osteolysis and/or proliferation of osteoblasts with bone formation. Such bone remodelling stimulus acts on the osteocytes leading to the release of several growth factors that promote the proliferation of stromal, haematopoietic and neoplastic cells.

Metastatic cancer cells, moreover, produce metalloproteases (MMPs) that degrade the matrix (type I collagen), and this stimulates the osteocytes to produce other factors, such as the sclerostin, that activate bone remodelling in a vicious circle (Fig. 1.3).

Initially, it was thought that only osteoblasts and osteoclasts were directly activated by meta-

static cancer cells, but to date it has been shown that osteocytes also are involved in bone turnover induced by cancer cell through the Wnt pathway and sclerostin secretion [15, 16]. Moreover several studies suggested that osteocytes not only play a key role in the regulation of bone marrow microenvironment [17–20] but also are involved in the proliferation of metastatic tumour cells [21, 22] through the production of cytokines and growth factors (Fig. 1.4).

1.2.1 Diagnosis of Bone Metastasis

Metastases are the most common type of secondary bone malignant tumour. Any malignant tumour can give rise to bone metastases [23–27]. In 25–30% of cases, the bone lesions may be the first manifestation of malignancy [27–29]. In the latest years, new technologies allowed an early detection of metastasis and helped to identify primary tumour site through imaging techniques and tumour marker identification [23, 27, 28, 30, 31]. Usually, histological examinations are not performed on bone metastasis of known origin. However, this was used to define prognostic and/or predictive markers for target cancer therapy (Fig. 1.5).

Fig. 1.3 (HE 20X) The intimate relationship between this bony trabecula resorption and metastatic cancer cells strongly suggests a crosstalk between bone cells and tumour cells involved in remodelling

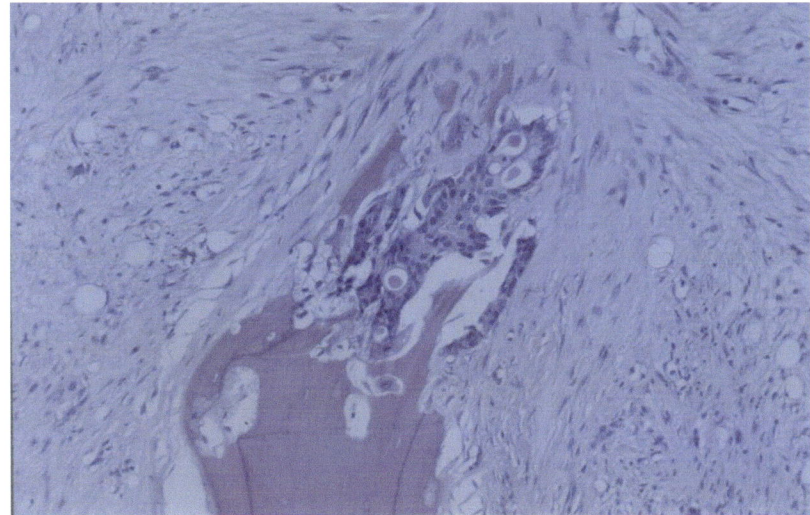

Fig. 1.4 (HE 10X) This metastatic squamous carcinoma grows up in marrow spaces permeating the bony trabeculae. Cytokines and growth factors are certainly involved in such extensive invasion without important bone destruction

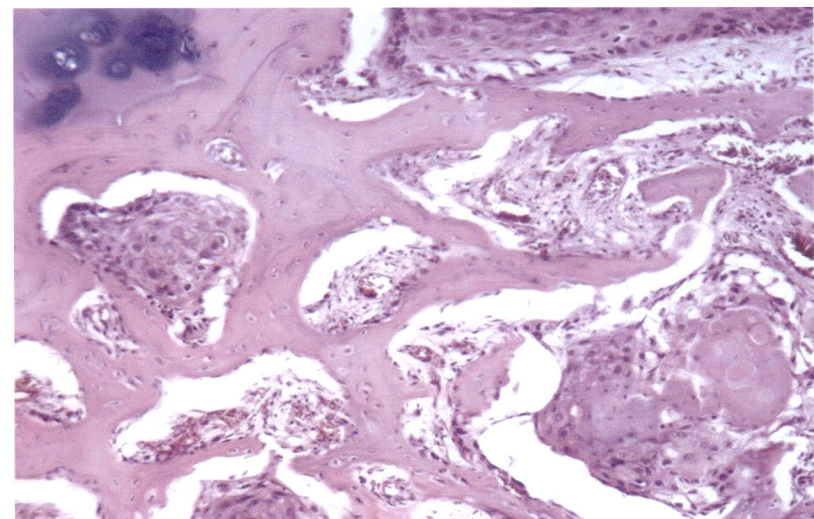

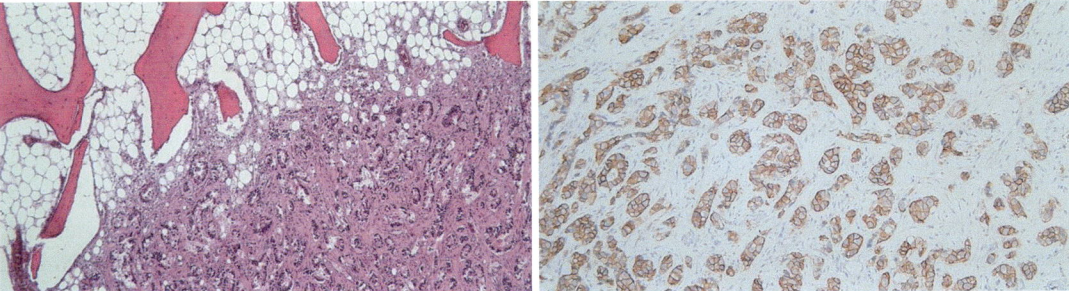

Fig. 1.5 (Left HE 20X, right Her2 40) This bone metastatic breast carcinoma is tested for Her2 expression as a predictive and prognostic indicator

Fig. 1.6 (HE 20X)
Peculiar morphology in
this case of metastatic
follicular thyroid
carcinoma allows an
easy diagnosis of the
primary location to be
performed

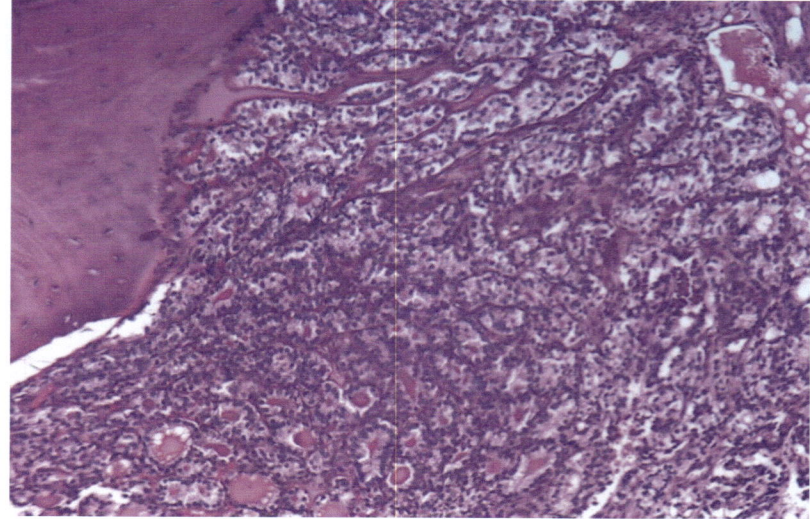

Fig. 1.7 (Oestrogen
20X)
Immunohistochemical
detection of the presence
of oestrogen receptors in
this bone metastatic
breast carcinoma allows
a diagnosis of the
primary location to be
supposed

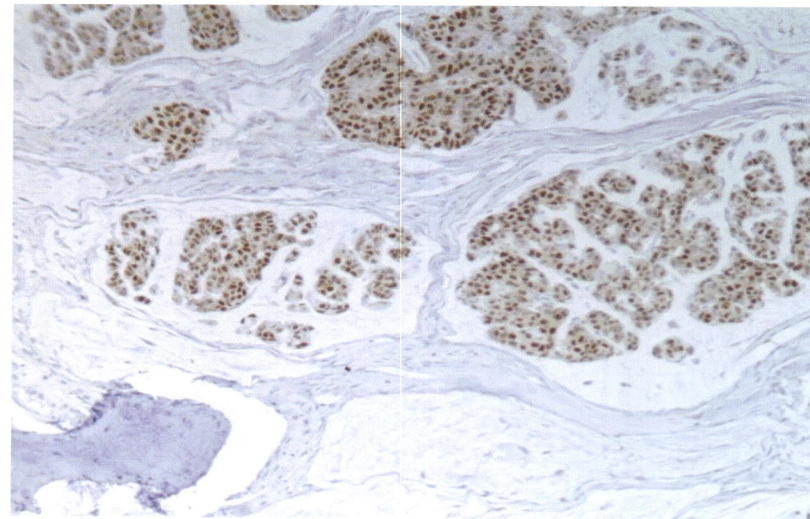

At the time of diagnosis, in 10–30% of patients with bone metastases, the primary tumour is not identified [24, 31–35]; despite clinical history, physical examinations and routine laboratory or imaging exams, the site of the primary tumour is not detected [35]. Therefore, in these cases the histologic findings derived from bone biopsy could be diagnostic (Fig. 1.6).

Sometimes, a metastatic bone lesion could have such a histological appearance of undifferentiated tumours not to allow a precise pathological classification using haematoxylin-eosin stain. Therefore, using the immunohistochemistry method (IHC) with labelled antibodies, it is possible to identify the immunophenotype of metastatic cells and to determine the origin of primary tumour [34, 36].

For example, oestrogen receptor, progesterone receptor and gross cystic disease fluid protein (GCDFP) are positive in breast carcinoma (Fig. 1.7), thyroid transcription factor-1 (TTF-1) in lung carcinoma, prostate-specific antigen (PSA) in prostatic carcinoma, renal cell carcinoma marker (RCCMA) and CD10 in renal carcinoma and thyroglobulin in thyroid carcinoma [37]. A simplified correspondence among immunohistochemical markers and possible primary tumour in bone metastasis of unknown origin is reported in Table 1.1 [38].

Table 1.1 Immunohistochemical panel in bone metastasis of unknown origin

Primary tumour	Ck	LCA	Vim.	Ck7	Ck20	TTF1	GCDFP	ER	CDX2	PSA	S100	CD56	Synap.	P63	MiTF	PSA	RCCma	Thyr	Urop	WT1
Lung carcinoma	+	−	−	+	−	+	−	−	−	−	−	−	−	+/−	−	−	−	−	−	−
Breast carcinoma	+	−	−	+	−	+	+	+	−	−	−	−	−	−	−	−	−	−	−	−
Gastrointestinal carcinoma	+	−	−	+/−	+	−	−	−	+	−	−	−	−	−	−	−	−	−	−	−
Prostate carcinoma	+	−	−	−	−	−	−	−	−	+	−	−	−	−	−	+	−	−	−	−
Melanoma	−	−	+	−	−	−	−	−	−	−	+	−	−	−	+	−	−	−	−	−
Ovarian serous carcinoma	+	−	−	+	−	−	−	+	−	−	−	−	−	−	−	−	−	−	−	+
Renal clear cell carcinoma	+	−	+	−	−	−	−	−	−	−	−	−	−	−	−	−	+	−	−	−
Thyroid carcinoma	+	−	+	+	−	−	−	−	−	−	−	−	−	−	−	−	−	+	−	−
Squamous cell carcinoma	+	−	−	−	−	−	−	−	−	−	−	−	−	+	−	−	−	−	−	−
Transitional cell carcinoma	+	−	−	+/−	+	−	−	−	−	−	−	−	−	+	−	−	−	−	+	−
Neuroendocrine carcinoma	+	−	−	−	+/−	−	−	−	−	−	−	+	+	−	−	−	−	−	−	−
Sarcoma	−	−	+	−	−	−	−	−	−	−	−	−	−	−	−	−	−	−	−	−
Lymphoma	−	+	+	−	−	−	−	−	−	−	−	−	−	−	−	−	−	−	−	−

CK pan-cytokeratin, *LCA* leukocyte common antigen, *Vim* vimentin, *TTF1* thyroid transcription factor 1, *GCD* gross cystic disease fluid protein 15, *ER* oestrogen receptor, *CDX2* caudal type homeobox 2, *MiTF* microphthalmia-associated transcription factor, *PSA* prostate-specific antigen, *Synap* Synaptophysin, *RCCma* renal cell carcinoma marker, *Thyr* thyroglobulin, *Urop* uroplakin and *WT1* Wilms tumour 1

Acknowledgements The authors are grateful to Dr. Martina Leopizzi for helping in building iconography and to Dr. Carmen Mazzitelli and Dr. Caterina Chiappetta for the critical review of the manuscript.

References

1. Stopeck AT, Lipton A, Body JJ, Steger GG, Tonkin K, de Boer RH, et al. Denosumab compared with zoledronic acid for the treatment of bone metastases in patients with advanced breast cancer: a randomized, double-blind study. J Clin Oncol. 2010;28:5132–9.
2. Fizazi K, Lipton A, Mariette X, Body JJ, Rahim Y, Gralow JR, et al. Randomized phase II trial of denosumab in patients with bone metastases from prostate cancer, breast cancer, or other neoplasms after intravenous bisphosphonates. J Clin Oncol. 2009;27:1564–71.
3. Ulrich U, Rhiem K, Schmolling J, Flaskamp C, Paffenholz I, Salzer H, et al. Cross-linked type I collagen C- and N-telopeptides in women with bone metastases from breast cancer. Arch Gynecol Obstet. 2001;264:186–90.
4. Brown JE, Cook RJ, Major P, Lipton A, Saad F, Smith M, et al. Bone turnover markers as predictors of skeletal complications in prostate cancer, lung cancer, and other solid tumors. J Natl Cancer Inst. 2005;97:59–69.
5. Coleman R, Body JJ, Aapro M, Hadji P, Herrstedt J. Bone health in cancer patients: ESMO clinical practice guidelines. Ann Oncol. 2014;25(Suppl 3):iii124–37.
6. Van Poznak CH, Temin S, Yee GC, Janjan NA, Barlow WE, Biermann JS, et al. American Society of Clinical Oncology executive summary of the clinical practice guideline update on the role of bone-modifying agents in metastatic breast cancer. J Clin Oncol. 2011;29:1221–7.
7. Parker C, Nilsson S, Heinrich D, Helle SI, O'Sullivan JM, Fossa SD, et al. Alpha emitter radium-223 and survival in metastatic prostate cancer. N Engl J Med. 2013;369:213–23.
8. Martin RB. Does osteocyte formation cause the nonlinear refilling of osteons? Bone. 2000;26:71–8.
9. Robling AG, et al. Mechanical stimulation of bone in vivo reduces osteocyte expression of Sost/sclerostin. J Biol Chem. 2008;283:5866–75.
10. Tu X, et al. Sost downregulation and local Wnt signaling are required for the osteogenic response to mechanical loading. Bone. 2012;50:209–17.
11. Leupin O, et al. Bone overgrowth-associated mutations in the LRP4 gene impair sclerostin facilitator function. J Biol Chem. 2011;286:19489–500.
12. Bellido T, Plotkin LI, Bruzzaniti A. Bone cells. In: Burr D, Allen M, editors. Basic and applied bone biology. Atlanta: Elsevier; 2014. p. 27–45.
13. Teitelbaum SL. Bone resorption by osteoclasts. Science. 2000;289:1504–8.
14. Khosla S. Minireview: the OPG/RANKL/RANK system. Endocrinology. 2001;142:5050–5.
15. Dallas SL, Prideaux M, Bonewald LF. The osteocyte: an endocrine cell and more. Endocr Rev. 2013;34:658–90.
16. Bonewald LF. The amazing osteocyte. J Bone Miner Res. 2011;26:229–38.
17. Xiong J, et al. Matrix-embedded cells control osteoclast formation. Nat Med. 2011;17:1235–41.
18. Nakashima T, et al. Evidence for osteocyte regulation of bone homeostasis through RANKL expression. Nat Med. 2011;17:1231–4.
19. Suva LJ. Sclerostin and the unloading of bone. J Bone Miner Res. 2009;24:1649–50.
20. Wijenayaka AR, et al. Sclerostin stimulates osteocyte support of osteoclast activity by a RANKL-dependent pathway. PLoS One. 2011;6:e25900.
21. Compton JT, Lee FY. A review of osteocyte function and the emerging importance of sclerostin. J Bone Joint Surg Am. 2014;96:1659–68.
22. Zhou JZ, et al. Differential impact of adenosine nucleotides released by osteocytes on breast cancer growth and bone metastasis. Oncogene. 2015;34:1831–42.
23. Vandecandelaere M, Flipo RM, Cortet B, Catanzariti L, Duquesnoy B, Delcambre B. Bone metastases revealing primary tumors. Comparison of two series separated by 30 years. Joint Bone Spine. 2004;71(3):224–9.
24. Nottebaert M, Exner GU, von Hochstetter AR, Schreiber A. Metastatic bone disease from occult carcinoma: a profile. Int Orthop. 1989;13(2):119–23.
25. Cooke KS, Kirpekar M, Abiri MM, Shreefter C. US case of the day. Skeletal metastasis from poorly differentiated carcinoma of unknown origin. Radiographics. 1997;17(2):542–4.
26. Piccioli A. Breast cancer bone metastases: an orthopedic emergency. J Orthop Traumatol. 2014;15(2):143–4.
27. Katagiri H, Takahashi M, Inagaki J, Sugiura H, Ito S, Iwata H. Determining the site of the primary cancer in patients with skeletal metastasis of unknown origin: a retrospective study. Cancer. 1999;86(3):533–7.
28. Piccioli A, Capanna R. Il trattamento delle metastasi ossee. Linee Guida S.I.O.T; 2008.
29. Wedin R, Bauer HC, Skoog L, Söderlund V, Tani E. Cytological diagnosis of skeletal lesions. Fine-needle aspiration biopsy in 110 tumours. J Bone Joint Surg Br. 2000;82(5):673–8.
30. Xu DL, Zhang XT, Wang GH, Li FB, Hu JY. Clinical features of pathological confirmed metastatic bone tumors—a report of 390 cases. Ai Zheng. 2005;24(11):1404.
31. Conroy T, Platini C, Troufleau P, Dartois D, Lupors IE, Malissard L, et al. Presentation clinique et facteur-spronostics au diagnostic de metastases osseuses. A propos de d'uneserie de 578 observations. Bull Cancer. 1993;80:S16e22.
32. Papagelopoulos P, Savvidou O, Galanis E, et al. Advances and challenges in diagnosis and management of skeletal metastases. Orthopedics. 2009;29(7):609–20.

33. Shih LY, Chen TH, Lo WH. Skeletal metastasis from occult carcinoma. J Surg Oncol. 1992;51(2):109–13.
34. Airoldi G. Cancer of unknown primary origin: utility and futility in clinical practice. Ital J Med. 2012;6:315–26.
35. Hemminki K, Riihimäki M, Sundquist K, Hemminki A. Site-specific survival rates for cancer of unknown primary according to location of metastases. Int J Cancer. 2013;133(1):182–9.
36. Bitran JD, Ultmann JE. Malignancies of undetermined primary origin. Dis Mon. 1992;38(4):213–60.
37. Oien KA, Dennis JL. Diagnostic work-up of carcinoma of unknown primary: from immunohistochemistry to molecular profiling. Ann Oncol. 2012;23(Suppl 10):271–7.
38. Simon MA, Karluk MB. Skeletal metastases of unknown origin. Diagnostic strategy for orthopedic surgeons. Clin Orthop Relat Res. 1982;166:96–103.

Bone-Modifying Agents and Anticancer Agents with Bone Effects

2

Daniele Santini, Francesco Pantano,
Michele Iuliani, Giulia Ribelli, Paolo Manca,
Bruno Vincenzi, and Giuseppe Tonini

Abstract

Bone metastases are virtually incurable resulting in significant disease morbidity, reduced quality of life, and mortality. Bone provides a unique microenvironment whose local interactions with tumor cells offer novel targets for therapeutic interventions. Increased understanding of the pathogenesis of bone disease has led to the discovery and clinical utility of bone-targeted agents other than bisphosphonates and denosumab, currently the standard of care in this setting.

In this chapter, we present the recent advances in molecular-targeted therapies focusing on therapies that inhibit bone resorption and/or stimulate bone formation and novel antitumor agents that exert significant effects on skeletal metastases, nowadays available in clinical practice or in phase of development.

2.1 Biological Background: The Bone Niche

Bone, particularly trabecular bone, is one of the most preferential metastatic target sites for malignancies such as breast, prostate, and lung cancers. Bone metastases are associated with a reduced quality of life and an increased risk of complications arising from bone weakness or deregulated calcium homeostasis. These complications (such as pathological fractures, spinal cord compression, or radiation, or surgery to the bone) are collectively defined as skeletal-related events (SREs). Additionally, the patient with metastatic bone disease frequently experiences significant pain that may be difficult to treat.

Depending on their radiographic appearance, bone metastases can be predominantly osteolytic, involving bone destruction, or osteoblastic characterized by large amounts of newly deposed woven bone. The lesion phenotype reflects the local interaction between tumor cells and the bone remodeling system [1–3].

Cross talk between tumor and bone cells, both through direct cell-cell contact and through soluble fàctors, is considered critical for the development and progression of bone metastases. Although tumor cells secrete proteolytic enzymes and can directly destroy bone matrix in vitro, the main mediators of bone destruction within a metastatic lesion are the osteoclasts (OCLs) [4]. Osteolysis activity causes the release of growth

D. Santini (✉) · F. Pantano · M. Iuliani · G. Ribelli
P. Manca · B. Vincenzi · G. Tonini
Medical Oncology Department, Campus Bio-Medico
University of Rome, Rome, Italy
e-mail: d.santini@unicampus.it

factors, stored in the bone matrix, into tumor microenvironment. These factors stimulate the growth of tumor cells and alter their phenotype, thus promoting a vicious cycle of metastasis and bone pathology. Physical factors within the bone microenvironment, including low oxygen levels, acid pH, and high extracellular calcium concentrations, may also enhance tumor growth [5]. Furthermore, there is evidence that osteolytic lesions are linked not only with increased OCL activity but also with impaired osteoblast (OBL) differentiation, activity [6, 7], and apoptosis [8]. OBL metastases are characterized by a higher OBL proliferation and bone matrix deposition associated with an increased OCL activity [9, 10]. The net result is a raise of OBL proliferation and differentiation that increases the deposition of abnormal, woven bone.

Anatomically, the bone areas most frequently colonized by disseminated tumor cells (DTCs) are the axial skeleton, including the spine, ribs, and pelvic bones. Bone stromal cells, such as osteoblasts, osteoclasts, mesenchymal stem/stromal cells (MSCs), endothelial cells, macrophages, neutrophils, lymphocytes, and hematopoietic stem/progenitor cells (HSPCs), have been shown to either expedite or impede the progression of cancer cell metastases [11, 12]. Furthermore, a series of trophic factors, cytokines, and chemokines serve as bone stroma-derived mediators that play critical roles in building the specialized bone metastatic niche. Of these known regulators, CX-chemokine ligand 12 (CXCL12), integrins, osteopontin (OPN), vascular cell adhesion molecule-1 (VCAM-1), transforming growth factor beta (TGF-β), Jagged 1, and the receptor activator of nuclear factor kappa-B ligand (RANKL) display the greatest influence in specifying the metastatic niche. Taken together, these bone marrow (BM) niche cells and factors constitute a finely organized network that promotes DTC homing, seeding, hibernation, and proliferation while facilitating the progressive breakdown of normal hematopoiesis and osteogenesis [5, 13, 14]. These tumor-stroma interactions could lead to the development of effective therapeutic agents, such as osteoclast-targeting bisphosphonates and the monoclonal antibody, which inhibits activation of the receptor activator of nuclear factor kappa-B ligand (RANKL) denosumab for controlling cancer-induced bone complications [15].

In the last two decades, the bisphosphonates and denosumab, a monoclonal antibody that inhibits activation of the receptor activator of nuclear factor kappa-B ligand (RANKL), have become established as a valuable additional approach to the range of current treatments. Multiple randomized controlled trials have clearly demonstrated that they are effective in reducing skeletal morbidity from metastatic cancer [16]. Moreover, radiopharmaceuticals are other interesting agents targeting bone metastases able to improve overall survival in patients with prostate cancer bone metastases. Finally, several molecules that are already approved as anticancer agents (such as antiandrogens, mTOR inhibitors, and c-Met inhibitors) are now in clinical evaluation for their potential beneficial effects on bone metabolism.

2.2   Bisphosphonates

Bisphosphonates are well established as successful agents for the management of osteoporosis as well as bone metastases in patients with solid cancer and multiple myeloma [17].

Bisphosphonates are analogues of pyrophosphate with a strong affinity for divalent metal ions, such as calcium ions, and for the skeleton. Indeed bisphosphonates are incorporated into the bone matrix by binding to exposed hydroxyapatite crystals that provide a barrier to osteoclast-mediated bone resorption and have direct inhibitory effects on osteoblasts. In particular, bisphosphonates are embedded in bone at active remodeling sites, released in the acidic environment of the resorption lacunae under active osteoclasts and are taken up by them. There are two classes of bisphosphonates, nonnitrogen-containing and nitrogen-containing bisphosphonates (N-BPs). The nitrogen-containing biphosphonates (alendronic, ibandronic, pamidronic, risedronic, and zoledronic acid) are more   potent   osteoclast   inhibitors   than nonnitrogen-containing bisphosphonates (e.g., clodronic, etidronic, and tiludronic acid) [18]. Moreover, nitrogen-containing bisphosphonates inhibit farnesyl pyrophosphatase, an enzyme responsible for the prenylation of GTPases that are essential for osteoclast function, structural integrity, and the prevention of apoptosis [18–20]. The inhibition of farnesyl pyrophosphatase also results in the accumulation of isopentenyl diphosphate that is incorporated into a cytotoxic nucleotide metabolite, ApppI [19]. Therefore, bisphosphonates affect osteoclast differentiation and maturation and thereby act as potent inhibitors of bone resorption. Preclinical evidence demonstrated that bisphosphonates do not affect only the bone microenvironment but have also a direct effect on macrophages, gamma delta T cells, osteoblasts, and cancer cells showing antitumor and/or antiangiogenic effects [21].

Strong evidence supports the role of bisphosphonates in the treatment of advanced breast cancer. A Cochrane Collaboration systematic review and meta-analysis of nine studies, which included 2806 patients, demonstrated that bisphosphonates decreased the SRE rate by 15% compared with placebo in women with breast cancer who had bone metastasis [22]. All bisphosphonates were effective (clodronic, pamidronic, ibandronic, and zoledronic acid) and reduced SREs by 20–40%, depending on the agent [20, 23–29]. The Cochrane Collaboration meta-analysis did not show an overall survival benefit for the use of bisphosphonates in women with breast cancer and bone metastasis. In addition, the review did not show consistent improvement in global quality of life or improvement in bone pain associated with bisphosphonate therapy. In a large randomized controlled trial that included more than 1000 patients, the effectiveness of zoledronic acid was compared with that of denosumab. This study showed the superiority of denosumab in delaying the time-to-first SRE and time-to-subsequent SREs [30]. However, overall survival, disease progression, and rate of adverse events were similar between the groups. Only a very modest improvement in health-related quality of life was noted, favoring the use of denosumab [31]. The National Comprehensive Cancer Network (NCCN), the American Society of Clinical Oncology (ASCO), and the European Society of Medical Oncology (ESMO) are consistent in recommending either zoledronic acid or denosumab [32–34].

Currently zoledronic acid is also used in men with bone metastatic prostate cancer that has progressed after initial hormone therapy. In this setting zoledronic acid reduced the frequency of SREs, prolonged median time-to-develop SREs, and decreased pain and analgesic scores [35, 36]. Moreover, zoledronic acid efficacy in preventing bone fractures was demonstrated in patients with high grade and/or locally advanced, nonmetastatic prostate adenocarcinoma receiving luteinizing hormone-releasing hormone (LHRH) agonist and radiotherapy (RT) [37].

Currently, the key question is: what is the role of zoledronic acid in hormone-sensitive prostate cancer? In the STAMPEDE trial, the addition of zoledronic acid to docetaxel did not improve survival outcomes or delay the SRE incidence [38]. In the CALGB/ALLIANCE 90202 study comparing early treatment in hormone-sensitive prostate cancer versus delayed treatment in castration-resistant prostate cancer (CRPC), no difference in SRE-free survival and no change in survival outcomes were noted. Thus, zoledronic acid did not improve SRE in hormone-sensitive disease (median time-to-first SRE was 31.9 months in the zoledronic acid group and 29.8 months in the placebo group) but showed, as previously described, benefit in SRE in castration-resistant disease [39].

2.3   Denosumab

The development and approval of denosumab, a fully monoclonal antibody against RANKL, have heralded a new era in the treatment of bone diseases by providing a potent, targeted, and reversible inhibitor of bone resorption.

The RANKL/RANK/OPG are members of the TNF and TNF-receptor superfamily and act as essential mediators of OCL formation, function, and survival. In particular, RANKL in normal process is secreted by OBLs and binds to its receptor

RANK, expressed by OCL precursors and mature OCLs stimulating bone resorption activity; at contrast osteoprotegerin (OPG), the decoy receptor for RANKL, prevents OCL activation [40]. Moreover, RANKL acts as a key paracrine effector for the mitogenic action of progesterone in mouse mammary epithelium and modulating estrogen-dependent expansion and regenerative potential of mammary stem cells [41, 42], mechanisms known to be important for mammary tumorigenesis. Murine in vivo models showed RANKL as a potent chemoattractant in tumors and supports the pro-migratory activity of RANK-expressing breast and prostate cancer cell lines; moreover in an in vivo melanoma model of bone metastases, the inhibition of RANKL results in a reduction of bone lesions and tumor burden [43]. RANKL is also expressed in some cancer cells, while in other case, cell-to-cell contact of tumor cells with OBLs enhances its expression; this contextually promotes the entry of cancer cells into the vicious cycle where the interaction with RANK-expressing OCLs stimulate their activation [43].

Recently evidences suggest an important role for RANKL/RANK in the immune system including in lymph node development, lymphocyte differentiation, dendritic cell survival, and T-cell activation and tolerance induction [44–46].

Denosumab was developed for the treatment of osteoporosis, cancer treatment-induced bone loss, bone metastases, and other skeletal pathologies mediated by OCLs. Denosumab showed superiority to zoledronic acid in delaying time-to-first SRE and time-to-first-and-subsequent SRE in bone metastatic breast cancer patients, as previously described [30]. In a castration-resistant prostate cancer patient population presenting bone metastases, the median time-to-first on-study SRE for the denosumab arm was significantly prolonged (21 months) compared to the zoledronic acid ones (17 months) with no improvements in the overall survival or progression of disease [47]. Another trial enrolled 1776 patients with myeloma-induced osteolysis and solid tumors other than breast and prostate cancers [48]. The results showed a median time-to-first on-study SRE of 21 months in the denosumab group and 16 months in the arm receiving zole-

dronic acid demonstrating a non-inferiority for denosumab versus zoledronic acid but neither a superiority after adjustment for multiple comparisons nor an advantage in the overall survival of denosumab over zoledronic acid.

Nevertheless, a post hoc analysis of these three phase III trials in patients with breast cancer [30], prostate cancer [47], or other solid tumors [48] (excluding multiple myeloma patients) showed that denosumab was superior to zoledronic acid in preventing SREs in patients with bone metastases, regardless of ECOG performance status, bone metastasis number, baseline visceral metastasis presence/absence, and urine N-telopeptide (uNTX) level [49].

In another phase III trial, 1432 men with non-metastatic castration-resistant prostate cancer were randomly assigned to denosumab or placebo. Denosumab increased the time-to-development of first bone metastasis by a median of 4.2 months compared with placebo, in a population of men deemed to be at a high risk for the development of metastatic disease. No difference in the overall survival (OS) was noted [50].

2.4   Antiandrogen Agents

Recent advances demonstrated that androgen-based pathways continue to have a clinically significant role in the progression of castrate-resistant prostate cancer (CRPC). In addition to androgen production by the adrenal gland and the testis, several enzymes involved in the synthesis of testosterone and dihydrotestosterone, including cytochrome P450 17 alpha hydroxysteroid dehydrogenase (CYP17), are highly expressed in tumor tissue [51].

Persistent androgen signaling is a validated therapeutic target in metastatic CRPC (mCRPC). Preclinical and clinical findings confirm that transition from endocrine-dependent to intracrine androgen signaling progression is a milestone in the lethal progression of prostate cancer and resistance to standard androgen deprivation therapy [52, 53]. Moreover, over the course of mCRPC progression, androgen receptor (AR) changes ensue. These include overexpression, mutation, alternative splicing, posttranslational modifications, or interactions with other pathways (nonclassical AR signaling) [54, 55].

Randomized trials that led to regulatory approval of CYP17 inhibitor, abiraterone acetate, and antiandrogen, enzalutamide, in mCRPC have also demonstrated that these drugs decreased the time-to-first SRE onset and radiological skeletal progression [56–60].

2.4.1   Abiraterone

Abiraterone acetate is an orally administered selective androgen biosynthesis inhibitor derived from the structure of pregnenolone. It potently and irreversibly inhibits both the hydroxylase and lyase activity of CYP17A with approximately 10–30-fold greater potency than ketoconazole [61] resulting in virtually undetectable serum and intratumoral androgen production in the adrenals, testes, and prostate cancer cells [62, 63]. Because adrenal inhibition of CYP17A results in blockade of glucocorticoid as well as adrenal androgen synthesis, abiraterone is co-administered with prednisone to ameliorate the secondary rise in adrenocorticotropic hormone (ACTH) that can lead to excess mineralocorticoid synthesis [64].

In phase III studies in mCRPC patients, it was demonstrated that abiraterone treatment is associated not only with a significant survival advantage in both chemotherapy-treated [64] and chemotherapy-naive patients [65] but also with a better pain control from skeletal metastases, a delay in time-to-develop SREs and in radiological skeletal progression in chemotherapy-treated patients. In this group, 25% of patients developed a skeletal event in 9.9 months when treated with abiraterone and 4.9 months with placebo, and the time-to-first SRE was 25.0 months with abiraterone compared to 20.3 months with placebo [64]. The benefits of abiraterone on metastatic bone disease may be not only secondary to a systemic control of the disease due to a direct antitumor effect but also due to a specific effect on bone microenvironment. Indeed, recently direct bone anabolic and an anti-resorptive effect of abiraterone both in vitro and in mCRPC patients was found. In particular, abiraterone was found to be able to specifically mod-

ulate OCLs and OBLs leading to direct anabolic and anti-resorptive effects both in the presence and absence of steroids, suggesting a noncanonical mechanism of action that seems to be, at least in part, androgen-independent [65].

2.4.2   Enzalutamide

Another promising oral AR inhibitor that targets multiple steps in the AR signaling pathway is enzalutamide. In the randomized phase III AFFIRM study, significant improvements in survival versus placebo were observed when enzalutamide was used as a treatment for patients with mCRPC following prior treatment with docetaxel. Additional benefits included significant delay in time-to-first SREs and improvement in several measures of pain and health-related quality of life [60]. Furthermore, in the phase III PREVAIL study evaluating enzalutamide versus placebo in patients with mCRPC, who had not received chemotherapy, the antiandrogen significantly decreased the risk of radiographic progression and death. There were also significant improvements in all secondary and prespecified exploratory endpoints, including delayed initiation of chemotherapy and a high percentage of patients with objective response compared with placebo [66]. Moreover, median time-to-first skeletal-related event was longer in the enzalutamide group than in the placebo group. Finally, treatment with enzalutamide was associated with a reduction in the risk of a first skeletal-related event, which was not dependent on bisphosphonate or denosumab use at baseline [67]. Ongoing and planned trials will help further define the optimal use of both abiraterone acetate and enzalutamide in the treatment of metastatic prostate cancer.

2.5   mTOR Inhibitors

Preclinical analyses show that mTOR pathway is involved in bone remodeling [68–74]. These effects are likely exerted via signal transduction by cytokines through the mTOR pathway, which decreases osteoclast apoptosis and promotes osteoclast survival [69, 70]. One cytokine pathway influenced by mTOR that is critical for osteoclast growth and differentiation is the RANK/osteo-protegerin pathway [69, 70, 75]. Notably, down-regulating mTOR via suppression of mTOR phosphorylation in the ST2 bone marrow-derived stromal cell line led to upregulation of osteopro-tegerin [72].

Other factors that reflect osteoclast activity may also be influenced by mTOR inhibition including cathepsin K, the main osteoclast-derived protease responsible for digesting colla-gen type I in the bone [71]. Cathepsin K mRNA expression and protein levels in human osteo-clasts decreased substantially after treatment with everolimus, an inhibitor of mTOR signaling [71]. Moreover, a study in bone marrow cells of cultured rabbit demonstrated that treatment with the mTOR inhibitor rapamycin decreased pro-duction of CTX, a bone resorption marker [69]. Finally, inhibiting mTOR in mice decreased osteoclast maturation and increased osteoclast apoptosis [69], suggesting that blocking the mTOR pathway may lead to a protective effect on the bone.

The phase III study BOLERO-2 showed a sta-tistically significant benefit in progression-free survival (PFS) adding everolimus to nonsteroidal aromatase inhibitor therapy in postmenopausal women with estrogen receptor-positive breast cancer progressing despite nonsteroidal aroma-tase inhibitor therapy [74]. Moreover an explor-atory analyses in this trial evaluating the effect of everolimus on bone marker levels and bone dis-ease progression showed a significant decrease of bone marker level at 6 months and 12 months from baseline and a reduction in bone disease progression in the combination arm (everolimus plus exemestane) [75]. As demonstrated by Gnant et al. [75], differences in the incidence of bone disease progression became evident between the treatment arms by week 12, with a lower cumula-tive incidence rate of bone disease progression for the combination arm (3.5%) versus the exemestane-only arm (6.6%) in the overall popu-lation. Bone disease progression remained nearly twofold lower in the combination arm versus the exemestane-only arm through week 30 (8.1% vs

15.0%, respectively), and similar trends contin-ued beyond 30 weeks [75]. The influence of bisphosphonate use on bone marker level changes was also examined in both treatment arms. At 12 weeks, bone marker levels were lower in the combination arm versus the exemestane-only arm and differences in changes from baseline to week 12 between treatment arms at this timepoint were larger in patients who received baseline bisphosphonates versus those who did not [75].

In a double-blind, placebo-controlled, phase II, randomized discontinuation study (RADAR) in breast cancer patients with HER2-negative breast cancer patients with bone metastases only, patients were randomized to everolimus-continuation or placebo, after being stable on 8 weeks of everolimus. Time to progression in patients with everolimus-continuation was 37.0 versus 12.6 weeks (95% CI 7.1–17.9) with pla-cebo suggesting that patients with bone metasta-ses only may retrieve long-term benefit from everolimus if they do not progress within 8 weeks of treatment [76].

Finally, in an ongoing phase II study, symp-tomatic skeletal event-free survival (SSE-FS) are evaluated in metastatic breast cancer patients treated with radium-223 dichloride in combina-tion with exemestane and everolimus versus pla-cebo in combination with exemestane and everolimus (NCT02258451).

These evidences from phase III clinical trial suggest that mTOR inhibition in combination with exemestane may have a beneficial effect on bone health in patients with bone metastases, reducing the incidence of bone metastases mor-bidity and mortality.

2.6   Radiopharmaceutical

Radiopharmaceuticals are other interesting agents targeting bone metastases; several studies showed how beta-emitting radiopharmaceuticals allow bone pain relief in mCRPC patients due to their similarity to calcium, emitting radiation when they are taken up at the site of osteoblastic activity.

Strontium-89 and samarium-153 were the first radiopharmaceuticals approved for bone metastases pain relief in patients with mCRPC [77, 78]. Although these radiopharmaceuticals are useful tool for pain palliations, no study showed impact on the overall survival, but only one randomized control trial showed that strontium-89 after six cycles of docetaxel improved clinical progression-free survival (CPFS) despite frequent hematological adverse events [79], limiting their use only in symptomatic patients with multiple bone sites.

Radium-223 is an alpha emitter that differs from beta emitter agents since it delivers a highly localized radiation to bone surface, causing double-stranded DNA breaks that lead to cell death, giving less irradiation to healthy bone marrow than beta emitters [80]. In particular it is a calcium-mimetic molecule that forms complex with hydroxyapatite, which forms 50% of the bone matrix; their linking allows radium-223 to be incorporated to the bone matrix emitting alpha particle preserving the health of bone tissue and bone marrow and limiting distribution to soft tissue [81].

Radium-223 was recently approved by FDA in men with symptomatic mCRPC with bone and no visceral metastases, presenting a significant impact on the overall survival in patients who progress with docetaxel or unfit to docetaxel. The rationale of its beneficial use as a bone target comes from several phase I and II trials that show safety and tolerability of Alpharadin, radium-223 chloride in solution, in mCRPC patients, with significant effects on bone turnover markers such as bone alkaline phosphatase (bALP) and uNTX [82, 83]. These encouraging data allowed investigators to conduct a randomized open-label, multicenter phase III trial evaluating the impact on the overall survival of radium-223 in mCRPC patients with bone metastases previously treated with docetaxel or unfit to receive docetaxel. This phase III trial was early stopped after preplanned efficacy interim analysis, since OS was significantly improved in the radium-223 arms versus placebo control arm (median, 14.0 vs 11.2 months), respectively; updated analyses in all 921 patients, performed before crossover from placebo to radium-223, showed a similar survival advantage for radium-223 treatment (median, 14.9 vs 11.3 months) [84]. Moreover radium-223 showed efficacy in all secondary end points including time-to-first symptomatic skeletal events (median, 15.6 months vs 9.8 months, respectively).

Furthermore, a prespecified subgroup analysis from this trial showed that radium-223 is effective and well tolerated irrespective of previous docetaxel use [85]. Starting from these promising results, new trials are under investigation to better understand combination therapy with docetaxel and other new emergent therapies, such as abiraterone acetate, that will improve the overall survival in this subset of patients (NCT01106352 and NCT02097303). Furthermore, several studies are also under evaluation in order to better understand the potential role of Alpharadin in patients with other cancers that have the tendency to metastasize to the bone (e.g., lung cancer, NCT 02283749).

Finally, data exist to support the co-administration of radium-223 with bisphosphonates. Indeed in ALSYMPCA, 41% of patients were on bisphosphonates at registration, and there was a clear delay in symptomatic skeletal events (SSEs) in these patients (19.6 vs 10.2 months). Although only a hypothesis-generating subset analysis, this observation suggests a possible positive interaction between radium-223 and osteoclast-targeted agents [86].

2.7 Agents Targeting Dikkopf-1/WNT Pathway

Dikkopf-1 (DKK1) is an inhibitory signal belonging to the WNT pathway. It performs a critical role in the onset of osteolytic skeletal metastases. In this setting the inhibition of OBL activity has been linked to the production of this soluble protein by tumor cells. DKK1 produced by tumor cells (breast, prostate) induces osteolytic lesions in in vivo animal models and sustains the formation of osteolytic cancer metastases. In addition elevated DKK1 levels are observed in serum of patients with multiple myelomas and in women with breast cancer metastatic to bone. Compelling evidences in humans and mice show that WNT signaling pathway increases bone mass stimulating, at least in part, OBL proliferation and activity. In particular WNT signaling acts by upregulating OPG and downregulating OBL RANKL expression [87] suggesting a mechanism by which WNT indirectly regulates osteoclastogenesis. In this axis the role of DKK1 inhibits OBL activity by blocking the action of WNT proteins on these cells [15]. Several data report that DKK1 promotes the formation of osteolytic metastases and may facilitate the conversion of osteoblastic metastases into an osteolytic phenotype. Preclinical data suggest that DKK1-neutralizing antibodies restored the bone mineral density (BMD) of the implanted myelomatous bone, increased the number of osteocalcin-expressing OBLs, and reduced the number of multinucleated tartrate-resistant acid phosphatase (TRAP)-expressing OCLs. Furthermore, the anti-DKK1-treated mice showed reduced tumor burden [15].

Treatment with a DKK-1-neutralizing antibody, BHQ880, resulted in increased osteoblast numbers and trabecular bone and inhibition of multiple myeloma cells growth in murine MM models [88]. This led to the evaluation of BHQ880 in a number of clinical trials of which the complete results have yet to be reported (NCT00741377, NCT01302886, and NCT01337752). The phase Ib trial showed that BHQ880 in combination with zoledronic acid and anti-myeloma therapy was well tolerated and demonstrated potential clinical activity in patients with relapsed/refractory multiple myeloma [89].

2.8 Agents Targeting c-MET/HGF Pathway

The receptor tyrosine kinase MET and its ligand hepatocyte growth factor (HGF) signaling pathway promote stemness phenotype, tumor growth, invasion, and metastases in several malignancies. Prominent expression of MET has been observed in primary and metastatic prostate carcinomas; in particular, it has been demonstrated that bone metastases have higher levels of expression of MET oncogene compared with lymph node metastases or primary tumors [90, 91].

Furthermore it is known that both HGF and MET are expressed by OBLs and OCLs, mediating cellular responses such as proliferation, migration, and differentiation. In OCLs, HGF and M-CSF signals, through tyrosine kinase receptors, lead to phosphorylation of common transducers and effectors such as Src, Grb2, and PI3-kinase. Additionally it has been demonstrated that HGF is able to support monocyte-OCL differentiation in the presence of RANKL as evidenced by the formation of numerous multinucleated TRAP and vitronectin receptor-positive cells which formed F-actin rings and which were capable of lacunar resorption [92]. On the other hand, HGF activates many signaling cascades in human mesenchymal stem cells, including rapid phosphorylation of ERK, p38, and AKT/PI3K, promoting OBL differentiation [93]. Moreover c-Met activation increases osteopontin (OPN) expression in human OBLs via the PI3K, Akt, c-Src, c-Jun, and AP-1 signaling pathway [94]. Interestingly, OCLs are found to synthesize and secrete biologically active HGF. These data strongly suggest the possibility of an autocrine regulation of the OCLs by HGF and a paracrine regulation of the OBLs by the HGF produced by OCLs [95].

Cabozantinib (XL184) is an orally bioavailable tyrosine kinase inhibitor with potent activity against MET and VEGF receptor 2 (VEGFR2).

In a multicenter, phase II, nonrandomized expansion study of men with CRPC, bone metastases, and disease progression despite docetaxel treatment, cabozantinib was associated with improvements in bone scans, patient-reported pain and analgesic use, measurable disease, CTCs, and bone biomarkers. The randomization was stopped because of these improvements in bone response, and a group of 31 patients had been randomly assigned. In this group, there was a marked improvement in the primary end point of progression-free survival (PFS) in patients receiving cabozantinib compared with placebo (median, 23.9 vs 5.9 weeks, respectively) [96]. Anyway in a following phase III trial (COMET-1), cabozantinib did not meet its primary end point of demonstrating a statistically significant increase in the overall survival (OS) compared to prednisone. COMET-1 yielded a median overall survival (OS) for men treated with cabozantinib of 11 months, compared with 9.8 months for the prednisone arm, which was not statically significant [97]. However, cabozantinib was associated with an improvement in bone scan responses at week 12 (42% for cabozantinib vs 3% for prednisone), in progression-free survival (median of 5.5 months in cabozantinib group vs 2.8 months in prednisone group), and with a reduction of skeletal-related event (SRE) rates (14% among patients on cabozantinib and 21% in patients on prednisone) [97]. Recently, a phase III study (METEOR) showed that cabozantinib reduced the risk of disease progression or death compared to everolimus in patients with metastatic renal cell carcinoma (RCC) [98]. Furthermore, in a prespecified analysis in the subgroup of patients with metastatic bone disease treated with cabozantinib (23%), a marked prolongation of PFS was observed (7.4 months in the cabozantinib arm vs 2.7 months in the everolimus arm). Moreover, SRE, in men who showed previous events, was observed in 15 of 91 patients (16%) in the cabozantinib arm and in 31 of 90 patients (34%) in the everolimus arm [99, 100].

Our group has previously demonstrated that cabozantinib inhibits OCL functions "directly" and "indirectly," reducing the RANKL/osteoprotegerin ratio in OBLs [101]. In particular, cabozantinib significantly inhibited OCL differentiation and bone resorption activity and downmodulated the expression of osteoclast marker genes in primary human OCLs. Differently, cabozantinib treatment had no effect on osteoblast viability or differentiation but increased osteoprotegerin mRNA and protein levels and downmodulated receptor activator of nuclear factor kappa-B ligand (RANKL) at both mRNA and protein levels.

Conclusions

Recent advances showed the important role played by adaptation of metastatic cells in the bone environment and the subsequent cross talk between tumor and host tissue, underlining their involvement in skeletal metastasis growth.

Despite the different approaches investigated to target this cross talk, up to now, only denosumab and bisphosphonates demonstrated to be a changing practice agent in delaying SRE. Moreover translational evidence seems to indicate some kind of efficacy of these compounds as direct anticancer agents. Anyway, currently, we are still far from fully understanding what really happens when disrupting the RANK/RANKL axis in the "real world," and, at the same time, we do not know which patients could benefit from this approach over and above the effects of denosumab as an antiresorptive agent.

Radium-223 is the first radiopharmaceutical with an overall survival benefit approved for the palliation of pain in patients with prostate cancer bone metastases. The significant efficacy in a hard-to-treat setting such as CRPC makes this compound worth of further exploration either in prostate cancer (hormone-sensitive setting, combination with chemotherapy or androgen deprivation therapy) or bone metastases from other solid tumors.

Recent interesting evidences demonstrated that antiandrogen molecules such as abiraterone and enzalutamide may simultaneously target prostate cancer cells and bone microenvironment. This could significantly influence future therapeutic approaches evaluating the possibility to combine antiandrogen treatment with bone-modifying agents (bisphosphonates, denosumab) in order to achieve a better disease control and management of prostate cancer bone metastases.

One of the most promising pathways, which deserves to be investigated more in detail, is mTOR signaling. Indeed the mechanisms underlying the anabolic antiresorptive effects of mTOR inhibition remain unknown as well as the biological elucidation of potential synergism with other bone target therapies.

Due to the extremely new mechanisms of the action of cabozantinib, it will be interesting to design novel clinical trials in order to investigate the activity of cabozantinib on skeletal disease-related end points and its potential synergism with standard antiresorptive agents in patients with bone metastatic solid tumors.

In the future, a more comprehensive understanding of the bone metastatic niche will facilitate the development of novel therapeutic strategies for preventing or curing otherwise fatal bone complications.

References

1. Keller ET, Zhang J, Cooper CR, et al. Prostate carcinoma skeletal metastases: cross-talk between tumor and bone. Cancer Metastasis Rev. 2001;20:333–49.
2. Mundy GR. Metastasis to bone: causes, consequences and therapeutic opportunities. Nat Rev Cancer. 2002;2:584–93.
3. Yin JJ, Pollock CB, Kelly K. Mechanisms of cancer metastasis to the bone. Cell Res. 2005;15:57–62.
4. Kozlow W, Guise TA. Breast cancer metastasis to bone: mechanisms of osteolysis and implications for therapy. J Mammary Gland Biol Neoplasia. 2005;10:169–80.
5. Kingsley LA, Fournier PG, Chirgwin JM, et al. Molecular biology of bone metastasis. Mol Cancer Ther. 2007;6:2609–17.
6. Mercer RR, Miyasaka C, Mastro AM. Metastatic breast cancer cells suppress OBL adhesion and differentiation. Clin Exp Metastasis. 2004;21:427–35.
7. Bu G, Lu W, Liu CC, et al. Breast cancer-derived Dickkopf1 inhibits OBL differentiation and osteoprotegerin expression: implication for breast cancer osteolytic bone metastases. Int J Cancer. 2008;123:1034–42.
8. Mastro AM, Gay CV, Welch DR, et al. Breast cancer cells induce OBL apoptosis: a possible contributor to bone degradation. J Cell Biochem. 2004;91:265–76.
9. Hall CL, Bafico A, Dai J, et al. Prostate cancer cells promote osteoblastic bone metastases through Wnts. Cancer Res. 2005;65:7554–60.
10. Hall CL, Kang S, MacDougald OA, et al. Role of Wnts in prostate cancer bone metastases. J Cell Biochem. 2006;97:661–72.
11. Kaplan RN, Psaila B, Lyden D. Bone marrow cells in the 'pre-metastatic niche': within bone and beyond. Cancer Metastasis Rev. 2006;25:521–9. https://doi.org/10.1007/s10555-006-9036-9.
12. Park SI, Soki FN, McCauley LK. Roles of bone marrow cells in skeletal metastases: no longer bystanders. Cancer Microenviron. 2011;4:237–46. https://doi.org/10.1007/s12307-011-0081-8.
13. Shen Y, Nilsson SK. Bone, microenvironment and hematopoiesis. Curr Opin Hematol. 2012;19:250–5. https://doi.org/10.1097/MOH.0b013e328353c714.
14. Psaila B, Lyden D. The metastatic niche: adapting the foreign soil. Nat Rev Cancer. 2009;9:285–93. https://doi.org/10.1038/nrc2621.
15. Weilbaecher KN, Guise TA, McCauley LK. Cancer to bone: a fatal attraction. Nat Rev Cancer. 2011;11:411–25.
16. Coleman RE, McCloskey EV. Bisphosphonates in oncology. Bone. 2011;49:71–6.
17. Roelofs AJ, Thompson K, Gordon S, et al. Molecular mechanisms of action of bisphosphonates: current status. Clin Cancer Res. 2006;12:6222s–30s.
18. Luckman SP, Hughes DE, Coxon FP, et al. Nitrogen-containing bisphosphonates inhibit the mevalonate pathway and prevent post-translational prenylation of GTP-binding proteins, including Ras. J Bone Miner Res. 1998;13:581–9.
19. Mönkkönen H, Auriola S, Lehenkari P, et al. A new endogenous ATP analog (ApppI) inhibits the mitochondrial adenine nucleotide translocase (ANT) and is responsible for the apoptosis induced by nitrogen-containing bisphosphonates. Br J Pharmacol. 2006;147:437–45.
20. Body JJ, Diel IJ, Lichinitzer M, et al. Oral ibandronate reduces the risk of skeletal complications in breast cancer patients with metastatic bone disease: results from two randomised, placebo-controlled phase III studies. Br J Cancer. 2004;90:1133–7.
21. Coleman R, Gnant M, Morgan G, et al. Effects of bone-targeted agents on cancer progression and mortality. J Natl Cancer Inst. 2012;104:1059–67.
22. Wong MH, Stockler MR, Pavlakis N. Bisphosphonates and other bone agents for breast cancer. Cochrane Database Syst Rev. 2012;2:CD003474.
23. Kohno N, Aogi K, Minami H, et al. Zoledronic acid significantly reduces skeletal complications compared with placebo in Japanese women with bone metastases from breast cancer: a randomized, placebo-controlled trial. J Clin Oncol. 2005;23:3314–21.
24. Lipton A, Theriault RL, Hortobagyi GN, et al. Pamidronate prevents skeletal complications and is effective palliative treatment in women with breast carcinoma and osteolytic bone metastases: long term follow-up of two randomized, placebo-controlled trials. Cancer. 2000;88:1082–90.
25. Body JJ, Diel IJ, Lichinitser MR, et al. Intravenous ibandronate reduces the incidence of skeletal com-

plications in patients with breast cancer and bone metastases. Ann Oncol. 2003;14:1399–405.

26. Heras P, Kritikos K, Hatzopoulos A, Georgopoulou AP. Efficacy of ibandronate for the treatment of skeletal events in patients with metastatic breast cancer. Eur J Cancer Care (Engl). 2009;18:653–6.

27. Kristensen B, Ejlertsen B, Groenvold M, et al. Oral clodronate in breast cancer patients with bone metastases: a randomized study. J Intern Med. 1999;246:67–74.

28. Paterson AH, Powles TJ, Kanis JA, et al. Double-blind controlled trial of oral clodronate in patients with bone metastases from breast cancer. J Clin Oncol. 1993;11:59–65.

29. Tubiana-Hulin M, Beuzeboc P, Mauriac L, et al. Double-blinded controlled study comparing clodronate versus placebo in patients with breast cancer bone metastases. Bull Cancer. 2001;88:701–7.

30. Stopeck AT, Lipton A, Body JJ, et al. Denosumab compared with zoledronic acid for the treatment of bone metastases in patients with advanced breast cancer: a randomized, double-blind study. J Clin Oncol. 2010;28:5132–9.

31. Martin M, Bell R, Bourgeois H, et al. Bone-related complications and quality of life in advanced breast cancer: results from a randomized phase III trial of denosumab versus zoledronic acid. Clin Cancer Res. 2012;18:4841–9.

32. Van Poznak CH, Von Roenn JH, Temin S. American Society of Clinical Oncology clinical practice guideline update: recommendations on the role of bone-modifying agents in metastatic breast cancer. J Oncol Pract. 2011;7:117–21.

33. Coleman R, Body JJ, Aapro M, et al. Bone health in cancer patients: ESMO clinical practice guidelines. Ann Oncol. 2014;25(suppl 3):iii124–i37.

34. Gralow JR, Biermann JS, Farooki A, et al. NCCN Task Force report: bone health in cancer care. J Natl Compr Cancer Netw. 2013;11(suppl 3):S1–50. quiz S51

35. Saad F, Gleason DM, Murray R, et al. A randomized, placebo-controlled trial of zoledronic acid in patients with hormone refractory metastatic prostate carcinoma. J Natl Cancer Inst. 2002;94(19):1458–68.

36. Saad F, Gleason DM, Murray R, et al. Long term efficacy of zoledronic acid for the prevention of skeletal complications in patients with metastatic hormone refractory prostate carcinoma. J Natl Cancer Inst. 2004;96(11):879–82.

37. Kachnic LA, Pugh SL, Tai P, Smith M, Gore E, Shah AB, Martin AG, Kim HE, Nabid A, Lawton CA. RTOG 0518: randomized phase III trial to evaluate zoledronic acid for prevention of osteoporosis and associated fractures in prostate cancer patients. Prostate Cancer Prostatic Dis. 2013;16(4):382–6. https://doi.org/10.1038/pcan.2013.35. Epub 2013 Oct 1

38. James ND, Sydes MR, Clarke NW, Mason MD, STAMPEDE investigators, et al. Addition of docetaxel, zoledronic acid, or both to first-line long-term hormone therapy in prostate cancer (STAMPEDE): survival results from an adaptive, multiarm, multistage, platform randomised controlled trial. Lancet. 2016;387:1163–77.

39. Smith MR, Halabi S, Ryan CJ, Hussain A, et al. Randomized controlled trial of early zoledronic acid in men with castration-sensitive prostate cancer and bone metastases: results of CALGB 90202 (alliance). J Clin Oncol. 2014;32(11):1143–50.

40. Liu XH, Kirschenbaum A, Yao S, et al. Cross-talk between the interleukin-6 and prostaglandin E(2) signaling systems results in enhancement of osteoclastogenesis through effects on the osteoprotegerin/receptor activator of nuclear factor-{kappa}B (RANK) ligand/RANK system. Endocrinology. 2005;146:1991–8.

41. Gonzalez-Suarez E, Jacob AP, Jones J, et al. RANK ligand mediates progestin-induced mammary epithelial proliferation and carcinogenesis. Nature. 2010;468:103–7.

42. Schramek D, Leibbrandt A, Sigl V, et al. OCL differentiation factor RANKL controls development of progestin-driven mammary cancer. Nature. 2010;468:98–102.

43. Nguyen DX, Bos PD, Massagu J. Metastasis: from dissemination to organ-specific colonization. Nat Rev Cancer. 2009;9:274–84.

44. Loser K, Mehling A, Loeser S, et al. Epidermal RANKL controls regulatory T-cell numbers via activation of dendritic cells. Nat Med. 2006;12:1372–9.

45. Akiyama T, Shimo Y, Yanai H, et al. The tumor necrosis factor family receptors RANK and CD40 cooperatively establish the thymic medullary microenvironment and self-tolerance. Immunity. 2008;29:423–37.

46. Knoop KA, Kumar N, Butler BR, et al. RANKL is necessary and sufficient to initiate development of antigen-sampling M cells in the intestinal epithelium. J Immunol. 2009;183:5738–47.

47. Fizazi K, Carducci M, Smith M, et al. Denosumab versus zoledronic acid for treatment of bone metastases in men with castration-resistant prostate cancer: a randomised, double-blind study. Lancet. 2011;377:813–22.

48. Henry DH, Costa L, Goldwasser F, et al. Randomized, double-blind study of denosumab versus zoledronic acid in the treatment of bone metastases in patients with advanced cancer (excluding breast and prostate cancer) or multiple myeloma. J Clin Oncol. 2011;29:1125–32.

49. Lipton A, Fizazi K, Stopeck AT, et al. Effect of denosumab versus zoledronic acid in preventing skeletal-related events in patients with bone metastases by baseline characteristics. Eur J Cancer. 2016;53:75–83.

50. Smith MR, Saad F, Oudard S, Shore N, et al. Denosumab and bone metastasis-free survival in men with nonmetastatic castration-resistant prostate cancer: exploratory

analyses by baseline prostate-specific antigen doubling time. J Clin Oncol. 2013;31(30):3800–6.

51. Montgomery RB, Mostaghel EA, Vessella R, et al. Maintenance of intratumoral androgens in metastatic prostate cancer: a mechanism for castration-resistant tumor growth. Cancer Res. 2008;68:4447–54.

52. Coffey K, Robson CN. Regulation of the androgen receptor by post-translational modifications. J Endocrinol. 2012;215:221–37.

53. Liu LL, Xie N, Sun S, et al. Mechanisms of the androgen receptor splicing in prostate cancer cells. Oncogene. 2014;33:3140–50.

54. Waltering KK, Urbanucci A, Visakorpi T. Androgen receptor (AR) aberrations in castration-resistant prostate cancer. Mol Cell Endocrinol. 2012;360:38–43.

55. Drake JM, Graham NA, Stoyanova T, et al. Oncogene-specific activation of tyrosine kinase networks during prostate cancer progression. Proc Natl Acad Sci U S A. 2012;109:1643–64.

56. De Bono S, Logothetis CJ, Molina A, et al. Abiraterone and increased survival in metastatic prostate cancer. N Engl J Med. 2011;364:1995–2005.

57. Scher HI, Beer TM, Higano CS, et al. Antitumour activity of MDV3100 in castration-resistant prostate cancer: a phase 1-2 study. Lancet. 2010;375:1437–46.

58. Fizazi K, Scher HI, Molina A, et al. Abiraterone acetate for treatment of metastatic castration-resistant prostate cancer: final overall survival analysis of the COU-AA-301 randomised, double-blind, placebo-controlled phase 3 study. Lancet Oncol. 2012;13:983–92.

59. Ryan CJ, Smith MR, de Bono JS, et al. Abiraterone in metastatic prostate cancer without previous chemotherapy. N Engl J Med. 2013;368:138–48.

60. Scher HI, Fizazi K, Saad F, et al. Increased survival with enzalutamide in prostate cancer after chemotherapy. N Engl J Med. 2012;367:1187–97.

61. Rowlands MG, Barrie SE, Chan F, et al. Esters of 3-pyridylacetic acid that combine potent inhibition of 17 alpha-hydroxylase/C17,20-lyase (cytochrome P45017 alpha) with resistance to esterase hydrolysis. J Med Chem. 1995;38:4191–7.

62. O'Donnell A, Judson I, Dowsett M, et al. Hormonal impact of the 17alpha-hydroxylase/C(17,20)-lyase inhibitor abiraterone acetate (CB7630) in patients with prostate cancer. Br J Cancer. 2004;90:2317–25.

63. Barrie SE, Potter GA, Goddard PM, et al. Pharmacology of novel steroidal inhibitors of cytochrome P450(17) alpha (17 alpha-hydroxylase/C17-20 lyase). J Steroid Biochem Mol Biol. 1994;50:267–73.

64. Attard G, Reid AH, Auchus RJ, et al. Clinical and biochemical consequences of CYP17A1 inhibition with abiraterone given with and without exogenous glucocorticoids in castrate men with advanced prostate cancer. J Clin Endocrinol Metab. 2012;97:507–16.

65. Iuliani M, Pantano F, Buttigliero C, et al. Biological and clinical effects of abiraterone on anti-resorptive

and anabolic activity in bone microenvironment. Oncotarget. 2015;6(14):12520–8.

66. Beer TM, Armstrong AJ, Rathkopf DE, et al. Enzalutamide in metastatic prostate cancer before chemotherapy. N Engl J Med. 2014;371:424–33.

67. Loriot Y, Miller K, Sternberg CN, et al. Effect of enzalutamide on health-related quality of life, pain, and skeletal-related events in asymptomatic and minimally symptomatic, chemotherapy-naive patients with metastatic castration-resistant prostate cancer (PREVAIL): results from a randomised, phase 3 trial. Lancet Oncol. 2015;16:509–21.

68. Moriceau G, Ory B, Mitrofan L, et al. Zoledronic acid potentiates mTOR inhibition and abolishes the resistance of osteosarcoma cells to RAD001 (everolimus): pivotal role of the prenylation process. Cancer Res. 2010;70:10329–39.

69. Glantschnig H, Fisher JE, Wesolowski G, Rodan GA, Reszka AA. M-CSF, TNF-alpha and RANK ligand promote osteoclast survival by signaling through mTOR/S6 kinase. Cell Death Differ. 2003;10:1165–77.

70. Bertoldo F, Silvestris F, Ibrahim T, et al. Targeting bone metastatic cancer: role of the mTOR pathway. Biochim Biophys Acta. 2014;1845(2):248–54.

71. Kneissel M, Luong-Nguyen NH, Baptist M, et al. Everolimus sup-presses cancellous bone loss, bone resorption, and cathepsin K expression by osteoclasts. Bone. 2004;35:1144–56.

72. Mogi M, Kondo A. Down-regulation of mTOR leads to up-regulation of osteoprotegerin in bone marrow cells. Biochem Biophys Res Commun. 2009;384:82–6.

73. Ory B, Moriceau G, Redini F, Heymann D. mTOR inhibitors(rapamycin and its derivatives) and nitrogen containing bisphosphonates: bi-functional compounds for the treatment of bone tumours. Curr Med Chem. 2007;14:1381–7.

74. Baselga J, Campone M, Piccart M, et al. Everolimus in postmenopausal hormone-receptor-positive advanced breast cancer. N Engl J Med. 2012;366:520–9.

75. Gnant M, Baselga J, Rugo HS, et al. Effect of everolimus on bone marker levels and progressive disease in bone in BOLERO-2. J Natl Cancer Inst. 2013;105:654–63.

76. Maass N, Harbeck N, Mundhenke C, et al. Everolimus as treatment for breast cancer patients with bone metastases only: results of the phase II RADAR study. J Cancer Res Clin Oncol. 2013;139:2047–56.

77. Sartor O, Reid RH, Bushnell DL, et al. Safety and efficacy of repeat administration of samarium Sm-153 lexidronam to patients with metastatic bone pain. Cancer. 2007;109:637–43.

78. Silberstein EB. Dosage and response in radiopharmaceutical therapy of painful osseous metastases. J Nucl Med. 1996;37:249–52.

79. James ND, Pirrie S, Barton D, et al. Clinical outcomes in patients with castrate-refractory prostate cancer (CRPC) metastatic to bone randomized in the

factorial TRAPEZE trial to docetaxel (D) with strontium-89 (Sr89), zoledronic acid (ZA), neither, or both (ISRCTN 12808747). ASCO meeting abstract. J Clin Oncol. 2013;31(Suppl).

80. Allen BJ. Clinical trials of targeted alpha therapy for cancer. Rev Recent Clin Trials. 2008;3:185–91.

81. Henriksen G, Breistol K, Bruland OS, et al. Significant antitumor effect from bone-seeking, alpha-particle-emitting (223)Ra demonstrated in an experimental skeletal metastases model. Cancer Res. 2002;62:3120–5.

82. Nilsson S, Franzen L, Parker C, et al. Bone-targeted radium-223 in symptomatic, hormone-refractory prostate cancer: a randomised, multicentre, placebo-controlled phase II study. Lancet Oncol. 2007;8:587–94.

83. Larsen RH, Saxtorph H, Skydsgaard M, et al. Radiotoxicity of the alpha-emitting bone-seeker 223Ra injected intravenously into mice: histology, clinical chemistry and hematology. In Vivo. 2006;20:325–31.

84. Parker C, Nilsson S, Heinrich D, et al. Alpha emitter radium-223 and survival in metastatic prostate cancer. N Engl J Med. 2013;369:213–23.

85. Hoskin P, Sartor O, O'Sullivan JM, et al. Efficacy and safety of radium-223 dichloride in patients with castration-resistant prostate cancer and symptomatic bone metastases, with or without previous docetaxel use: a prespecified subgroup analysis from the randomised, double-blind, phase 3 ALSYMPCA trial. Lancet Oncol. 2014;15:1397–406.

86. Gartrell BA, Coleman R, Efstathiou E, et al. Metastatic prostate cancer and the bone: significance and therapeutic options. Eur Urol. 2015;68(5):850–8.

87. Spencer GJ, Utting JC, Etheridge SL, et al. Wnt signalling in OBLs regulates expression of the receptor activator of NFkappaB ligand and inhibits osteoclastogenesis in vitro. J Cell Sci. 2006;119:1283–96.

88. Fulciniti M, Tassone P, Hideshima T, et al. Anti-DKK1 mAb (BHQ880) as a potential therapeutic agent for multiple myeloma. Blood. 2009;114(2):371–9.

89. Iyer SP, Beck JT, Stewart AK, et al. A phase IB multicentre dose-determination study of BHQ880 in combination with anti-myeloma therapy and zoledronic acid in patients with relapsed or refractory multiple myeloma and prior skeletal-related events. Br J Haematol. 2014;167:366–75.

90. Zhang S, Zhau HE, Osunkoya AO, et al. Vascular endothelial growth factor regulates myeloid cell leukemia-1 expression through neuropilin-1-dependent activation of c-MET signaling in human prostate cancer cells. Mol Cancer. 2010;9:9.

91. Knudsen BS, Gmyrek GA, Inra J, et al. High expression of the Met receptor in prostate cancer metastasis to bone. Urology. 2002;60:1113–7.

92. Adamopoulos IE, Xia Z, Lau YS, et al. Hepatocyte growth factor can substitute for M-CSF to support osteoclastogenesis. Biochem Biophys Res Commun. 2006;350:478–83.

93. Aenlle KK, Curtis KM, Roos BA, et al. Hepatocyte growth factor and p38 promote osteogenic differentiation of human mesenchymal stem cells. Mol Endocrinol. 2014;28:722–30.

94. Chen HT, Tsou HK, Chang CH, et al. Hepatocyte growth factor increases osteopontin expression in human OBLs through PI3K, Akt, c-Src, and AP-1 signaling pathway. PLoS One. 2012;7:e38378.

95. Grano M, Galimi F, Zambonin G, et al. Hepatocyte growth factor is a coupling factor for OCLs and OBLs in vitro. Proc Natl Acad Sci U S A. 1996;93:7644–8.

96. Smith DC, Smith MR, Sweeney C, et al. Cabozantinib in patients with advanced prostate cancer: results of a phase II randomized discontinuation trial. J Clin Oncol. 2013;31:412–9.

97. Smith MR, De Bono JS, Sternberg CN, et al. Final analysis of COMET-1: cabozantinib (Cabo) versus prednisone (Pred) in metastatic castration-resistant prostate cancer (mCRPC) patients (pts) previously treated with docetaxel (D) and abiraterone (A) and/or enzalutamide (E). In: 2015 genitourinary cancers symposium.

98. Choueiri TK, Escudier B, Powles T, Mainwaring PN, Rini BI, Donskov F, Hammers H, Hutson TE, Lee JL, Peltola K, Roth BJ, Bjarnason GA, Geczi L, et al. Cabozantinib versus everolimus in advanced renal-cell carcinoma. N Engl J Med. 2015;373:1814–23. https://doi.org/10.1056/NEJMoa1510016.

99. Santini D, Tonini G. Treatment of advanced renal-cell carcinoma. N Engl J Med. 2016;374:888–9. https://doi.org/10.1056/NEJMc1515613#SA2.

100. Motzer RJ, Escudier B, Choueiri TK. Treatment of advanced renal-cell carcinoma. N Engl J Med. 2016;374:889–90. https://doi.org/10.1056/NEJMc1515613.

101. Fioramonti M, Santini D, Iuliani M, et al. Cabozantinib targets bone microenvironment modulating human osteoclast and osteoblast functions. Oncotarget. 2017;8(12):20113–21. https://doi.org/10.18632/oncotarget.15390.

Bone-Targeted Therapies in Adjuvant Setting

3

Toni Ibrahim and Federica Recine

Abstract

Improvement in the understanding of bone disease biology has led to the development of bone-targeted agents (BTAs). The most widely used BTAs are bisphosphonates, which are inhibitors of osteoclastogenesis and osteoclast activation, and the new bone-targeted therapy, which is denosumab, an inhibitor of receptor activator of nuclear factor kappa-B ligand (RANKL).

Breast cancer and prostate cancer represent the most common cancers with a high incidence of bone metastasis in their disease clinical course and in which there are several trials investigating bone health in adjuvant setting. Furthermore, it has become clear that the bone homeostasis is fundamental for the optimal management of breast cancer and prostate cancer at any stages, to prevent skeletal fractures.

The routine clinical use of BTAs in adjuvant setting is still controversial, even though evidences showed that targeting bone-cell function can provide a potential additional approach to preventing systemic relapse as a component of standard adjuvant therapy.

Keywords

Breast cancer · Prostate cancer Bisphosphonates · Denosumab · Adjuvant therapy · Skeletal fractures · Bone health

3.1 Introduction

The normal homeostasis of the bone is a dynamic and complex process involving a balance between osteolysis mediated by osteoclasts and osteogenesis induced by osteoblasts. The bone represents the most common site of metastasis in neoplastic disease, including breast and prostate cancer. These tumours are among the most frequent malignancies in which bone metastases can have a strong clinical impact, affecting quality of life and overall survival [1].

Alterations in the bone homeostasis and metabolism, due to the presence of cancer cells, lead to a disruption of bone integrity, which can result in skeletal morbidity, identifying the so-called skeletal-related events (SREs): bone pain, pathological fractures, need for orthopaedic surgery to prevent or repair major structural damage, spinal cord compression and hypercalcaemia [2].

In addition to the effects of cancer cells in the bone, there are relevant effects on bone health induced by cancer treatments. The cancer treatment-induced bone loss (CTIBL) represents another bone condition caused by anti-tumoural agents, which is correlated to an increased bone

T. Ibrahim · F. Recine (✉)
Osteoncology and Rare Tumors Center,
Istituto Scientifico Romagnolo per lo Studio e la
Cura di Tumori (IRST) IRCCS, Meldola,
Forlì-Cesena, Italy
e-mail: federica.recine@irst.emr.it

turnover, and risk of skeletal fractures. All of these conditions are related to a considerable morbidity and negatively impact on patients' quality of life, affecting also healthcare resources [3].

The introduction of bone-targeted therapies showed to improve the clinical outcomes of patients with bone metastases, with the aim to prevent skeletal complications and to relieve bone pain; moreover these agents can have a role in the early stages of the disease to preserve the bone health [1, 4].

In the adjuvant setting, the use of bone-targeted therapies has the primary purpose to inhibit bone loss and to prevent adverse effects of cancer treatments on bone health. Ovarian suppression with luteinizing hormone-releasing hormone (LHRH) agonists and the use of aromatase inhibitors (AIs) in early breast cancer patients, as well as androgen deprivation therapy in high-risk prostate cancer patients, are the principal adjuvant therapies that can affect bone health. Chemotherapy can also have a direct negative impact on bone health. Interestingly, some evidences suggest that treatment with bone-targeted therapies can also prevent bone metastasis and also reduce recurrences outside the bone [5, 6].

In these recent years, it has become clear that the bone microenvironment plays an important role in the bone homeostasis and metastasization process. The improvement in the understanding of bone biology has led to the identification of the crosstalk between primitive and metastatic cancer cells, cellular components of the bone marrow microenvironment and bone matrix that appears to be critical for the development and progression of bone metastases [7].

In the bone microenvironment, there are several factors with autocrine and paracrine actions that keep the balance between bone resorption and new bone formation, including transforming growth factors (TGFs), insulin-like growth factors (IGFs), platelet-derived growth factors (PDGFs), tumour necrosis factors (TNFs), interleukins (ILs), receptor activator of nuclear factor kappa-B ligand (RANK-L), RANK receptor and osteoprotegerin. These factors can also act as growth tumour factors that can cause the interactions between tumour cells and bone cells, identi-

fying a vicious cycle in which tumour cells stimulate the bone cells to cause both bone destruction and bone formation. As a consequence, the bone microenvironment provides tumour cells with growth factors which cause tumour growth in bone.

In this scenario, the so-called pre-metastatic bone niche shows the unique characteristic to provide homing signals to cancer cells and to create a specific microenvironment for the colonization by the cancer cells [8–10].

Bone-targeted treatments, including bisphosphonates and denosumab, are indicated in the management of cancer patients in various settings throughout the course of the disease, including the adjuvant setting for the prevention of bone loss. They can interact with growth factors and cytokine signalling between tumour and bone cells, showing direct and indirect inhibitory effects on the vicious cycle [11].

Bisphosphonates are antiresorptive agents that inhibit specifically osteoclasts, blocking bone resorption and increasing of mineralization. They are characterized by a chemical structure of analogues of pyrophosphate, with carbon replacing the central oxygen, which promotes their binding to the mineralized bone matrix [12, 13]. There are two groups of bisphosphonates, non-nitrogen-containing and nitrogen-containing, which exhibit different effects on osteoclasts. The non-nitrogen-containing bisphosphonates are etidronate, clodronate and tiludronate, while the class of nitrogen-containing bisphosphonates, which are more potent osteoclast inhibitors, includes pamidronate, alendronate, ibandronate, risedronate and zoledronic acid.

The new bone-targeted therapy, represented by denosumab, is a fully human monoclonal antibody that specifically inhibits receptor activator of nuclear factor kappa-B ligand (RANKL) and has been demonstrated to inhibit bone destruction mediated by osteoclasts [14, 15]. RANK-L is a TNF member that is expressed by osteoblasts and is released by activated T cells. The activity of RANK-L is correlated by osteoprotegerin (OPG), another TNF family member that binds and subsequently prevents activation of its receptor,

RANK. When RANK binds to RANK-L, there is an osteoclast formation, activation and survival, stimulating the bone resorption. Denosumab received the approval by the Food and Drug Administration (FDA) in November 2010 for the prevention of SREs in patients with bone metastases from solid tumours, including those from prostate cancer.

Preclinical models suggest a potential antitumoural activity of bone-targeted therapy, with direct and indirect effects. The direct anticancer activity consists in the inhibition of tumour cell growth, induction of tumour cell apoptosis and synergistic action with anti-tumoural treatments. The indirect anticancer effect includes the inhibition of tumour migration, invasion and metastasis, but also the inhibition of angiogenesis, the stimulation of immune surveillance and the suppression of growth factors produced by the bone [16–19].

Despite a lack of regulatory approval in most healthcare systems, the routine use of bisphosphonate as part of adjuvant therapy is considerably increasing. Current guidelines underline the importance of bone health to prevent skeletal fractures in patients with early-stage breast cancer in treatment with AIs or ovarian suppression and men with prostate cancer receiving ADT and suggest the use of bone-targeted therapy to improve clinical outcomes in these cancer populations [20–24].

3.2 The Role of Bone-Targeted Therapy on Early-Stage Breast Cancer

Breast cancer is the most frequently diagnosed cancer in women, and it is the second major cause of cancer-related death [25]. Breast cancer commonly spreads to the bone and may result in skeletal complications due to bone fragility caused by an alteration in the balance of bone homeostasis with an increase of osteoclastic activation and bone resorption. Bone-targeted therapies are routinely used in the setting of bone metastasis with the aim to prevent most of the skeletal complications.

However, the role of bone-targeted therapies in the early-stage breast cancer is less defined, even though attention to the bone status represents an important issue in this setting, because of the increased risk of fracture for the bone fragility caused by anti-tumoural treatments.

The impact of bone-targeted therapies in the setting of adjuvant breast cancer has been evaluated in several randomized clinical trials, and results depend on the type of hormonal therapy and the menopausal setting [2, 24].

Adjuvant endocrine therapy is routinely used in patients with hormone-responsive early breast cancer with the aim to prevent growth of residual tumour cells and to extend patient survival. Hormonal treatments, such as LHRH analogues with tamoxifen and AIs, may affect bone health, leading to bone metabolism changes, resulting in a rapid loss of bone mass in both premenopausal and postmenopausal women with breast cancer. These alterations in the bone structure, including osteoporosis and CTIBL, can increase the incidence of skeletal fractures [26].

Ovarian suppression in premenopausal women represents a major risk of bone loss in this population, due to the almost complete elimination of circulating oestrogens, which normally maintain bone mass with a direct action to the bone. The association with LHRH agonist, which affects the hypothalamic-pituitary-gonadal axis, causing amenorrhoea, and tamoxifen seems to be correlated to a lower impairment of bone health compared to the combination with AIs [27].

Tamoxifen, which is a selective oestrogen receptor modulator (SERM), represents the most commonly adjuvant endocrine therapy in premenopausal women with hormone receptor-positive breast cancer. This drug exhibits positive and negative effects on bone, depending on the menopausal state; in the premenopausal setting, tamoxifen can lead to a bone loss, especially in combination with LHRH agents, while in postmenopausal women, it seems to have a bone-protective effects [28–31].

Two randomized trials in postmenopausal breast cancer patients showed statistically significant increases in BMD in the groups receiving tamoxifen versus placebo. In a randomized double-blind placebo-controlled trial, including 140 postmenopausal women with negative lymph nodes breast cancer, it has been shown that tamoxifen resulted in a 0.61% increase in lumbar spine BMD compared with a 1% decrease in lumbar spine BMD for placebo-treated women ($p < 0.001$). Another study, evaluating postmenopausal patients with low-risk breast cancer, demonstrated an increase of about 2% in BMD in the group treated with tamoxifen compared with a 5% decrease in BMD in the group receiving placebo ($p = 0.00074$) [32, 33].

Treatment with AIs, such as letrozole, anastrozole or exemestane, has become a standard therapy for endocrine-responsive breast cancer in high-risk premenopausal and postmenopausal patients. These drugs prevent the conversion of androgens to oestrogen by the aromatase enzyme, reducing circulating hormonal levels. It was demonstrated that in several large trials, treatment with steroidal or nonsteroidal AIs is associated with significant bone loss that is more rapid than the one associated with menopause, with a significant increased incidence of fractures. Furthermore, the AIs treatment duration is correlated to the severity of the alteration of bone turnover [34].

The anastrozole tamoxifen alone or in combination (ATAC) study in postmenopausal women with early-stage breast cancer demonstrated the superiority of AIs over tamoxifen in terms of disease-free survival (hazard ratio [HR], 0.86; $p = 0.03$) and time to disease recurrence (HR, 0.83; $p = 0.015$). In this trial anastrozole therapy was associated with a higher incidence of fractures compared to tamoxifen alone (11% versus 7.7%) [35–37].

The Intergroup Exemestane Study (IES) investigated the role of exemestane in the adjuvant treatment of postmenopausal breast cancer. In this trial patients with breast cancer after 2–3 years of adjuvant tamoxifen were randomized to continue tamoxifen to 5 years or switch to exemestane until the completion of 5 years of adjuvant treatment, showing an improvement in terms of disease-free survival (DFS) and distant recurrence-free survival (RFS) in the exemestane arm. These results were confirmed also by subsequent analysis [38–41].

Moreover, results from some real-life trials suggested that the prevalence of bone fractures can be under-reported in the pivotal hormonal studies. In particular, the ABCSG-18 trial focusing on bone health, reported that the rates of bone fractures in the placebo group were higher than in previous reports from large trials of AIs [42–44].

Similarly, chemotherapy can have detrimental effects on the bone health by the primary ovarian dysfunction, resulting in low levels of circulating oestrogens. Moreover, chemotherapy can have both direct and indirect effects on the bone microenvironment, leading to the reduction of BMD [45].

3.2.1 BTAs and Prevention of Bone Loss

Many modern guidelines and recommendations suggest that patients with breast cancer in treatment with endocrine therapy should be monitored for bone loss and considered for anti-resorptive therapies [20–24].

The assessment of BMD, which is the most important parameter in the monitoring of bone status, is performed with routine dual-energy X-ray absorptiometry scan (DXA scan) and should be integrated with the evaluation of other risk factors, such as lack of vitamin D, and lifestyle factors, including smoking and alcohol intake, and laboratory assessment to exclude secondary causes of osteoporosis [46].

The role of bone-targeted therapies, including bisphosphonates, in the adjuvant breast cancer setting has been extensively studied in large clinical trials, with doses and schedules similar to those used in osteoporosis, showing to prevent bone loss.

An intravenous therapy with zoledronic acid every 6 months, monthly oral ibandronate and weekly oral risedronate has demonstrated to prevent bone loss in patients receiving AIs therapy for postmenopausal breast cancer [47, 50].

The Austrian Breast and Colorectal Cancer Study Group trial-12 (ABCSG-12) was designed to assess the clinical efficacy of goserelin-induced ovarian suppression plus tamoxifen or anastrozole with or without zoledronic acid in 1803 early breast cancer patients. A substudy was included in the study design with the aim to evaluate the long-term effects of endocrine therapy and the concomitant zoledronic acid every 6 months on BMD, which showed significant bone loss in patients who received endocrine therapy alone, and maintenance of BMD in patients who received endocrine therapy in combination with zoledronic acid [48].

The ARIBON trial analyzed the prevention of anastrozole-induced bone loss with monthly oral Ibandronate. This trial is a double-blind, randomized, placebo-controlled study evaluated the impact of bisphosphonate treatment on BMD in high-risk patients for osteoporosis during 5 years of anastrozole therapy. Results showed that oral ibandronate was able to prevent bone loss and reduce markers of bone turnover in patients with osteopenia and osteoporosis [49, 50].

In the study of anastrozole with the bisphosphonate risedronate (SABRE), breast cancer patients in treatment with anastrozole with a T score of between −1 and −2 were randomized to receive weekly risedronate or placebo. After 2 years, BMD increased by 2.2% at the lumbar spine and by 1.8% at the hip [51].

The new bone protection option, denosumab, for postmenopausal women with early breast cancer showed to be an effective intervention to prevent skeletal fractures.

In postmenopausal osteoporosis, denosumab 60 mg was approved for use by subcutaneous injection administered every 6 months based on the results of the FREEDOM study in which denosumab reduced significantly the risk of vertebral, nonvertebral and hip fractures by 68%, 20% and 40%, respectively, compared to placebo [52].

3.2.2 BTAs and Clinical Benefit

In addition to their effects on treatment-induced bone loss, breast cancer bone-targeted treatments in the adjuvant setting also provide the potential benefit to improve the clinical outcomes with fewer relapses of metastatic disease in bone and survival. The majority of adjuvant clinical studies with BTAs in the early stage of breast cancer are summarized in Table 3.1.

Evidences of clinical benefit with bisphosphonates therapy were initially reported with clodronate, which showed to reduce relapses and to improve overall survival (OS) and disease-free survival (DFS) in high-risk breast cancer patients in association with standard therapy [53, 54].

Other clinical trials confirmed these observations, demonstrating that zoledronic acid in combination with standard adjuvant therapy can improve the clinical outcomes. In particular, the ABCSG-12 trial, reported an improvement of DFS with a 29% of reduction for recurrences in the combination group treated with endocrine therapy and zoledronic acid [55].

In the AZURE trial, 3360 patients with stage II or III breast cancer, unselected for menopausal status or hormonal receptors status, were randomized to receive standard adjuvant systemic therapy with or without zoledronic acid every 3–4 weeks for 6 cycles, then every 3–6 months, for a total of 5 years. The authors demonstrated a 25% improvement for DFS in the predefined subgroup of patients who were postmenopausal for at least 5 years before study entry [56].

Results from the ABCSG-12 and AZURE trials suggested the initial hypothesis that adjuvant bisphosphonates may have a benefit only in women with low levels of reproductive hormones, as a result of menopause or ovarian suppression therapy.

The Zometa-Femara Adjuvant Synergy Trial (ZO-FAST Trial) enrolled 301 postmenopausal patients to receive letrozole with immediate zoledronic acid 4 mg every 6 months for 5 years or delayed zoledronate, showing a 34% relative risk reduction for recurrence and a better DFS in upfront zoledronic acid arm, compared with the delaying therapy arm. These results were confirmed at a longer follow up [57, 58].

The German Adjuvant Intergroup Node-Positive (GAIN) study investigated adjuvant ibandronate, and although no differences in DFS were reported, there was a positive trend with respect to DFS in postmenopausal patients [59].

Table 3.1 Major clinical studies of bone-targeted therapies in adjuvant breast cancer setting

Clinical study	No. of patients	Hormonal status	Study design	Clinical outcomes
ABCSG12 [48]	1803	Premenopausal	Goserelin + hormonal therapy + ZA vs goserelin + hormonal therapy + placebo × 3 years	Primary end point: DFS positive Secondary endpoints: OS and RFS negative
AZURE [56]	3360	Pre- and postmenopausal	ZA every 3–4 weeks × 6 cycles then q3–6 months vs placebo × 5 years	– Primary end point: DFS negative in overall population; distant DFS positive for postmenopausal women – Secondary endpoints: BM-free survival positive; OS and IDFS negative
ZO-FAST [57, 58]	1035	Postmenopausal	Immediate ZA q6 months × 5 years, or delayed ZA	Secondary end points: DFS positive OS negative
GAIN [59]	2994	Pre- and postmenopausal	Ibandronate + dose-dense CT vs dose-dense CT + placebo × 2 years	Primary end points: OS and DSF negative
NSABP-34 [60]	3323	Pre- and postmenopausal	Adjuvant CT and/or hormonal therapy + oral clodronate vs adjuvant CT and/or hormonal therapy + placebo × 3 years	– Primary end point: DSF negative; (>50 years benefit in DSF, no in OS) – Secondary endpoints: OS, BM-free survival and RFS negative
ABCSG-18 [42]	3425	Postmenopausal	AI + denosumab 60 mg twice per year vs AI + placebo	Secondary end points: Positive DFS in tumour larger than 2 cm; ductal histology type and both ER-PR positive

OS overall survival, *DFS* disease-free survival, *IDFS* invasive disease-free survival, *RFS* recurrence-free survival, *DM* distant metastases, *BMFS* bone metastasis-free survival, *ZA* zoledronic acid, *AI* aromatase inhibitors, *CT* chemotherapy

Similar results have been shown in the National Surgical Adjuvant Breast and Bowel Project protocol B-34 (NSABP-34 Trial), in which there was a significant difference in the subgroup of patients older than 50 years of age, while the overall results did not show an outcome benefit for 3 years of oral clodronate [60].

Moreover, zoledronic acid is being investigated in the ongoing Italian multicentric HOBOE trial, which is evaluating the drug as adjuvant treatment in combination with letrozole for early breast cancer patients receiving adjuvant endocrine therapy.

Recently the meta-analysis of Early Breast Cancer Trials Collaborative Group (EBCTCG), based on individual patient data from 26 randomized trials, showed that among premenopausal women, treatment had no apparent effect on any outcome, but among 11,767 postmenopausal women, it produced highly significant reductions in recurrence (RR 0.86, 95% CI 0.78–0.94; $2p = 0.002$), distant recurrence (0.82, 0.74–0.92; $2p = 0.0003$), bone recurrence (0.72, 0.60–0.86; $2p = 0.0002$) and breast cancer mortality (0.82, 0.73–0.93; $2p = 0.002$). Even for bone recurrence, however, the heterogeneity of benefit was barely significant by menopausal status ($2p = 0.06$ for trend with menopausal status) or age ($2p = 0.03$), and it was non-significant by bisphosphonate class, treatment schedule, oestrogen receptor status, nodes, tumour grade or concomitant chemotherapy. No differences were seen in non-breast cancer mortality. Bone fractures were reduced (RR 0.85, 95% CI 0.75–0.97; $2p = 0.02$) [61].

The Southwest Oncology Group (SWOG) trial confirmed the evidence that there are not differences in disease recurrence according to different dosing schedules and type of adjuvant bisphosphonates, including oral clodronate, oral ibandronate or intravenous zoledronic acid [62].

Denosumab is also investigated in the adjuvant breast cancer population to evaluate the benefit of the anti-RANKL agent in this setting, even though there are only few reported data on disease recurrence with the use of denosumab.

Results from the randomized, double-blind, placebo-controlled ABCSG-18 trial showed that in postmenopausal patients with hormone receptor-positive early-stage breast cancer who receive adjuvant aromatase inhibitor therapy, treatment with denosumab 60 mg twice per year significantly reduced the risk of clinical fractures and disease recurrence in postmenopausal women with breast cancer receiving aromatase inhibitors. Moreover, denosumab also increased the bone mineral density at the total lumbar spine, total hip and femoral neck and reduced the incidence of new and the worsening of pre-existing vertebral fractures [42].

Moreover, denosumab is being investigated in the ongoing D-CARE trial that is evaluating the drug as adjuvant treatment for high-risk early breast cancer patients receiving neoadjuvant or adjuvant therapy (NCT01077154). Results have not yet been published at the time of this writing.

Currently, there are no trials which directly compared a bisphosphonate with denosumab for the prevention of bone fracture prevention. For this reason the choice of the bone-targeted therapy should be made considering every clinical situation and reimbursement criteria for the drugs.

3.3 Bone-Targeted Therapy on High-Risk Prostate Cancer

Prostate cancer is the most common cancer in men in industrialized countries and the second cause of cancer-related death in this population [25]. Since the seminal work of Huggins in 1940, it is known that the pathogenesis of prostate cancer (PC) is primarily driven by androgens and biochemical castration obtained with androgen deprivation therapy is the cornerstone of treatment for patients with prostate cancer [63].

Androgen deprivation therapy (ADT), which consists in bilateral orchiectomy or a luteinizing hormone-releasing hormone (LHRH) agonist or antagonist, with or without an antiandrogen, represents the standard therapy for metastatic prostate cancer that can be used also in high-risk prostate cancer patients [64–66].

High-risk prostate cancer can occur in approximately 15% of all new diagnoses [67]. The definition of high risk can vary widely, and the most significant predictive factors of disease relapse in prostate cancer include clinical tumour stage, PSA level, Gleason score and nodal status [68, 69].

ADT achieves a benefit in terms of disease-free and overall survival in various clinical settings, including adjuvant treatment in locally advanced prostate cancer patients receiving radiation therapy [65].

However, since androgens are important for the preservation of bone mass, exerting anti-apoptotic effects on osteoblasts and pro-apoptotic effects on osteoclasts, the ADT leads testosterone to castration levels ($\leq$50 ng/dL) and determines a significant reduction of BMD with a consequent increase in bone fractures risk [70].

More than 70% of men with prostate cancer are older than 65, and already at risk for osteoporosis or fragility fracture. A correlation between bone loss and increased susceptibility to metastasis was reported in prostate cancer patients, underlining the importance to preserve bone health in high-risk prostate cancer [71]. Non-metastatic prostate cancer patients in treatment with continuous or intermittent ADT can show a significant bone loss within the first 6–12 months after starting hormonal therapy [72].

Moreover, bone fragility fractures may be associated with decreased survival and quality of life in this cancer population, and with an increased mortality [73].

In a large study included more than 50,000 patients from the Surveillance, Epidemiology and End Results database, a higher number of patients receiving ADT had osteoporosis compared to the group not receiving hormonal therapy. The risk of bone fracture at 5 years in patients receiving ADT was almost double that in patients without hormone deprivation [74].

In this context, the use of bone-targeted treatments is crucial, even though no approved therapy is indicated for the reduction of the risk of fracture in prostate cancer patients. The benefit of bone-targeted therapies in prostate cancer depends on the hormone-sensitive or castration-resistant disease status.

3.3.1 Hormone-Sensitive Prostate Cancer

In a randomized placebo-controlled study, intravenous pamidronate 60 mg administered every 3 months showed to reduce bone loss over 48 weeks of treatment in men receiving leuprolide [75]. However, despite the benefit in preventing osteoporosis/CTIBL in men receiving ADT for PC, intravenous pamidronate therapy was not correlated to an improvement of BMD values [76].

Interestingly, treatment with zoledronic acid every 3–12 months is able to prevent bone loss associated with therapy and also to increase BMD compared with baseline values [77].

Two placebo-controlled studies, the PR04 and PR05 trials, evaluated oral clodronate in patients with non-metastatic and metastatic PC, respectively. Treatment with clodronate was associated with an OS benefit among men with metastatic disease compared with placebo (HR for death = 0.77, 95% CI = 0.60–0.98, p = 0.032). However, among men without metastatic disease, there was no evidence of an OS benefit with clodronate compared with placebo (HR for death = 1.12; 95% CI = 0.89–1.42, p = 0.94) [66]. These trials have reported 10-year survival rates in patients with prostate cancer with (n = 311 patients) or without metastatic disease (n = 508 patients) [78].

The multi-arm and multicentre trial conducted by the Medical Research Council called the Systemic Therapy in Advanced or Metastatic Prostate Cancer: Evaluation of Drug Efficacy (STAMPEDE) is a large trial with a multistage design. This trial evaluated several drugs in combination with hormonal therapy in patients with high-risk localized or metastatic prostate cancer with the aim to investigate whether the addition of treatments at the time of long-term hormone therapy initiation improves overall survival.

The different arms comparing several treatments include docetaxel, zoledronic acid, celecoxib, abiraterone, enzalutamide and radiotherapy (only among the patients with metastatic disease) in combination with ADT versus only ADT. Recently the results of the comparison between the addition of zoledronic acid, docetaxel, or their combination to the standard of care versus the standard of care alone have been published, showing that zoledronic acid was not correlated to survival improvement, failure-free survival and skeletal-related events, while docetaxel chemotherapy, given at starting of hormone therapy, determined a benefit in overall survival, as well as improvements in prostate-cancer-specific survival, failure-free survival and skeletal-related events. The combination of zoledronic acid and docetaxel was associated with similar improvements, with a smaller benefit. Authors concluded that zoledronic acid should not become part of the standard of care [79].

Similarly, an early treatment with zoledronic acid in metastatic setting hormone-sensitive prostate cancer showed a non-decreased risk for SREs compared with the same treatment initiated after progression to castration-resistant disease [80].

Moreover, the randomized open-label multinational Zometa European Study (ZEUS) showed that treatment with zoledronic acid every 3 months was ineffective for the prevention of bone metastases in high-risk non-metastatic patients at 4 years [81].

However, in prostate cancer the role of bisphosphonates in the prevention of bone metastasis remains undefined.

The efficacy of denosumab in patients in treatment with ADT was reported in the Denosumab HALT Prostate Cancer Study Group. In this trial, patients with non-metastatic PC receiving ADT were randomized to 60 mg of denosumab or placebo every 6 months. At 24 months, the treatment arm showed a statistically significant improvement in BMD at the total hip, the femoral neck, radium and the whole body [82].

3.3.2 Castration-Resistant Prostate Cancer (CRPC)

The majority of patients will become resistant to the initial hormonal approach with ADT, despite castrate levels of serum androgens, developing CRPC. A considerable number of patients with CRPC continue to respond to second generation hormonal treatments, suggesting the persistence of the activity of androgen receptor (AR) in the pathogenesis of prostate cancer, also during the progression of the disease.

The AR represents the principal driver of tumour growth and the most important therapeutic target in the prostate cancer [83].

There is a particular clinical condition characterized by a progressive CRPC with no evidence of bone metastases, in which higher baseline value of PSA and shorter PSA doubling time are correlated with time to the first bone metastasis and death.

The optimal management of M0 CRPC is challenging and may represent the most interesting clinical setting in which BATs can have an important impact for the prevention of bone metastases.

Among bone-targeted therapies, denosumab reported a benefit in delaying bone metastases in non-metastatic CRPC patients. Indeed, a randomized controlled trial was designed to evaluate the effects of zoledronic acid on the time to the first bone metastasis in non-metastatic CRPC patients. It was terminated before completion of accrual after interim analyses showing that the observed event occurred less frequently than expected [84].

A randomized, double-blind, placebo-controlled, phase 3 study evaluated the efficacy of denosumab in non-metastatic CRPC. Denosumab significantly increased bone metastasis-free survival by a median of 4.2 months over placebo (HR 0.85; $p = 0.028$) and delayed time to symptomatic first bone metastases, but had no impact on OS [85].

These results pointed out the importance of targeting the bone microenvironment to prevent bone metastasis in prostate cancer.

3.4 Safety Considerations

Overall, bone-targeted therapies are well tolerated, with a low incidence of adverse effects.

Adverse effects of bisphosphonates include flu-like symptoms such as fatigue, myalgia and fever, particularly with the first infusions (44%). Other adverse effects are hypocalcaemia (6%) and osteonecrosis of the jaw (ONJ) (1–2%) [86].

Zoledronic acid has been associated with renal impairment, and dose adjustments are necessary for patients with reduced renal function. In contrast to zoledronic acid, denosumab is not correlated to renal impairment, but denosumab is associated with a higher risk of hypocalcaemia [87].

During treatment with bone-targeted therapies, patients should receive an oral intake of calcium and vitamin D, and a condition of pre-existing hypocalcaemia must also be corrected before initiating therapy.

Bisphosphonates and denosumab treatments have been associated with the development of osteonecrosis of the jaw (ONJ).

The incidence of ONJ is about 1.3% when monthly intravenous somministration for bisphosphonates is used in the setting of advanced cancer, while it is less frequent with 6 monthly somministration of intravenous bisphosphonates or with oral bisphosphonates given in adjuvant setting to preserve bone health.

Nevertheless, before bisphosphonates and denosumab are initiated, it is recommended that patients undergo a dental examination, maintaining good oral hygiene and avoiding invasive dental surgical procedures while on treatment [88, 89].

Conclusion

Bone-targeted therapies, including bisphosphonates and denosumab, are important in the management of cancer patients even in adjuvant setting for the preservation of bone health. Over the past 30 years, a prolongation in survival was reported to be correlated to an improvement of diagnostic and therapeutic interventions, and the long-term effects of treatment on the skeleton have become a relevant concern and a rationale for the use of

BTAs. In addition, these therapies showed to improve clinical outcomes in patients with postmenopausal breast cancer and men with prostate cancer. The survival benefit associated with the use of adjuvant BTAs provides an important additional strategy in the treatment of early stages in breast cancer and prostate cancer.

Based on these evidences, adjuvant bisphosphonates or denosumab should be part of the standard of care, in particular for early postmenopausal breast cancer and non-metastatic CRPC.

However, the absence of adequate biomarkers and a direct comparison in clinical trials can create difficulties in the selection of patients who may benefit from a specific bone-targeted therapy.

In this context, translational and clinical research is clearly needed.

References

1. Ibrahim T, Farolfi A, Mercatali L, Ricci M, Amadori D. Metastatic bone disease in the era of bone-targeted therapy: clinical impact. Tumori. 2013;99(1):1–9.
2. Coleman RE. Risks and benefits of bisphosphonates. Br J Cancer. 2008;98(11):1736–40.
3. D'Oronzo S, Stucci S, Tucci M, Silvestris F. Cancer treatment-induced bone loss (CTIBL): pathogenesis and clinical implications. Cancer Treat Rev. 2015;41(9):798–808.
4. Brown JE, Cook RJ, Major P, Lipton A, Saad F, Smith M, Lee K-A, Zheng M, Hei Y-J, Coleman RE. Bone turnover markers as predictors of skeletal complications in prostate cancer, lung cancer, and other solid tumors. J Natl Cancer Inst. 2005;97:59–69.
5. Gnant M, Mlineritsch B, Stoeger H, et al. Zoledronic acid combined with adjuvant endocrine therapy of tamoxifen versus anastrozol plus ovarian function suppression in premenopausal early breast cancer: final analysis of the Austrian Breast and Colorectal Cancer Study Group trial 12. Ann Oncol. 2015;26:313–20.
6. Gnant M. Role of bisphosphonates in postmenopausal women with breast cancer. Cancer Treat Rev. 2014;40:476–84.
7. Yoneda T, Hiraga T. Crosstalk between cancer cells and bone microenvironment in bone metastasis. Biochem Biophys Res Commun. 2005;328(3):679–87.
8. Ibrahim T, Flamini E, Mercatali L, Sacanna E, Serra P, Amadori D. Pathogenesis of osteoblastic bone metastases from prostate cancer. Cancer. 2010;116(6):1406–18. Erratum in: Cancer. 2010 May 15;116(10):2503
9. Lories RJ, Luyten FP. Osteoprotegerin and osteoprotegerin-ligand balance: a new paradigm in bone metabolism providing new therapeutic targets. Clin Rheumatol. 2001;20:3–9.
10. Hofbauer LC, Neubader A, Heufelder AE. Receptor activator of nuclear factor-kb ligand and osteoprotegerin. Cancer. 2001;92:460–70.
11. Shapiro CL. Bisphosphonates in breast cancer patients with skeletal metastases. Hematol Oncol Clin North Am. 1994;8:153–63.
12. Rogers MJ, Gordon S, Benford HL, et al. Cellular and molecular mechanisms of action of bisphosphonates. Cancer. 2000;88:2961–78.
13. Roelofs AJ, Thompson K, Gordon S, Rogers MJ. Molecular mechanisms of action of bisphosphonates: current status. Clin Cancer Res. 2006;12:6222s–30s.
14. Bekker PJ, Holloway DL, Rasmussen AS, et al. A single-dose placebo-controlled study of AMG 162, a fully human monoclonal antibody to RANKL, in postmenopausal women. J Bone Miner Res. 2004;19:1059–66.
15. Body JJ, Facon T, Coleman RE, et al. A study of the biological receptor activator of nuclear factor-kappa B ligand inhibitor, denosumab, in patients with multiple myeloma or bone metastases from breast cancer. Clin Cancer Res. 2006;12:1221–8.
16. Fromigue O, Lagneaux L, Body JJ. Bisphosphonates induce breast cancer cell death in vitro. J Bone Miner Res. 2000;15:2211–21.
17. Senaratne SG, Pirianov G, Mansi JL, Arnett TR, Colston KW. Bisphosphonates induce apoptosis in human breast cancer cell lines. Br J Cancer. 2000;82:1459–68.
18. Verdijk R, Franke HR, Wolbers F, Vermes I. Differential effects of bisphosphonates on breast cancer cell lines. Cancer Lett. 2007;246:308–12.
19. Mercatali L, Spadazzi C, Miserocchi G, Liverani C, De Vita A, Bongiovanni A, Recine F, Amadori D, Ibrahim T. The effect of everolimus in an in vitro model of triple negative breast cancer and osteoclasts. Int J Mol Sci. 2016;17(11):E1827.
20. Associazione Italiana di Oncologia Medica (AIOM) guidelines 2016.
21. Body JJ, Bergmann P, Boonen S, et al. Management of cancer treatment-induced bone loss in early breast and prostate cancer—a consensus paper of the Belgian Bone Club. Osteoporos Int. 2007;18:1439–50.
22. Reid DM, Doughty J, Eastell R, et al. Guidance for the management of breast cancer treatment-induced bone loss: a consensus position statement from a UK Expert Group. Cancer Treat Rev. 2008;34(Suppl 1):S3–S18.
23. Lee CE, Leslie WD, Czaykowski P, et al. A comprehensive bone-health management approach for men with prostate cancer receiving androgen deprivation therapy. Curr Oncol. 2011;18:e163–72.
24. Coleman R, Body JJ, Aapro M, Hadji P, J. Herrstedt on behalf of the ESMO Guidelines Working Group Bone health in Cancer Patients. ESMO clinical prac-

tice guidelines. Ann Oncol. 2014;25(Supplement 3):iii124–37.

25. Siegel RL, Miller KD, Jemal A. Cancer statistics, 2016. CA Cancer J Clin. 2016;66(1):7–30.

26. Brufsky A. Cancer treatment-induced bone loss: pathophysiology and clinical perspectives. Oncologist. 2008;13:187–95.

27. Gnant M, et al. Adjuvant endocrine therapy plus zole-dronic acid in premenopausal women with early-stage breast cancer: 5-year follow-up of the ABCSG-12 bone-mineral density substudy. Lancet Oncol. 2008;9:840–9.

28. Hirbe A, Morgan EA, Uluçkan Ö, Weilbaecher K. Skeletal complications of breast cancer therapies. Clin Cancer Res. 2006;12(20 Pt 2):6309s–14s.

29. Cuzick J, Forbes J, Edwards R, et al. First results from the International Breast Cancer Intervention Study (IBIS-I): a randomised prevention trial. Lancet. 2002;360:817–24.

30. Cosman F. Selective estrogen-receptor modulators. Clin Geriatr Med. 2003;19:371–9.

31. Powles TJ, Hickish T, Kanis JA, Tidy A, Ashley S. Effect of tamoxifen on bone mineral density measured by dual-energy x-ray absorptiometry in healthy premenopausal and postmenopausal women. J Clin Oncol. 1996;14:78–84.

32. Love RR, Mazess RB, Barden HS, et al. Effects of tamoxifen on bone mineral density in postmeno-pausal women with breast cancer. N Engl J Med. 1992;326:852–6.

33. Kristensen B, Ejlertsen B, Dalgaard P, et al. Tamoxifen and bone metabolism in postmenopausal low-risk breast cancer patients: a randomized study. J Clin Oncol. 1994;12:992–7.

34. Eastell R, Adams JE, Coleman RE, et al. Effect of anastrozole on bone mineral density: 5-year results from the anastrozole, tamoxifen, alone or in combination trial 18233230. J Clin Oncol. 2008;26:1051–7.

35. Baum M, Buzdar A, Cuzick J, et al. Anastrozole alone or in combination with tamoxifen versus tamoxifen alone for adjuvant treatment of postmeno-pausal women with early-stage breast cancer: results of the ATAC (Arimidex, Tamoxifen Alone or in Combination) trial efficacy and safety update analy-ses. Cancer. 2003;98:1802–10.

36. Eastell R, Hannon RA, Cuzick J, et al. Effect of an aromatase inhibitor on BMD and bone turnover mark-ers: 2-year results of the Anastrozole, Tamoxifen, Alone or in Combination (ATAC) trial (18233230). J Bone Miner Res. 2006;21:1215–23.

37. Eastell R, Adams J. Results of the 'Arimidex' (anas-trozole, A), Tamoxifen (T), Alone or in Combination (C) (ATAC) trial: Effects on bone mineral density (BMD) and bone turnover (ATAC Trialists' Group). In: Presented at the 27th Congress of the European Society for Medical Oncology, Nice, 711, 18–22 Oct 2002.

38. Coleman RE, Body J-J, Gralow JR, Lipton A. Bone loss in patients with breast cancer receiving aromatase inhibitors and associated treatment strategies. Cancer Treat Rev. 2008;34(Suppl 1):S31–42.

39. Coombes RC, Hall E, Gibson L, et al. A randomized trial of exemestane after two to three years of tamoxi-fen therapy in postmenopausal women with primary breast cancer. N Engl J Med. 2004;350:1081–92.

40. Coombes RC, Hall E, Snowdon CF, Bliss JM. The Intergroup Exemestane Study: a randomized trial in postmenopausal patients with early breast cancer who remain disease-free after two to three years of tamoxifen-updated survival analysis. Breast Cancer Res Treat. 2004;88(suppl 1):S7.

41. Coombes RC, Kilburn LS, Snowdon CF, et al. Survival and safety of exemestane versus tamoxi-fen after 2–3 years' tamoxifen treatment (Intergroup Exemestane Study): a randomised controlled trial. Lancet. 2007;369:559–70.

42. Gnant M, Pfeiler G, Dubsky PC, et al. Adjuvant deno-sumab in breast cancer (ABCSG-18): a multicentre, randomised, double-blind, placebo-controlled trial. Lancet. 2015;386:433–43.

43. Soiland H, Hagen KB, Gjerde J, Lende TH, Lien EA. Breaking away: high fracture rates may merit a new trial of adjuvant endocrine therapy in Scandinavian breast cancer patients. Acta Oncol. 2013;52:861–2.

44. Early Breast Cancer Trialists Collaborative Group (EBCTCG). Aromatase inhibitors versus tamoxifen in early breast cancer: patient-level meta-analysis of the randomised trials. Lancet. 2015;386:1341–52.

45. Lester J, Dodwell D, McCloskey E, Coleman R. The causes and treatment of bone loss associ-ated with carcinoma of the breast. Cancer Treat Rev. 2005;31:115–42.

46. Wilson C, Coleman R. Adjuvant bone-targeted thera-pies for postmenopausal breast cancer. JAMA Oncol. 2016;2(4):423–4.

47. Cheung AM, Tile L, Cardew S, et al. Bone density and structure in healthy postmenopausal women treated with exemestane for the primary prevention of breast cancer: a nested substudy of the MAP.3 randomised controlled trial. Lancet Oncol. 2012;13:275–84.

48. Gnant MF, Mlineritsch B, Luschin-Ebengreuth G, Grampp S, Kaessmann H, Schmid M, Menzel C, Piswanger-Soelkner JC, Galid A, Mittlboeck M, Hausmaninger H, Jakesz R. Zoledronic acid prevents cancer treatment-induced bone loss in premenopausal women receiving adjuvant endocrine therapy for hormone-responsive breast cancer: a report from the Austrian Breast and Colorectal Cancer Study Group. J Clin Oncol. 2007;25:820–8.

49. Lester JE, Dodwell D, Purohit O, Gutcher SA, Ellis SP, Thorpe R. Prevention of anastrozole-induced bone loss with oral monthly ibandronate during aromatase inhibitor therapy for breast cancer. Clin Cancer Res. 2008;14:6336–42.

50. Lester JE, Dodwell D, et al. Prevention of anastrozole induced bone loss with monthly oral ibandronate: final 5 year results from the ARIBON trial. J Bone Oncol. 2012;1(2):57–62.

51. Van Poznak C, Hannon RA, Clack G, Campone M, Mackey JR, Apffelstaedt J, Eastell R. The SABRE (Study of Anastrozole with the Bisphosphonate RisedronatE) study: 12 month analysis. Breast Cancer Res Treat. 2007;106(suppl 1):S37.

52. Cummings SR, San Martin J, McClung MR, et al. Denosumab for prevention of fractures in postmenopausal women with osteoporosis. N Engl J Med. 2009;361:756–65.

53. Diel IJ, Jaschke A, Solomayer EF, et al. Adjuvant oral clodronate improves the overall survival of primary breast cancer patients with micrometastases to the bone marrow-a long-term follow-up. Ann Oncol. 2008;19:2007–11.

54. Powles TJ, Paterson A, McCloskey E, et al. Reduction in bone relapse and improved survival with oral clodronate for adjuvant treatment of operable breast cancer. Breast Cancer Res Treat. 2006;8:R13.

55. Gnant M, Mlineritsch B, Schippinger W, et al. Endocrine therapy plus zoledronic acid in premenopausal breast cancer. N Engl J Med. 2009;360:679–91.

56. Coleman RE, Marshall H, Cameron D, AZURE Investigators, et al. Breast-cancer adjuvant therapy with zoledronic acid. N Engl J Med. 2011;365(15):1396–405.

57. Brufsky AM, Bosserman LD, Caradonna RR, et al. Zoledronic acid effectively prevents aromatase inhibitor-associated bone loss in postmenopausal women with early breast cancer receiving adjuvant letrozole: Z-FAST study 36-month follow-up results. Clin Breast Cancer. 2009;9:77–85.

58. Coleman R, de Boer R, Eidtmann H, et al. Zoledronic acid (zoledronate) for postmenopausal women with early breast cancer receiving adjuvant letrozole (ZO-fast study): final 60-month results. Ann Oncol. 2013;24:398–405.

59. von Minckwitz G, et al. German adjuvant intergroup node-positive study: a phase III trial to compare oral ibandronate versus observation in patients with high-risk early breast cancer. J Clin Oncol. 2013;31:3531–9.

60. Paterson AH, Anderson SJ, Lembersky BC, Fehrenbacher L, Falkson CI, King KM, Weir LM, Brufsky AM, Dakhil S, Lad T, Baez-Diaz L, Gralow JR, Robidoux A, Perez EA, Zheng P, Geyer CE Jr, Swain SM, Costantino JP, Mamounas EP, Wolmark N. Oral clodronate for adjuvant treatment of operable breast cancer (National Surgical Adjuvant Breast and Bowel Project protocol B-34): a multicentre, placebo-controlled, randomised trial. Lancet Oncol. 2012;13(7):734–42.

61. Early Breast Cancer Trialists' Collaborative Group (EBCTCG). Adjuvant bisphosphonate treatment in early breast cancer: meta-analyses of individual patient data from randomised trials. Lancet. 2015;386:1353–61.

62. Gralow JBW, Paterson AHG, Lew D, et al. Phase III trial of bisphosphonates as adjuvant therapy in primary breast cancer: SWOG/Alliance/ECOG-ACRIN/NCIC Clinical Trials Group/NRG oncology study S0307 [abstract 558]. J Clin Oncol. 2014;32(5(suppl)).

63. Huggins C, Hodges CV. Studies on prostatic cancer. I. The effect of castration, of estrogen and of androgen injection on serum phosphatases in metastatic carcinoma of the prostate. Cancer Res. 1941;1:293–7.

64. Heidenreich A, Pfister D, Ohlmann CH, Engelmann UH. Androgen deprivation for advanced prostate cancer. Urol A. 2008;47(3):270–83.

65. Denis LJ, Keuppens F, Smith PH, EORTC Genito-Urinary Tract Cancer Cooperative Group and the EORTC Data Center, et al. Maximal androgen blockade: final analysis of EORTC phase III trial 30853. Eur Urol. 1998;33:144–51.

66. Sharifi N, Gulley JL, Dahut WL. Androgen deprivation therapy for prostate cancer. JAMA. 2005;294(2):238–44.

67. Bastiana PJ, Boorjian SA, Bossi A, et al. High-risk prostate cancer: from definition to contemporary management. Eur Urol. 2012;61(6):1096.

68. D'Amico AV, Cote K, Loffredo M, et al. Determinants of prostate cancer specific survival after radiation therapy for patients with clinically localized prostate cancer. J Clin Oncol. 2002;20:4567–73.

69. Kattan MW, Eastham JA, Stapleton AM, Wheeler TM, Scardino PT. A preoperative nomogram for disease recurrence following radical prostatectomy for prostate cancer. J Natl Cancer Inst. 1998;90:766–71.

70. Manolagas SC. Birth and death of bone cells: basic regulatory mechanisms and implications for the pathogenesis and treatment of osteoporosis. Endocr Rev. 2000;21(2):115–37.

71. Higano CS. Bone loss and the evolving role of bisphosphonate therapy in prostate cancer. Urol Oncol. 2003;21(5):392–8.

72. Galvão DA, Spry NA, Taaffe DR, et al. Changes in muscle, fat and bone mass after 36 weeks of maximal androgen blockade for prostate cancer. BJU Int. 2008;102:44–7.

73. Center JR, Nguyen TV, Schneider D, Sambrook PN, Eisman JA. Mortality after all major types of osteoporotic fracture in men and women: an observational study. Lancet. 1999;353(9156):878–82.

74. Shahinian VB, Kuo YF, Freeman JL, Goodwin JS. Risk of fracture after androgen deprivation for prostate cancer. N Engl J Med. 2005;352(2):154–64.

75. Smith MR, McGovern FJ, Zietman AL, Fallon MA, Hayden DL, Schoenfeld DA, Kantoff PW, Finkelstein JS. Pamidronate to prevent bone loss during androgen-deprivation therapy for prostate cancer. N Engl J Med. 2001;345(13):948–55.

76. Lipton A, Small E, Saad F, et al. The new bisphosphonate, zometa (zoledronic acid), decreases skeletal complications in both osteolytic and osteoblastic lesions: a comparison to pamidronate. Cancer Investig. 2002;20(suppl 2):45–54.

77. Smith MR, Eastham J, Gleason DM, Shasha D, Tchekmedyian S, Zinner N. Randomized controlled trial of zoledronic acid to prevent bone

loss in men receiving androgen deprivation therapy for nonmetastatic prostate cancer. J Urol. 2003;169(6):2008–12.

78. Dearnaley DP, Mason MD, Parmar MK, Sanders K, Sydes MR. Adjuvant therapy with oral sodium clodronate in locally advanced and metastatic prostate cancer: long-term overall survival results from the MRC PR04 and PR05 randomised controlled trials. Lancet Oncol. 2009;10(9):872–6.

79. James ND, Sydes MR, Clarke NW, Mason MD, Dearnaley DP, et al. Addition of docetaxel, zoledronic acid, or both to first-line long-term hormone therapy in prostate cancer (STAMPEDE): survival results from an adaptive, multiarm, multistage, platform randomised controlled trial. Lancet. 2016;387:1163–77.

80. Smith MR, Halabi S, Ryan CJ, et al. Randomized controlled trial of early zoledronic acid in men with castration-sensitive prostate cancer and bone metastases: results of CALGB 90202 (alliance). J Clin Oncol. 2014;32:1143–50.

81. Wirth M, Tammela T, Cicalese V, Gomez Veiga F, Delaere K, Miller K, Tubaro A, Schulze M, Debruyne F, Huland H, Patel A, Lecouvet F, Caris C, Witjes W. Prevention of bone metastases in patients with high-risk nonmetastatic prostate cancer treated with zoledronic acid: efficacy and safety results of the Zometa European Study (ZEUS). Eur Urol. 2015;67(3):482–91.

82. Smith MR, Egerdie B, Hernández Toriz N, Feldman R, Tammela TL, Saad F, Heracek J, Szwedowski M, Ke C, Kupic A, Leder BZ, Goessl C, Denosumab HALT Prostate Cancer Study Group. Denosumab in men receiving androgen-deprivation therapy for prostate cancer. N Engl J Med. 2009;361(8):745–55.

83. Chen Y, Sawyers CL, Scher HI. Targeting the androgen receptor pathway in prostate cancer. Curr Opin Pharmacol. 2008;8(4):440–8.

84. Smith MR, Kabbinavar F, Saad F, Hussain A, Gittelman MC, Bilhartz DL, Wynne C, Murray R, Zinner NR, Schulman C, Linnartz R, Zheng M, Goessl C, Hei YJ, Small EJ, Cook R, Higano CS. Natural history of rising serum prostate-specific antigen in men with castrate nonmetastatic prostate cancer. J Clin Oncol. 2005;23(13):2918–25.

85. Smith MR, Saad F, Coleman R, et al. Denosumab and bone-metastasis-free survival in men with castration-resistant prostate cancer: results of a phase 3, randomised, placebo-controlled trial. Lancet. 2012;379:39–46.

86. Ibrahim T, Barbanti F, Giorgio-Marrano G, et al. Osteonecrosis of the jaw in patients with bone metastases treated with bisphosphonates: a retrospective study. Oncologist. 2008;13(3):330–6.

87. European Medicines Agency. Xgeva (denosumab) summary of product characteristics. 2014. http://www.ema.europa.eu/docs/en_GB/document_library/EPAR_Product_Information/human/002173/WC500110381.pdf.

88. Saad F, Brown JE, Van Poznak C, et al. Incidence, risk factors, and outcomes of osteonecrosis of the jaw: integrated analysis from three blinded active-controlled phase III trials in cancer patients with bone metastases. Ann Oncol. 2012;23:1341–7.

89. Migliorati CA, Epstein JB, Abt E, Berenson JR. Osteonecrosis of the jaw and bisphosphonates in cancer: a narrative review. Nat Rev Endocrinol. 2011;7:34–42.

Part II

Approach to the Patient

Estimating Survival in Patients with Skeletal Metastases Using PATHFx: An Adaptive, Validated, Clinical Decision Support Tool

4

Jonathan A. Forsberg and Rikard Wedin

Abstract

We are in the middle of a healthcare revolution. Big data including demographics, molecular markers, and physiologic indicators are

One of the authors (JAF) is an employee of the US Government. This work was prepared as part of his official duties. Title 17 USC § 105 provides that "Copyright protection under this title is not available for any work of the United States Government." Title 17 USC § 101 defined a US Government work as a work prepared by a military service member or employees of the US Government as part of that person's official duties. The opinions or assertions contained in this paper are the private views of the authors and are not to be construed as reflecting the views, policy, or positions of the Department of the Navy, Department of Defense, nor the US Government. Each author certifies that all investigations were conducted in conformity with ethical principles of research. This work was performed at the Karolinska University Hospital, Stockholm Sweden.

J. A. Forsberg (✉)
Orthopaedic Oncology, Orthopaedics, Walter Reed Department of Surgery, Uniformed Services University of the Health Sciences,
Bethesda, MD, USA

Department of Molecular Medicine and Surgery, Karolinska Institute, Stockholm, Sweden

Orthopaedic Oncology, Department of Orthopaedic Surgery, Johns Hopkins University,
Baltimore, MD, USA
e-mail: jforsbe1@jhmi.edu

R. Wedin
Department of Molecular Medicine and Surgery, Karolinska Institute, Stockholm, Sweden

Department of Orthopaedics, Karolinska University Hospital, Stockholm, Sweden

being codified by advanced techniques in information technology. The result is an explosion in the number of prognostic models that have been applied to a variety of clinical problems. Given that mobile or otherwise interconnected applications are ubiquitous in modern society, physicians may be tempted to confuse fingertip availability and relative ease of use with a tool that has been properly vetted for clinical use. It would seem that tech-savvy doctors are abandoning their healthy skepticism that has been ingrained by years of journal clubs, academic medicine, and/or clinical practice. However, this should not be the case. When using an "app," physicians should demand the same level of scrutiny and apply the same healthy skepticism as they do for the literature they read, the implants they select, and the medications they prescribe [1].

Preface: A Word of Caution

We are in the middle of a healthcare revolution. Big data including demographics, molecular markers, and physiologic indicators are being codified by advanced techniques in information technology. The result is an explosion in the number of prognostic models that have been applied to a variety of clinical problems. Given that mobile or otherwise interconnected applications are ubiquitous in modern society, physicians may be tempted to confuse fingertip availability and relative ease of use with a tool that has been properly vetted for clinical use. It would seem that tech-savvy doctors are abandoning their healthy skepticism that has been ingrained by years of journal clubs, academic medicine, and/or clinical practice. However, this should not be the case. When using an "app," physicians should demand the same level of scrutiny and apply the same healthy skepticism as they do for the literature they read, the implants they select, and the medications they prescribe [1].

As we look toward personalized or precision medicine, there is perhaps no better application than in the treatment of advanced cancer. At the end of life, patients must balance the reality of dying, with a desire for self-preservation. In addition, survival estimates made by members of the treatment team can help set patient, family, and physician expectations. Since no two patients present with exactly the same clinical characteristics or disease burden, these estimates can be difficult to make. Nevertheless, their importance cannot be understated, when approaching patients who are terminal—but necessarily terminally ill. Unfortunately, our ability as clinicians to provide detailed survival estimates is generally inaccurate, which has spurred concerted efforts to improve [2, 3].

To complicate matters, most physicians refuse to prognosticate, or knowingly withhold information from their patients. Lamont and Christakis [4] describe this phenomenon in a study of 311 patients with terminal cancer. They show that physicians were perfectly able to derive estimates of survival in nearly all (97%) cases. However, physicians communicated *actual* estimates to only 37%. They misled patients by providing a *different* estimate in 40% and knowingly *withheld* the survival estimate from the remaining 23%. For the group who were misled, estimates were almost always optimistic, and the patient would then make decision-based, overly optimistic survival information. On the one hand, optimism is healthy and important for cancer treatment. However, physicians who present *overly* optimistic estimates are likely to generate unanticipated consequences.

Receiving an overly optimistic prognosis from a treating physician can have a dramatic influence on treatment decisions. Patients in this setting are more likely to opt for more aggressive treatment, rather than perhaps more appropriate

palliative measures. This, in turn, leads to higher complication rates, ad lower patient satisfaction [5]. Clearly, better communication between patients and their physicians could lead to improved shared decision-making regarding end-of-life care.

For the orthopedic surgeon, the question of life expectancy may be less philosophical but is certainly no less important. In fact, the goals of orthopedic surgery in terminally ill patients are to relieve pain and preserve function for the maximum amount of time [6, 7]. Surgical considerations in this setting are dependent on several factors, described in the Chap. 5. However, when making treatment decisions, it is critical that orthopedic surgeons refrain from basing treatment decisions solely on the appearance of imaging and understand that survival plays a crucial role [8].

Many have identified independent predictors of survival in patients with bony metastases, operative, or otherwise [9–16]. These include the specific oncologic diagnosis; the subjective Eastern Cooperative Oncology Group (ECOG) performance status [17]; the number of bone metastases; the presence of visceral metastases [18], serum hemoglobin [14], and serum albumin [15]; the senior surgeon's estimate of survival [13]; the speed of tumor growth [16]; a diagnosis of lung cancer [14]; the appendicular bone metastases [9]; the type of reconstructive procedure performed [12]; and the time from oncologic diagnosis to total hip arthroplasty (for proximal femoral metastases) [10]. Despite the large number of covariates that have been associated with survival in this patient population, there exists no consensus as to which ones should be routinely used. As such, their ability to predict survival as part of a cohesive model is unacceptably inaccurate, at 5–15% in the best of the reported series [13]. Nevertheless, this body of work demonstrated that it was possible to derive generalized estimations of survival based on an individual's disease-related and laboratory parameters. However, more accurate, personalized estimations were not yet possible.

In an attempt to develop a prognostic tool useful for surgical decision-making, Tokuhashi et al. [19] devised a scoring system to bin each patient's postoperative survival into one of three groups: <6 months, >6 months, or >1 year. He and his coauthors collected several prognostic variables including, for the first time, the Karnofsky score, a measure of performance status [20]. The investigators also documented the number of intra- and extraspinal bone metastases, the number and type of organ metastases, the primary oncologic diagnosis, and the Frankel classification that describes the degree of neurologic impairment. They then externally validated the model in 246 additional patients and observed that survival greater than, or less than, 6 months could be estimated in a reliable manner [21]. Independent external validation produced similar results [22]; however, Tokuhashi's scoring system applies only to patients with symptomatic spine metastases and therefore has limited value to the general orthopedic community.

Recognizing the value of a model that could be applied to all patients with skeletal metastases, several have developed nomograms, including Nathan et al. [13], Paulino Pereira et al. [23], and Sørensen et al. [16]. Despite widespread interest in a prognostic tool, these particular models have yet to undergo external validation.

Nevertheless, several prognostic models have undergone external validation and are available to orthopedic surgeons, worldwide. These include methods described by Tokuhashi et al. [19], Katagiri et al. [24], and Forsberg et al. [25]. Each is designed to estimate the likelihood of survival at time points useful for surgical decision-making. Specifically, survival estimates at 3, 6, and 12 months post-surgery can help surgeons determine which patients might benefit from surgical intervention (by estimating the probability of survival at 3 months) and also whether he or she should consider using a more durable implant (by estimating the probability of survival at 6 or 12 months). In addition, those considering palliative treatment for patients with metastatic bone disease may seek to estimate very short (1 month) life expectancy [26]. By the same token, more favorable estimates of between 1 and 6 months may help justify less-invasive approaches such as intramedullary fixation or plate and screw constructs. Finally, a survey of Musculoskeletal Tumor Society members [27] indicated that survival at 6 months is commonly used to determine whether to choose a more durable reconstruction option such as conventional or modular "tumor" prostheses. In addition, for patients that are likely to survive 12 months or longer, the evidence supporting more durable implants becomes stronger [28, 29]. Furthermore, applying the same approach to more complicated tumors, involving the sacrum, pelvis, and shoulder girdle, demands more extensive reconstructive options, which carry with them extended hospital stays and rehabilitation. In these settings, longer estimates of 18 or 24 months may be helpful in selecting appropriate patients.

Importantly, most prognostic models available to the orthopedic community are based on data that is decades old, in some cases. It is unclear which systemic treatment(s) were used; however, it is likely that modern patients with skeletal metastases are treated differently. In fact, most patients with advanced cancer now receive targeted immunotherapy, which may make designed conventional models estimate life expectancy as obsolete, unless the tools are designed to improve over time.

4.1   PATHFx (www.pathfx.org)

One application designed to deliver survival estimates, and improve over time, is PATHFx. Introduced in 2011 [30], this validated clinical decision-support tool [25, 31] uses clinical and physiologic variables to generate the probability of survival at 1, 3, 6, 12, 18, and 24 months after orthopedic surgery [32]. Suggested variables include age, sex, oncologic diagnosis, indication for surgery (impending or complete pathologic fracture), number of bone metastases (solitary or multiple), presence or absence of organ metastases, presence or absence of lymph node metastases, preoperative hemoglobin (g/dL; on admission, before transfusion, if applicable), absolute lymphocyte count (K/mL), and the senior surgeon's estimates of survival (postoperatively in months). Including the surgeon's estimate—a subjective assessment—may seem controversial. However, doing so allows surgeons with considerable expertise to provide a weighted estimate of survival that can be combined with the other, more objective, features within PATHFx. After using decision analysis to confirm that the tool is suitable for, clinical use [25, 31, 33], the authors made it freely available to orthopedic surgeons, worldwide, at www.pathfx.org (Fig. 4.1a, b), and the 1–12-month models have been validated around the world, including the USA, Scandinavia, and Italy [25, 31], with a planned external validation in Japan. In addition, external validation of the 18- and 24-month models, added to PATHFx in 2017, is currently underway in Scandinavia and Japan. Finally, although PATHFx is indicated for use in surgical candidates only, prospective validation in patients receiving palliative treatment for metastatic bone disease is currently underway.

Recognizing that survival tools must be applicable to orthopedic surgeons worldwide, we created an international metastatic bone disease registry, hosted in Sweden, designed to collect data from a variety of centers in the USA, Scandinavia, Italy, Japan, and Singapore. Importantly, PATHFx is integrated into the registry to ensure its estimates remain accurate, thereby validating the models in a prospective and perpetual manner. In addition, data from this registry may be exported into a development environment, so that the effect of new variables on the PATHFx models can be evaluated and

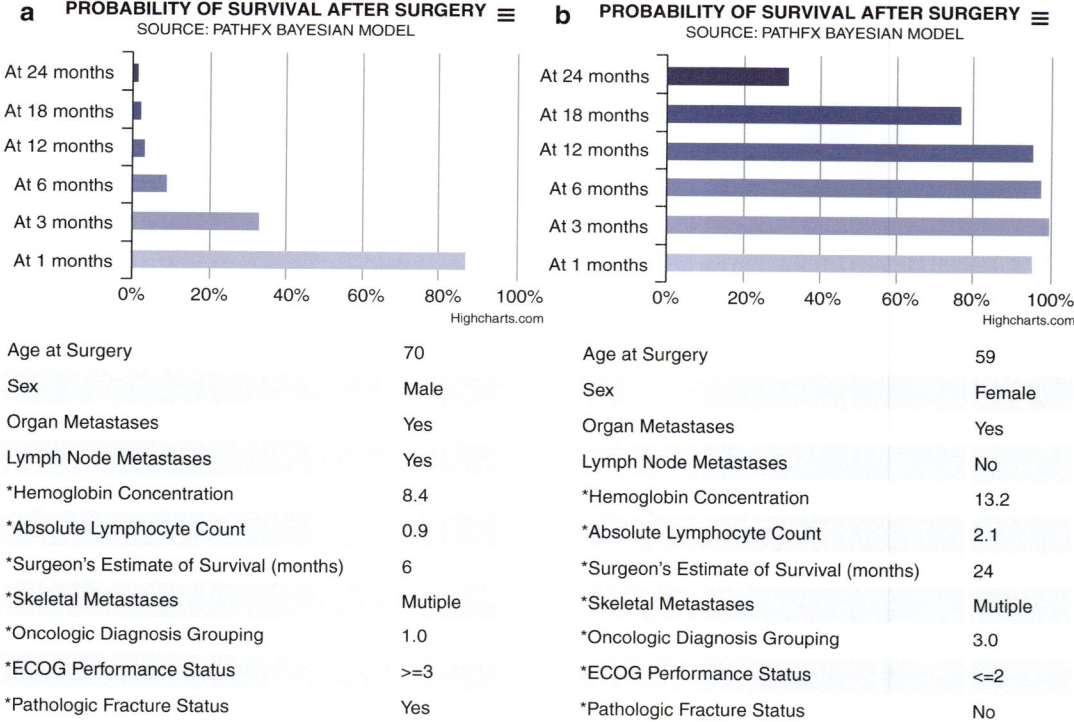

Fig. 4.1 (**a**, **b**) This screenshot of www.pathfx.org demonstrates two typical patient scenarios encountered by orthopedic surgeons. The patient's characteristics are shown below, and his or her personalized estimates of survival are presented as horizontal bar graphs above. (**a**) This graph demonstrates very poor survival trajectory that may help provide surgeons and caregivers with objective information. In this case, palliative therapy, or less-invasive means of surgical stabilization, such as intramedullary nails or plate/screw/cement constructs, may be appropriate. (**b**) By the same token, more favorable survival estimates, such as the one depicted here, can be used to justify the need for more durable, complicated, and expensive implants, such as conventional, or modular "tumor," or even custom prostheses

that disease-specific models can be developed. This may help ensure prognostic estimates remain personalized as much as possible.

In conclusion, survival estimates are important when treating patients with metastatic bone disease. Several methods designed to estimate life expectancy are available to orthopedic surgeons; however, as with any clinical decision support tool, one must ensure the method(s) used are applicable to one's patient population.

4.2 Recommendations for the Use of Clinical Decision Support Tools

1. Any clinical decision support tool must undergo external validation and decision analysis, in its intended patient population, prior to being used in a clinical manner.
2. Clinical decision support tools should be designed to accommodate uncertainty. Although most are not designed to be used with incomplete information, some, like PATHFx, retain accuracy when confronted with missing information.
3. As the name implies, clinical decision support tools are meant to support surgeons in their decision-making process and are no substitute for good clinical judgment.

References

1. Forsberg JA. Suggested guidelines. In: Wedin R, Bauer H, Weidenhielm L, editors. Turning data into decisions. Stockholm: Karolinska University Press; 2015. p. 1–74.
2. Glare P, Virik K, Jones M, et al. A systematic review of physicians' survival predictions in terminally ill cancer patients. BMJ. 2003;327(7408):195–8. https://doi.org/10.1136/bmj.327.7408.195.
3. Hartsell WF, Desilvio M, Bruner DW, et al. Can physicians accurately predict survival time in patients with metastatic cancer? Analysis of RTOG 97-14. J Palliat Med. 2008;11(5):723–8. https://doi.org/10.1089/jpm.2007.0259.
4. Lamont EB, Christakis NA. Prognostic disclosure to patients with cancer near the end of life. Ann Intern Med. 2001;134(12):1096–105.
5. Weeks JC, Cook EF, O'Day SJ, et al. Relationship between cancer patients' predictions of prognosis and their treatment preferences. JAMA. 1998;279(21):1709–14.
6. Clohisy DR, Le CT, Cheng EY, Dykes DC, Thompson RC. Evaluation of the feasibility of and results of measuring health-status changes in patients undergoing surgical treatment for skeletal metastases. J Orthop Res. 2000;18(1):1–9. https://doi.org/10.1002/jor.1100180102.
7. Harrington KD, Sim FH, Enis JE, Johnston JO, Dick HM, Gristina AG. Methyl methacrylate as an adjunct in internal fixation of pathological fractures. J Bone Joint Surg Am. 1976;58(8):1047–55.
8. Forsberg JA, Wedin R, Bauer H. Which implant is best after failed treatment for pathologic femur fractures? Clin Orthop Relat Res. 2013;471(3):735–40. https://doi.org/10.1007/s11999-012-2558-2.
9. Sugiura H, Yamada K, Sugiura T, Hida T, Mitsudomi T. Predictors of survival in patients with bone metastasis of lung cancer. Clin Orthop Relat Res. 2008;466(3):729–36.
10. Schneiderbauer MM, Knoch von M, Schleck CD, Harmsen WS, Sim FH, Scully SP. Patient survival after hip arthroplasty for metastatic disease of the hip. J Bone Joint Surg Am. 2004;86(8):1684–9.
11. Lin PP, Mirza AN, Lewis VO, et al. Patient survival after surgery for osseous metastases from renal cell carcinoma. J Bone Joint Surg Am. 2007;89(8):1794–801. https://doi.org/10.2106/JBJS.F.00603.
12. Narazaki D, Alverga Neto C, Baptista A, Camargo M. Prognostic factors in pathologic fractures secondary to metastatic tumors. Clinics. 2006;61:313–20.
13. Nathan S, Healey J, Mellano D, et al. Survival in patients operated on for pathologic fracture: implications for end-of-life orthopedic care. J Clin Oncol. 2005;23(25):6072–82.
14. Hansen BH, Keller J, et al. The Scandinavian Sarcoma Group Skeletal Metastasis Register. Survival after surgery for bone metastases in the pelvis and extremities. Acta Orthop Scand Suppl. 2004;75(311):11–5.
15. Stevenson JD, McNair M, Cribb GL, Cool WP. Prognostic factors for patients with skeletal metastases from carcinoma of the breast. Bone Joint J. 2016;98-B(2):266–70. https://doi.org/10.1302/0301-620X.98B2.36185.
16. Sørensen MS, Gerds TA, Hindsø K. Prediction of survival after surgery due to skeletal metastases in the extremities. Bone Joint J. 2016;98-B(2):271–7. https://doi.org/10.1302/0301-620X.98B2.
17. Oken MM, Creech RH, Tormey DC, et al. Toxicity and response criteria of the Eastern Cooperative Oncology Group. Am J Clin Oncol. 1982;5(6):649.
18. Bauer H, Wedin R. Survival after surgery for spinal and extremity metastases: prognostication in 241 patients. Acta Orthop. 1995;66(2):143–6.
19. Tokuhashi Y, Matsuzaki H, Toriyama S, Kawano H, Ohsaka S. Scoring system for the preoperative evaluation of metastatic spine tumor prognosis. Spine. 1990;15(11):1110–3.

20. Karnofsky DA. The clinical evaluation of chemotherapeutic agents in cancer. New York: Columbia University Press; 1949.

21. Tokuhashi Y, Matsuzaki H, Oda H, Oshima M, Ryu J. A revised scoring system for preoperative evaluation of metastatic spine tumor prognosis. Spine. 2005;30(19):2186–91.

22. Yamashita T, Siemionow KB, Mroz TE, Podichetty V, Lieberman IH. A prospective analysis of prognostic factors in patients with spinal metastases: use of the revised Tokuhashi score. Spine. 2011;36(11):910–7. https://doi.org/10.1097/BRS.0b013e3181e56ec1.

23. Paulino Pereira NR, Janssen SJ, van Dijk E, et al. Development of a prognostic survival algorithm for patients with metastatic spine disease. J Bone Joint Surg Am. 2016;98(21):1767–76. https://doi.org/10.2106/JBJS.15.00975.

24. Katagiri H, Takahashi M, Inagaki J, Sugiura H, Ito S, Iwata H. Determining the site of the primary cancer in patients with skeletal metastasis of unknown origin. Cancer. 2000;86(3):533–7.

25. Forsberg JA, Wedin R, Bauer HCF, et al. External validation of the Bayesian Estimated Tools for Survival (BETS) models in patients with surgically treated skeletal metastases. BMC Cancer. 2012;12(1):493. https://doi.org/10.1186/1471-2407-12-493.

26. Mavrogenis AF, Angelini A, Vottis C, et al. Modern palliative treatments for metastatic bone disease. Clin J Pain. 2016;32(4):337–50. https://doi.org/10.1097/AJP.0000000000000255.

27. Steensma M, Healey JH. Trends in the surgical treatment of pathologic proximal femur fractures among Musculoskeletal Tumor Society members. Clin Orthop Relat Res. 2013;471(6):2000–6. https://doi.org/10.1007/s11999-012-2724-6.

28. Wedin R, Bauer HC, Wersäll P. Failures after operation for skeletal metastatic lesions of long bones. Clin Orthop Relat Res. 1999;358:128–39.

29. Steensma M, Boland PJ, Morris CD, Athanasian E, Healey JH. Endoprosthetic treatment is more durable for pathologic proximal femur fractures. Clin Orthop Relat Res. 2012;470(3):920–6. https://doi.org/10.1007/s11999-011-2047-z.

30. Forsberg JA, Eberhardt J, Boland PJ, Wedin R, Healey JH. Estimating survival in patients with operable skeletal metastases: an application of a Bayesian belief network. PLoS One. 2011;6(5):e19956. https://doi.org/10.1371/journal.pone.0019956.

31. Piccioli A, Spinelli MS, Forsberg JA, et al. How do we estimate survival? External validation of a tool for survival estimation in patients with metastatic bone disease-decision analysis and comparison of three international patient populations. BMC Cancer. 2015;15(1):424. https://doi.org/10.1186/s12885-015-1396-5.

32. Forsberg JA, Wedin R, Boland PJ, Healey JH. Can we estimate short- and intermediate-term survival in patients undergoing surgery for metastatic bone disease? Clin Orthop Relat Res. 2017;475:1252–61. https://doi.org/10.1007/s11999-016-5187-3.

33. Forsberg JA, Sjoberg D, Chen Q-R, Vickers A, Healey JH. Treating metastatic disease: which survival model is best suited for the clinic? Clin Orthop Relat Res. 2013;471(3):843–50. https://doi.org/10.1007/s11999-012-2577-z.

How Expected Survival Influences the Choice of Surgical Procedure in Metastatic Bone Disease

Panagiotis Tsagozis, Jonathan Forsberg, Henrik C. F. Bauer, and Rikard Wedin

Abstract

Accurate estimation of expected survival is very helpful in the choice of patients that are good candidates for surgery, as well as in the choice of the surgical method and implant used. If we treat the short-time survivors and the long-time survivors with the same reconstruction, we will inevitably overtreat the short-time survivors and undertreat the long-time survivors. This translates to too extensive surgery and rehabilitation need in the short-time survivors. In this chapter we discuss our present general treatment recommendations based on prognosis.

Keywords

Skeletal metastasis · Bone metastasis Survival · Prognosis · PATHFx · Skeletal reconstruction · Surgical treatment

P. Tsagozis · H. C. F. Bauer · R. Wedin (✉)
Department of Orthopaedics, Karolinska University Hospital, Stockholm, Sweden

Department of Molecular Medicine and Surgery, Karolinska Institute, Stockholm, Sweden
e-mail: RIKARD.WEDIN@KAROLINSKA.SE

J. Forsberg
Department of Molecular Medicine and Surgery, Karolinska Institute, Stockholm, Sweden

Orthopaedic Oncology, Orthopaedics, Walter Reed Department of Surgery, Uniformed Services University of the Health Sciences, Bethesda, MD, USA

5.1 Introduction

Cancer patients with pathological fracture constitute a diverse population, characterized by notable variability in overall condition, expected survival, as well as presentation and expectations regarding treatment. The prognosis varies considerably and is dependent on the type of primary tumour and the extent of the disease [1–3]. The choice of treatment should be adapted to the local symptoms and degree of skeletal destruction, whether the pathological fracture is actual or impending, the biology of the primary neoplasm and ultimately by the expected survival of the patient. Ideally, the type of surgery and implant chosen should carry the least associated morbidity and risk for secondary complications, provide optimal pain relief and allow for adjuvant treatment. As the management of pathological fractures generally does not rely on bone healing, the reconstructive method should have an expected longevity that exceeds the patients expected survival.

5.2 When to Operate?

Skeletal metastases seldom require surgical treatment as most are managed by radiotherapy and medical oncological treatment. The decision to operate should take into account the level of pain, the performance status, the presence of a pathological fracture and the location as well as the radiological characteristics of the lesion (lytic or sclerotic, proportion of the bone involved). According to our experience, surgery is required in approximately 20% of patients referred with symptomatic skeletal metastatic lesions [4]. In the extremities, the principal indication for surgery is the presence of pathological fractures, as non-operative treatments will neither control pain nor restore function. In the case of bone lesions without fracture, our main indication for surgical treatment is pain on weight bearing. We have not found the scoring systems to assess the risk of fracture to be helpful, and we do not use the term *prophylactic fixation* [5]. If the patient has significant pain and loss of function, we treat surgically; if the patient has neither, we refer to radiotherapy. In solitary lesions of certain cancer types such as kidney cancer, there may be an indication for en bloc resection [6, 7]. However, as oncological treatments of previously refractory cancer types are becoming more effective, such surgical indications will probably become irrelevant.

In spinal metastases, the same indications apply, although it is the neurological compromise, rather than pain or pathological fracture which poses the surgical indication in this occasion. Hence, in our institution, most patients with epidural compression of the spinal cord but without major neurological symptoms will be referred for radiotherapy. The risk of wound-healing problems is higher, and the postoperative recovery period is longer after surgery for spinal metastases than for pathological fracture of extremities [8–11]. Therefore, patients with life expectancy of less than 3 months will in most cases not benefit from spinal surgery.

The goals of operative treatment are pain relief and restoration of function. Radiotherapy is almost never effective in ameliorating pain related to weight bearing or physical activity. Moreover, treatment of pathological fractures cannot rely on bone healing. First, only a minority of pathological fractures will heal, due to multifactorial poor bone-healing capability as well as short patient survival. Second, patients with pathological fractures need a reconstruction that provides prompt pain relief and allows immediate and full weight bearing.

5.3 Survival Estimation as a Tool to Guide Treatment

Survival estimates, both to identify those patients who will probably die within a couple of months and those who can be expected to survive more than a year, have an important bearing on treatment decision. Yet, they should only serve as an adjunct to sound clinical decision-making, and we should be aware that physicians generally have an overtly optimistic and unrealistic view of the patients' prospects [12, 13].

Our interest in prognosis as a tool for differentiating surgical treatment for patients with skeletal metastases started in the mid-1990s, and our first paper on the subject was published in 1995 [14]. At that time, we observed a very high complication rate and sought to understand the causes of it [8]. Indeed, in 1999, our complication rate was up to 20% and the reoperation rate 11%. Now, approximately two decades later, our group at Karolinska has published some 30 papers and mentored 3 dissertations in this field, but our complication rate is still not satisfying.

Analysis of patients treated in the 1990s showed that approximately two out of five were alive 1 year after surgery, and one out of five had died within 6 weeks from operation [14]. We realized that if we treated the short-time survivors and the long-time survivors with the same reconstruction, we will inevitably overtreat the short-time survivors and undertreat the long-time survivors. This translates to too extensive surgery and rehabilitation need in the short-time survivors. On the other hand, implant failures would be far too common in the long-time survivors. In fact, of the few who survived 5 years, one half was reoperated because of implant failure and/or local tumour progression [4]. It became evident that the choice of reconstruction should not be solely based on the radiographical appearance of the metastatic focus but rather be part of an individualized approach where a reliable estimation of the patients' survival plays a central role.

In 2011 Jonathan Forsberg developed PATHFx, a prognostic decision support, as a part of his thesis "Turning data into decisions: Clinical decision support in orthopaedic oncology" (Karolinska Institute, 2015) [15]. PATHFx is based on Bayesian belief network and calculates the probability of the patient surviving 1, 3, 6, 12, 18 and 24 months, based on variables that have previously shown to be important in risk stratification of patients with skeletal metastatic events. The tool is available online and has so far successfully been externally validated in a Scandinavian, an Italian and a Japanese patient population [16–18]. To improve the prognostic accuracy and to keep PATHFx updated as new cancer treatments emerge, a new web-based registry has been started. The "International Bone Metastasis Registry" has been developed in collaboration with the Regional Cancer Center in Stockholm, Sweden. The registry can also be used to find new prognostic variables and to compare treatment outcomes among various centres and countries.

Accurate estimation of expected survival is very helpful in the choice of patients that are good candidates for surgery, as well as in the choice of the surgical method and implant used, as discussed in the following section. Our hope is that the accuracy of PATHFx will improve as more patients are registered worldwide, and we advocate its use as an adjunct to sound medical judgement.

5.4 Which Implant Should Be Used? General Considerations

Treatment of pathological fractures should not rely on bone healing. On the contrary, the basic principle is that the implant used should provide maximum stability or, optimally, should bypass the skeletal lesion and transfer the mechanical loads to the uninvolved parts of the skeleton. Moreover, it should tolerate immediate weight bearing and should require a minimal period of rehabilitation. The surgical procedure should also carry an acceptable morbidity.

There is increasing evidence that prosthesis rather than osteosynthesis should be used in lesions around the hip and the proximal femur, as well as around the shoulder joint, as they seem to provide superior pain relief and have lower risk of failure [4, 19]. Indeed, plates and nails have a high risk for mechanical failure, presumably as they depend on normal bone healing to prevent long-term failure. Moreover, the morbidity associated with prosthetic surgery is not considerably higher compared to osteosynthesis. When it comes to the choice of prosthetic device, the use of a cemented one is an absolute requirement since no osseointegration is expected. Hemiarthroplasty is generally sufficient in hip replacements, when intraoperative inspection of the acetabular cartilage does not reveal any degenerative changes. In fit and physically active patients with excellent prognosis, total hip replacement should be considered. As mentioned above, in cases of solitary renal metastases, en bloc rather than intralesional resection is associated with improved patient survival [4, 6]. Thus, reconstruction of the skeletal defect with a tumour endoprosthesis is motivated, when the expected patient survival is excellent [4].

When the use of a plate is necessary, either due to technical reasons or poor expected survival, absolute stability should be the goal, since no healing will ensue. The principles of rigid osteosynthesis should be applied, and lytic lesions should be curetted and replaced with bone cement (polymethyl methacrylate), in order to both reduce the potential of progression of the metastasis and provide superior mechanical stability. Indeed, bone cement is an excellent material that has a direct thermal anti-tumoural effect due to the exothermic polymerization reaction [20] and provides for good purchase of screws.

5.5 Treatment Policy at the Karolinska University Hospital

In our Department, a long bone fracture will be surgically treated unless the patient is in the terminal phase of his disease. However, we are

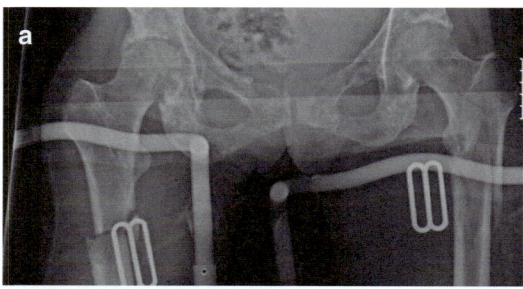

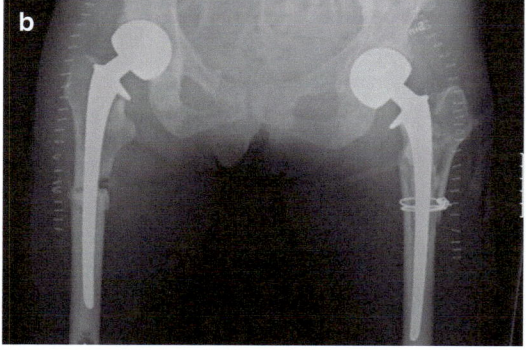

Fig. 5.1 A 54-year-old female with a history of breast cancer, presenting with spontaneous pathological femoral fracture bilaterally (**a**). Bilateral cemented hip hemiarthroplasty allowing immediate mobilization of full weight bearing (**b**)

cautious accepting patients for spinal or acetabular surgery if expected survival is shorter than 3 months. Our guidelines are partly based on our own experiences and complication rate for these two types of surgery [21–23].

In the subtrochanteric region of the femur, we prefer an endoprosthesis, especially if expected survival is longer than 6 months (Fig. 5.1) [24]. Plates and nails are prone to fatigue fractures and failure in the long term, and we try to avoid them in patients who have an expected survival longer than 6 months. Moreover, intramedullary nail osteosynthesis provides only relative stability and thus poor pain relief.

We advocate the use of a cemented hemiprosthesis for pathologic proximal humeral fractures and interlocked intramedullary nail for lesions in the diaphysis [19]. In the metastasis of the proximal humerus, a cemented reversed geometry total shoulder replacement is contemplated for patients surviving longer than 6 months. Reversed shoulder prosthesis, as compared to hemiprosthesis, probably provides a better shoulder function but is also technically more demanding and probably associated with higher risk of complications.

In spinal surgery we almost only operate patients with neurological deficits [25]. If the vertebrae at the level of spinal cord compression have not been fractured, we often only perform a laminectomy without stabilization, especially if survival is expected to be less than 6 months. A generalized outline of the above recommendations is shown in Fig. 5.2.

5.6   Post-operative Considerations

The goal of surgery should be immediate weight bearing, and anything less should be seen as a failure. Moreover, routine use of orthoses should be discouraged. Follow-up should be adjusted to the type of reconstruction and expected survival of the patient.

Routine post-operative radiotherapy is usually offered when the wound has healed. The goal is to prevent continued bone destruction and protect the implant from failure. However, radiotherapy may result in stress fractures, wound-healing problems and infections [26]. There is still uncertainty regarding the optimal schedule and dose of radiotherapy, even if single-dose treatments have shown comparable efficacy regarding pain relief as multiple-dose ones [27]. Moreover, there are no studies comparing the outcome of surgery with or without postoperative radiotherapy in the treatment of pathological fractures. In a previous study, we showed that the reoperation rate in irradiated fractures was 13% as compared to 10% in non-radiated ones, and the radiotherapy-associated complication rate was 10% [8]. Overall, patients with expected survival of less than 3 months probably do not need any adjuvant radiotherapy. Furthermore, the use of prostheses or cement augmentation after intralesional excision further weakens the indication for radiotherapy.

Fig. 5.2 Schematic outline of treatment recommendations for skeletal metastatic disease at the Karolinska University Hospital

General treatment recommendations based on prognosis as per PATHFx

< 50 % chance of surviving for 3 months

Intramedullary nail for metastasis of the long bone

No spinal or pelvic surgery

> 50 % chance of surviving for 6 months

Prosthesis rather than intramedullary nail

Reversed shoulder prosthesis

> 50 % chance of surviving for 12 months

Total hip replacement in the physically fit patient

Wide excision for solitary metastasis from kidney cancer

Advanced reconstructions of the pelvis and spinal column

References

1. Hansen BH, Keller J, Laitinen M, Berg P, Skjeldal S, Trovik C, et al. The Scandinavian Sarcoma Group Skeletal Metastasis Register. Survival after surgery for bone metastases in the pelvis and extremities. Acta Orthop Scand Suppl. 2004;75:11–5.
2. Kirkinis MN, Lyne CJ, Wilson MD, Choong PFM. Metastatic bone disease: a review of survival, prognostic factors and outcomes following surgical treatment of the appendicular skeleton. Eur J Surg Oncol. 2016. https://doi.org/10.1016/j.ejso.2016.03.036.
3. Ratasvuori M, Wedin R, Keller J, Nottrott M, Zaikova O, Bergh P, et al. Insight opinion to surgically treated metastatic bone disease: Scandinavian Sarcoma Group Skeletal Metastasis Registry report of 1195 operated skeletal metastasis. Surg Oncol. 2013;22:132–8. https://doi.org/10.1016/j.suronc.2013.02.008.
4. Wedin R. Surgical treatment for pathologic fracture. Acta Orthop Scand Suppl. 2001;72:2p., 1–29.
5. Mirels H. Metastatic disease in long bones: a proposed scoring system for diagnosing impending pathologic fractures. Clin Orthop. 1989;2003:S4–13. https://doi.org/10.1097/01.blo.0000093045.56370.dd.
6. Ratasvuori M, Wedin R, Hansen BH, Keller J, Trovik C, Zaikova O, et al. Prognostic role of en-bloc resection and late onset of bone metastasis in patients with bone-seeking carcinomas of the kidney, breast, lung, and prostate: SSG study on 672 operated skeletal metastases. J Surg Oncol. 2014;110:360–5. https://doi.org/10.1002/jso.23654.
7. Fukushima H, Hozumi T, Goto T, Nihei K, Karasawa K, Nakanishi Y, et al. Prognostic significance of intensive local therapy to bone lesions in renal cell carcinoma patients with bone metastasis. Clin Exp Metastasis. 2016;33:699–705. https://doi.org/10.1007/s10585-016-9805-y.
8. Wedin R, Bauer HC, Wersäll P. Failures after operation for skeletal metastatic lesions of long bones. Clin Orthop Relat Res. 1999;358:128–39.
9. Wise JJ, Fischgrund JS, Herkowitz HN, Montgomery D, Kurz LT. Complication, survival rates, and risk factors of surgery for metastatic disease of the spine. Spine. 1999;24:1943–51.
10. Bollen L, de Ruiter GCW, Pondaag W, Arts MP, Fiocco M, Hazen TJT, et al. Risk factors for survival of 106 surgically treated patients with symptomatic spinal epidural metastases. Eur Spine J. 2013;22:1408–16. https://doi.org/10.1007/s00586-013-2726-4.
11. Lau D, Leach MR, Than KD, Ziewacz J, La Marca F, Park P. Independent predictors of complication following surgery for spinal metastasis. Eur Spine J. 2013;22:1402–7. https://doi.org/10.1007/s00586-013-2706-8.
12. Viganò A, Dorgan M, Bruera E, Suarez-Almazor ME. The relative accuracy of the clinical estimation of the duration of life for patients with end of life cancer. Cancer. 1999;86:170–6.
13. Chow E, Harth T, Hruby G, Finkelstein J, Wu J, Danjoux C. How accurate are physicians' clinical predictions of survival and the available prognostic tools in estimating survival times in terminally ill cancer patients? A systematic review. Clin Oncol (R Coll Radiol). 2001;13:209–18.
14. Bauer HC, Wedin R. Survival after surgery for spinal and extremity metastases. Prognostication in 241 patients. Acta Orthop Scand. 1995;66:143–6.
15. Forsberg JA, Eberhardt J, Boland PJ, Wedin R, Healey JH. Estimating survival in patients with oper-

able skeletal metastases: an application of a Bayesian belief network. PLoS One. 2011;6:e19956. https://doi.org/10.1371/journal.pone.0019956.

16. Forsberg JA, Wedin R, Bauer HCF, Hansen BH, Laitinen M, Trovik CS, et al. External validation of the Bayesian Estimated Tools for Survival (BETS) models in patients with surgically treated skeletal metastases. BMC Cancer. 2012;12:493. https://doi.org/10.1186/1471-2407-12-493.

17. Piccioli A, Spinelli MS, Forsberg JA, Wedin R, Healey JH, Ippolito V, et al. How do we estimate survival? External validation of a tool for survival estimation in patients with metastatic bone disease-decision analysis and comparison of three international patient populations. BMC Cancer. 2015;15:424. https://doi.org/10.1186/s12885-015-1396-5.

18. Ogura K, Gokita T, Shinoda Y, Kawano H, Takagi T, Ae K, Kawai A, Wedin R, Forsberg JA. Can a multivariate model for survival estimation in skeletal metastases (PATHFx) be externally validated using Japanese patients? Clin Orthop Relat Res. 2017;475(9):2263–70. https://doi.org/10.1007/s11999-017-5389-3.

19. Wedin R, Hansen BH, Laitinen M, Trovik C, Zaikova O, Bergh P, et al. Complications and survival after surgical treatment of 214 metastatic lesions of the humerus. J Shoulder Elb Surg. 2012;21:1049–55. https://doi.org/10.1016/j.jse.2011.06.019.

20. Nelson DA, Barker ME, Hamlin BH. Thermal effects of acrylic cementation at bone tumour sites. Int J Hyperthermia. 1997;13:287–306.

21. Stark A, Bauer HC. Reconstruction in metastatic destruction of the acetabulum. Support rings and arthroplasty in 12 patients. Acta Orthop Scand. 1996;67:435–8.

22. Weiss RJ, Wedin R. Surgery for skeletal metastases in lung cancer. Acta Orthop. 2011;82:96–101. https://doi.org/10.3109/17453674.2011.552779.

23. Tsagozis P, Wedin R, Brosjö O, Bauer H. Reconstruction of metastatic acetabular defects using a modified Harrington procedure. Acta Orthop. 2015;86:690–4. https://doi.org/10.3109/17453674.2015.1077308.

24. Weiss RJ, Ekström W, Hansen BH, Keller J, Laitinen M, Trovik C, et al. Pathological subtrochanteric fractures in 194 patients: a comparison of outcome after surgical treatment of pathological and non-pathological fractures. J Surg Oncol. 2013;107:498–504. https://doi.org/10.1002/jso.23277.

25. Bauer HC. Posterior decompression and stabilization for spinal metastases. Analysis of sixty-seven consecutive patients. J Bone Joint Surg Am. 1997;79:514–22.

26. Tibbs MK. Wound healing following radiation therapy: a review. Radiother Oncol J Eur Soc Ther Radiol Oncol. 1997;42:99–106.

27. Tong D, Gillick L, Hendrickson FR. The palliation of symptomatic osseous metastases: final results of the study by the Radiation Therapy Oncology Group. Cancer. 1982;50:893–9.

The Role of Radiotherapy in Long Bone Metastases and Pelvis

6

Michele Fiore, Carla Germana Rinaldi, and Sara Ramella

Abstract

Bone metastases are a common complication of advanced cancer that can cause severe and debilitating effects. External beam radiation therapy (EBRT) provides significant palliation of painful bone metastases in around 70% of patients, induces remineralization, prevents impending fractures, and promotes healing of pathological fractures, reducing the skeletal-related events (SRE). Hypofractionated schedules are used for the treatment of bone metastases; the most commonly used are a single 8 Gy, 20 Gy in five daily treatments (4 Gy per treatment), and 30 Gy in ten daily treatments (3 Gy per treatment). Postoperative external beam irradiation can significantly reduce disease progression and subsequent loss of fixation. In the postoperative setting, the treatment field should include the entire interlocking device, nails, or prosthesis in order to remove any microscopic dissemination of disease. Two-dimensional or 3D conformal radiotherapy could be used for treatment planning. Simple field assessment (anteroposterior-posteroanterior AP-PA field) is often used for treatment planning of long bones, leading to a shorter treatment time. For pelvic bone metastases, a more complex field assessment could be considered to lessen the dose to the organs at risk, leading to a better tolerability of the treatment itself. Recent technological advances, such as intensity-modulated radiotherapy (IMRT) and stereotactic body radiotherapy (SBRT), can be used in a particular setting of oligometastatic patients to deliver a substantial dose of radiation to the tumor and spare healthy normal tissues.

6.1 Introduction

Bone metastases are a common complication of advanced cancer that can cause severe and debilitating effects including severe pain, reduced mobility, spinal cord compression, life-threatening electrolyte imbalances, and pathologic fracture [1].

The distribution of bone metastases approximately mirrors the distribution of red marrow, presumably reflecting increased blood flow in red marrow compared to yellow marrow.

The spine, pelvis, and ribs are the main sites of the bone metastases, and the extremities, especially the distal portions, are non-predilection sites. Of the extremities, proximal portions of femurs are the most frequently involved site [2].

Upper extremity metastases can cause critical functional impairment and can hinder personal

M. Fiore · C. G. Rinaldi · S. Ramella (✉)
Radioterapia Oncologica,
Università Campus Biomedico, Rome, Italy
e-mail: s.ramella@unicampus.it

© Springer International Publishing AG, part of Springer Nature 2019
V. Denaro et al. (eds.), *Management of Bone Metastases*, https://doi.org/10.1007/978-3-319-73485-9_6

hygiene, independent ambulation, the ability to use external aids, meal management, and general activities of daily living.

Massive metastases to the pelvis, especially to the periacetabular area, are still a difficult treatment problem. They inhibit patients' walking independently, leading to the need for crutches or a walking frame. Joint motion is usually significantly limited and related to pain. These infirmities are accompanied by imminent muscle atrophy. Bed-ridden patients are more likely to develop thromboembolism and infectious complications. The patients need constant care of the family or healthcare practitioners and require analgesic treatment [3–5].

Pain may be localized or diffuse and may worsen upon weight bearing [6]. As a consequence of bone pain, patients often have increased difficulty with activities of daily living and decreased quality of life (QOL) [7].

External beam radiation therapy (EBRT) provides significant palliation of painful bone metastases in around 70% of patients, with up to 10–35% of patients achieving complete pain relief at the treated site [8]. Moreover, radiotherapy induces remineralization for strengthening of the weakened bone – so it prevents impending fractures – and promotes the healing of pathological fractures, thus reducing the skeletal-related events (SRE). As a consequence, radiotherapy for painful bone metastases leads to a better quality of life [9].

The precise mechanism of action by which radiation induces pain control is still not fully known: the shrinkage of the tumor bulk, which is the removal of tumor from the bone, enables the osteoblastic repair and a restored integrity of the damaged bone, leading to pain relief and reducing the mechanical effects of the compression and infiltration of the bone tissue, and the relative production of cytokines that act on receptors responsible for the pain. However, the early period of pain relief seen (25% in 24–48 h), the absence of dose-response relationship (single vs multiple fractions), and the absence of a clear relationship to the primary tumor suggest that the tumor shrinkage itself is unlikely to account for the pain relief [10–12].

Therefore, the early response leads to the hypothesis that early reacting and very sensitive cells, and the molecules they produce, are involved in this answer. Obvious candidate cells are the inflammatory cells that are largely present in the bone metastasis microenvironment. Reduction of the inflammatory cells by ionizing radiation inhibits the release of chemical pain mediators and is probably responsible for the rapid reaction seen in some patients [13]. Other candidate cells are the osteoclasts. A clear dose-response relationship between the dose of ionizing radiations and the decrease in the number of osteoclasts in vitro has been observed [14]. The inhibitory effect on the osteoclast activity exerted by ionizing radiations was also shown in a study conducted by Vakaet et al., in which patients with greater benefit after radiation therapy had a lower concentration of urinary bone reabsorption markers compared to "non-responders" [15].

6.2 Radiotherapy Dose and Fractionation

The conventional fractionation of radiotherapy provides daily fractions of 1.8–2 Gy, from Monday to Friday, and the total dose is determined by the radiosensitivity of the tumor and the tolerance of healthy tissues involved in the radiation field. Hypofractionated radiotherapy is delivered with high dose per fraction, in few days [16].

Historically, hypofractionated schedules are used for the treatment of bone metastases, based on two types of considerations:

- Empirical: relatively low doses of radiation are sufficient to control the pain in 80% of patents [17].
- Utilitarian: a small number of sessions is more comfortable for patients in poor conditions, and it reduces waiting lists in radiotherapy centers.

Many randomized trials have been conducted on dose fractionation schedules of palliative radiotherapy [17].

Table 6.1 Randomized studies on hypofractionated treatment regimens

Study	No of Pz (No Eval.)	Dose (Gy/ fractions)	Complete response (%)	Overall response	Path fractures (%)
Tong et al., 1982, USA (solitary treatment site)	266 (146)	20/5	53	82	4
		40/15	61	85	18
Multiple site	750 (613)	15/5	49	87	5
		20/5	56	85	7
		25/5	49	83	9
		30/10	57	78	8
Hirokawa et al., 1988, Japan	128	25/5	NA	75	NA
		30/10		75	
Rasmusson et al., 1995, Danmark	217 (127)	15/3	NA	69	NA
		30/10		66	
Niewald et al., 1996, Germany	100	20/5	33	77	8
		30/10	31	86	13

From the 1980s to the 1990s, four randomized studies [18–21] evaluating different hypofractionated treatment regimens have been conducted (Table 6.1), showing no differences in terms of frequency and duration of palliation, functional recovery, and incidence of pathological fractures, and all the treatment dose schedules were equally effective.

In the past 15 years, especially in Northern Europe, the use of a single high-dose session of radiotherapy for bone metastases has been tested. In particular, the results of numerous randomized trials comparing a single dose of 8 Gy with more prolonged regimens are enclosed in four meta-analysis [22–25], which came to the same conclusion in terms of the effectiveness of a single fraction of radiotherapy for pain control with minimal side effects.

The first of these was published by Wu in 2003 [22]. Sixteen trials were divided into three categories: (1) studies comparing single fractions of different doses, (2) studies comparing single dose vs multiple fractions, and (3) comparison of multifraction schedules of varying durations. (1) The two trials comparing single fraction of 4 Gy vs 8 Gy showed that the overall palliative response was significantly lower with 4 Gy per fraction, although there were no differences in terms of complete response. (2) An analysis of comparative trials between single fraction and multifraction regimens did not reveal any difference in terms of complete (39.2 vs. 40%) and overall (62.1 vs. 58.7%) response. (3) No signifi-

cant difference was found in terms of acute toxicity between the different radiation schedules.

The meta-analysis of 11 randomized trials by Sze et al. [23] confirmed equal effectiveness in terms of overall (60% vs 59% of total 1769 pts) and complete (34% vs 32%) response to pain between monofractionated and multifractionated regimens. However, the rate of retreatments and pathological fractures was higher in patients undergoing single session of RT compared with multifractionated regimens. The same conclusion is reached by Chow et al. [24], in his meta-analysis of 16 randomized trials comparing single fraction radiotherapy and more prolonged regimes which showed no differences in terms of global response to pain, a trend toward more retreatments in the single fraction group, and an increased incidence of pathologic fractures and spinal cord compressions in the single-session group (p 0.75 and 0.13, respectively).

In 2012, the same group updated the meta-analysis [25] and evaluated five additional randomized trials that were compared to those included in the earlier study; they showed once again that there was no statistically significant difference in the analgesic response between the two fractionation modes. The overall response rate to the pain was 60% (1696/2818) in patients undergoing single session of 8 Gy and 61% (1711/2799) in those receiving multiple fractions. Seventeen trials reported the rate of complete responses to pain on a total of 5263 patients, and also in this case, there were no significant differences (23% in the case of single fraction-ation vs 24% more protracted schedules). A trend in favor of multiple fractionations as regards the incidence of pathologic fractures and spinal cord compression was furthermore confirmed, although the difference was not statistically significant. In addition, the authors suggested that the higher percentage of retreatments in the group subjected to the single fraction could be explained by a greater reluctance of the physicians to retreat patients already treated by multifraction schedules.

In conclusion, the longer course has the advantage of a lower incidence of repeat treatment to the same site, but the single fraction has been proved to be more convenient for patients and caregivers [1].

The fractionation of most commonly used palliative radiotherapy regimens is as follows: a single 8 Gy, 20 Gy in five daily treatments (4 Gy per treatment), and 30 Gy in ten daily treatments (3 Gy per treatment). Moreover, the choice of the most suitable fractionation schedule for each patient cannot be done without a careful assessment of the patients' clinical conditions. As a consequence, models to predict survival have been worked out in order to determine the patients' prognosis and consequently the best choice of fractionation. For example, Westhoff et al. [26] found that in predicting survival in patients with painful bone metastases, KPS combined with primary tumor was comparable to a more complex model. Considering the amount of variables in complex models and the additional burden on patients, the use of a simple model only taking into account KPS and primary tumor type is preferred for daily use.

6.3 Radiotherapy and Surgery

Metastatic bone disease involving the pelvis and femur is a common clinical occurrence. A pathologic fracture in this region is a catastrophic event that results in significant pain and loss of function. The major goal in the management of the patient is to relieve pain and to restore function and ambulation. A team effort is important to rec-ognize the full therapeutic potential of each situation [27].

When a fracture affects the long bones or other weight-bearing bones such as the pelvis, a surgical stabilization is suggested when possible to treat the pain and to retain a functional limb [28]. Surgery is also indicated as prophylaxis for patients with metastatic lesions at a considerable risk of fracture (impending fractures). After the performance of the surgical stabilization, the patient is often sent to the radiation oncologist to assess the opportunity for an adjuvant radiotherapy.

Postoperative external beam irradiation can significantly reduce disease progression and subsequent loss of fixation. In fact, multiple reviews advise a short course of radiotherapy (from five to ten fractions) after surgical treatment, since it would allow bone healing, prevent tumor progression, minimize the risk of implant failure, and decrease the rate of secondary procedures [29–35]. In the postoperative setting, the treatment field should include the entire interlocking device, nails, or prosthesis in order to remove any microscopic dissemination of disease as the entire bone is at risk for microscopic involvement, because during the rod placement, the procedure may seed neoplastic cells at other sites.

In a recent review by Willeumier et al. [36], the authors asserted that there was a lack of clinical evidence about postoperative radiotherapy after surgical fixation of impending or actual pathologic fractures at the long bones. Based on the results of the only two articles that met the inclusion criteria for inclusion in the analysis, a firm conclusion on the standard use of postoperative radiotherapy in the long bones could not be drawn. The authors concluded that a large, multicenter, randomized study would provide further insights and lead to a firmer substantiated treatment plan for patients with metastases to the long bones.

Furthermore, the life expectancy must be taken into account in determining the most suitable treatment since the adjuvant and prophylactic treatments require time and energy of the fragile patient and might negatively affect the quality of life.

6.4   Radiotherapy Technique

No formal immobilization is usually required for patient setup, but adequate analgesia should be available for the patient during the planning and treatment.

An X-ray simulator could be used; this would provide good localization for the pelvis and long bones.

When two-dimensional, or conventional, radiation therapy is used, planning can be done rapidly, and the patients can start the treatment very quickly, as opposed to other techniques that require more in-depth (and time consuming) planning. As a consequence, this type of treatment, when still available, is generally reserved for urgent palliative treatments.

Nowadays most hospitals use a CT simulator to plan the treatment for bone metastases in a process known as 3D conformal radiotherapy. The advantage of CT-guided therapy compared to conventional therapy is that CT-guided therapy allows to delineate the metastases and normal organs in three dimensions, as opposed to using the "flat" image of an X-ray.

The target volumes should be defined after the review of all the diagnostic imaging. Attention should be paid to soft-tissue masses, which are often associated to bone metastases and responsible for the observed symptoms. Such lesions are best assessed by CT or MRI [37]. An adequate margin around the bone should be used.

For long bones, the clinical target volume (CTV) should encompass the entire marrow cavity of the bone but should avoid articular surfaces, and despite the low dose, a corridor for lymph drainage should be used [38]. Although the pelvis is a typical metastatic site, little consensus exists regarding the target volume delineation for radiotherapy of pelvic bone metastases. Because the pelvis has a curved shape and encompasses bowel loops and the bladder, contouring the target volume and protecting the organs at risk are challenging. In fact, many organs such as the intestines, urinary bladder, and internal sex organs are located within or near the pelvis. During the treatment planning, it is advisable to avoid uninvolved sensitive tissues like perineum.

Simple field assessment (anteroposterior-posteroanterior AP-PA field) is often used for treatment planning of long bones, leading to a shorter treatment time (Fig. 6.1).

For pelvic bone metastases, a more complex field assessment could be considered to lessen the dose to the organs at risk leading to a better tolerability of the treatment itself.

Recent technological advances, such as the intensity-modulated radiotherapy (IMRT) and the stereotactic body radiotherapy (SBRT), have enabled more successful radiation treatments by delivering a substantial dose of radiations to the tumor, while sparing healthy normal tissues.

However, these techniques should be reserved to a particular setting of oligometastatic patients. This setting is identified by a new category of patients with good prognosis and life expectancy with a single or limited number of metastases, early detected by the improvement of imaging techniques and careful follow-up. These patients could benefit from more sophisticated and complex radiotherapy that can prevent long-term complications of the treatment itself and that allow an extended control of the disease and the symptoms.

Radiosurgery, stereotactic radiotherapy, intensity-modulated radiotherapy, etc., may represent valid therapeutic options for the treatment of long bones and pelvic metastases in well-selected clinical conditions.

IMRT is an advanced form of three-dimensional conformal radiotherapy. It is of particular value for target volumes with concave or complex shapes with close proximity to radiosensitive normal structures. It has two key additional features compared to conformal radiotherapy:

1. Nonuniform intensity of the radiation beams
2. Computerized inverse planning [39]

IMRT is useful in particular for pelvic bone metastases, since (1) standard conventional anteroposterior/posteroanterior (APPA) or box techniques often result in large volumes of bowel receiving the prescription dose, and the concave pelvic target volume encircling normal organs (bowel, bladder, and genital region) lends itself to

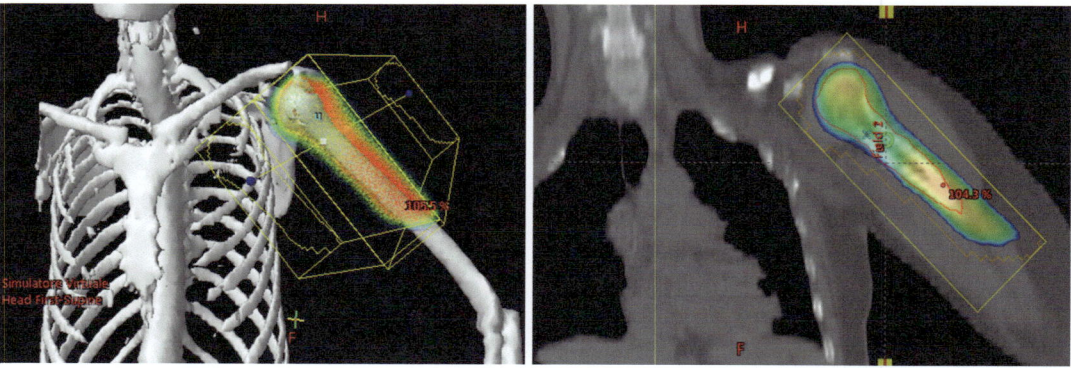

Fig. 6.1 AP-PA field assessment for humeral bone metastases

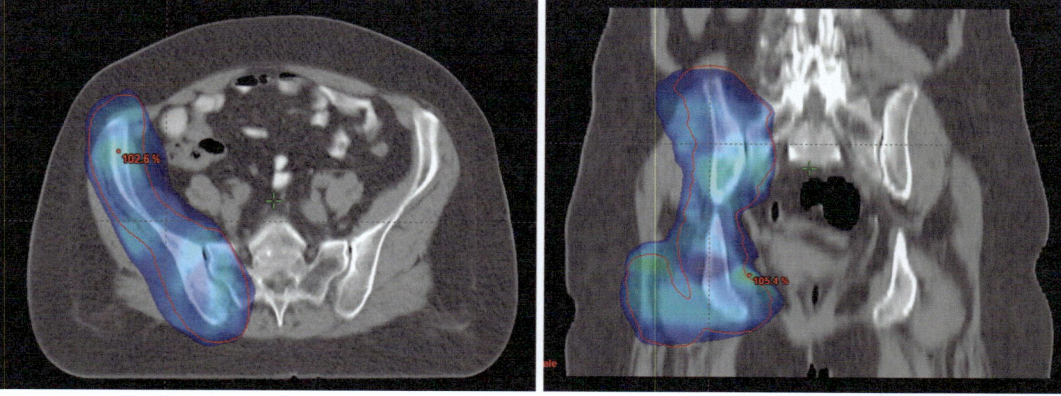

Fig. 6.2 IMRT dose distribution for the right ileum

IMRT, and the use of standard solutions to optimize planning target volume (PTV) coverage and spare central OARs; (2) gastrointestinal toxicity occurs frequently after large-field pelvic palliative RT; (3) indications for palliation of bone metastases often arise during ongoing systemic therapy; (4) the requirements for pelvic reirradiation may increase as systemic therapies improve; and (5) volumetric modulated arc delivery has been shown to be time-efficient and is well-suited to the fast irradiation of large volumes [40] (Figs. 6.2 and 6.3).

However, for IMRT the immobilization and treatment planning process is longer than 3D conformal radiotherapy, and the treatment delivery times are often prolonged; therefore, some patients could not be able to withstand the time necessary for treatment.

On the other hand, SBRT is a technique that allows to deliver high doses of radiation to the tumor in a single fraction (radiosurgery) or in few fractions (fractionated stereotactic radiotherapy), with a high dose gradient, to achieve a better disease control and simultaneously a considerable sparing of the surrounding normal tissues. Its use is increasingly widespread in the field of bone metastases, in particular for the treatment of spinal metastases, since the local recurrence can have irremediable consequences; moreover, there is little distance from critical organs like the spinal cord or the esophagus. But SBRT could be useful also for pelvic metastases since the pelvis has a curved shape and encompasses bowel loops and the bladder and internal sex organs.

However, as for IMRT, the immobilization and treatment planning process of SBRT is time

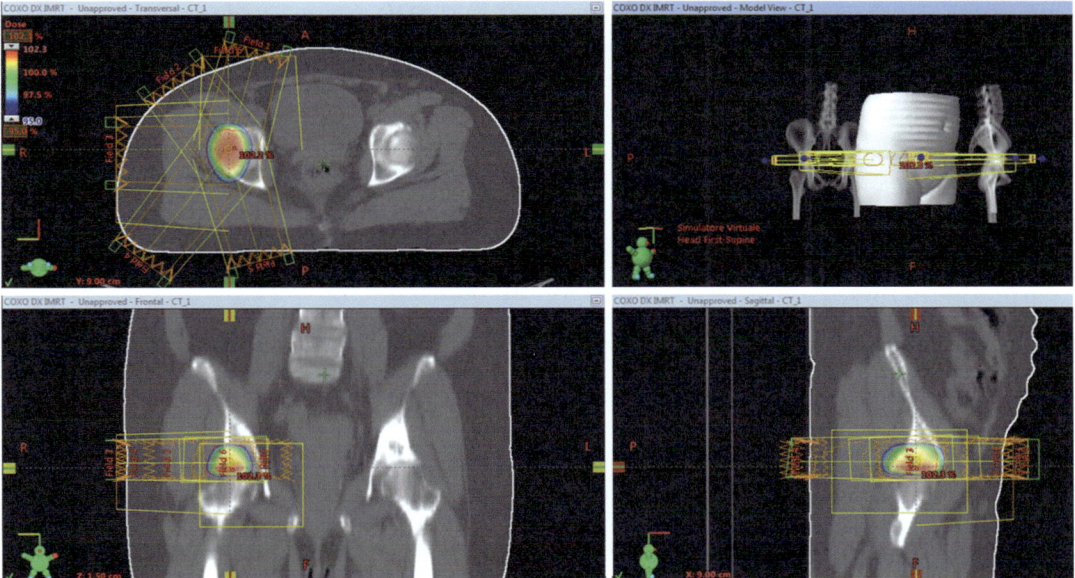

Fig. 6.3 IMRT treatment planning for acetabular metastasis

consuming and may delay the beginning of the treatment in a patient with severe bone pain. Patients must be able to lie immobilized and still for an extended period and should have a sufficiently good performance status [41]. Additionally, if the accuracy is compromised, the surrounding tissues will receive higher doses of radiation that could potentially lead to a more severe toxicity after treatment.

As an adjunctive matter, the economic impact of this complex technique should not be underestimated, and its role should be carefully evaluated in the management of patients with bone metastases. A recent area of research is in fact the one of cost-effectiveness of stereotactic radiotherapy in the palliative setting [42]. Therefore, the American Society for Radiation Oncology (ASTRO) Task Force recommends the use of SBRT only in clinical trials.

6.5   Radiotherapy Side Effects

The side effects of radiation therapy are specific to the treated area. Since patients with long bones or pelvic metastases often have a short life expectancy, they usually experience only the acute side effects of radiotherapy.

Even if a complete response of the pain could be achieved from 10 to 35% of patients, with overall pain response rates approaching 70%, some patients could experience an increase at the beginning of the treatment, due to radiation-induced edema and to the resulting compression of the neighboring healthy tissue. This event, known as "pain flare-up," is a common side effect of palliative radiotherapy for bone metastases and is more frequent for extensive lesions and/or higher fraction doses. Pain flare occurs in nearly 40% of the patients that receive palliative RT for symptomatic bone metastases and is not a predictor for pain response [43]. In a recent randomized placebo-controlled, phase 3 trial, Chow et al. [44] found that 4 mg dexamethasone tablets taken orally at least 1 h before the beginning of radiation treatment, and then every day for 4 days after radiotherapy (days 1–4), reduced the radiation-induced pain flare in the treatment of painful bone metastases.

For pelvic bone metastases, a gastrointestinal toxicity frequently occurs after large-field pelvic palliative RT. In patients treated by chemotherapy, the radiotherapy could also lead to a reduction in marrow reserves.

For long bones metastases, radiotherapy might cause lymphedema due to an alteration of lymph drainage if a low-dose corridor is not guaranteed.

Careful radiation treatment planning and the use of more sophisticated radiotherapy techniques for patients with long life expectancy can prevent most side effects. Patients should be reassured that the side effects that they could experience in most cases will resolve upon the completion of radiotherapy.

References

1. Lutz S, Berk L, Chang E, Chow E, Hahn C, Hoskin P, et al. Palliative radiotherapy for bone metastases: an ASTRO evidence-based guideline. Int J Radiat Oncol Biol Phys. 2011;79(4):965–76. https://doi.org/10.1016/j.ijrobp.2010.11.026.
2. Kakhki VR, Anvari K, Sadeghi R, Mahmoudian AS, Torabian-Kakhki M. Pattern and distribution of bone metastases in common malignant tumors. Nucl Med Rev Cent East Eur. 2013;16(2):66–9. https://doi.org/10.5603/NMR.2013.0037.
3. Bauer HC. Controversies in the surgical management of skeletal metastases. J Bone Joint Surg Br. 2005;87(5):608–17.
4. Canale ST, Beaty HJ. Campbell's operative orthopaedics. 12th ed. Oxford: Mosby Elsevier; 2013.
5. Coleman RE. Clinical features of metastatic bone disease and risk of skeletal morbidity. Clin Cancer Res. 2006;12(20 Pt 2):6243s–9s.
6. Mantyh P. Bone cancer pain: causes, consequences, and therapeutic opportunities. Pain. 2013;154(Suppl 1):S54–62. https://doi.org/10.1016/j.pain.2013.07.044. Epub 2013 Jul 31
7. Pituskin E, Fairchild A, Dutka J, Gagnon L, Driga A, Tachynski P, et al. Multidisciplinary team contributions within a dedicated outpatient palliative radiotherapy clinic: a prospective descriptive study. Int J Radiat Oncol Biol Phys. 2010;78(2):527–32.
8. Chow E, Wong R, Hruby G, Connolly R, Franssen E, Fung KW, et al. Prospective patient-based assessment of effectiveness of palliative radiotherapy for bone metastases. Radiother Oncol. 2001;61:77–82.
9. McDonald R, Chow E, Rowbottom L, Bedard G, Lam H, Wong E, et al. Quality of life after palliative radiotherapy in bone metastases: a literature review. J Bone Oncol. 2014;4(1):24–31. https://doi.org/10.1016/j.jbo.2014.11.001.
10. Hoskin PJ. Bisphosphonates and radiation therapy for palliation of metastatic bone disease. Cancer Treat Rev. 2003;29(4):321–7.
11. Saarto T, Janes R, Tenhunen M, Kouri M. Palliative radiotherapy in the treatment of skeletal metastases. Eur J Pain. 2002;6(5):323–30.
12. Poulsen HS, Nielsen OS, Klee M, Rørth M. Palliative irradiation of bone metastases. Cancer Treat Rev. 1989;16(1):41–8.
13. Mercadante S. Malignant bone pain: pathophysiology and treatment. Pain. 1997;69(1–2):1–18.
14. Tsay TP, Chen MH, Oyen OJ, Hahn SS, Marty JJ. The effect of cobalt-60 irradiation on bone marrow cellularity and alveolar osteoclasts. Proc Natl Sci Counc Repub China B. 1995;19(3):185–95.
15. Vakaet LA, Boterberg T. Pain control by ionizing radiation of bone metastasis. Int J Dev Biol. 2004;48(5–6):599–606.
16. Cliffoard Chao KS, Perez CA, Brady LW. Radiation oncology management decisions. Philadelphia: Lippincott Williams & Wilkins; 2002.
17. Fletcher GH. Textbook of radiotherapy. Philadelphia: Lea & Febiger; 1980. p. 943–6.
18. Tong D, Gillick L, Hendrickson FR. The palliation of symptomatic osseous metastases: final results of the study by the Radiation Therapy Oncology Group. Cancer. 1982;50(5):893–9.
19. Hirokawa Y, Wadasaki K, Kashiwado K, Kagemoto M, Katsuta S, Honke Y, et al. A multi-institutional prospective randomized study of radiation therapy of bone metastases. Nihon Igaku Hoshasen Gakkai Zasshi. 1988;48(11):1425–31.
20. Rasmusson B, Vejborg I, Jensen AB, Andersson M, Banning AM, Hoffmann T, et al. Irradiation of bone metastases in breast cancer patients: a randomized study with 1 year follow-up. Radiother Oncol. 1995;34(3):179–84.
21. Niewald M, Tkocz HJ, Abel U, Scheib T, Walter K, Nieder C, et al. Rapid course radiation therapy vs. more standard treatment: a randomized trial for bone metastases. Int J Radiat Oncol Biol Phys. 1996;36(5):1085–9.
22. Wu JS, Wong R, Johnston M, Bezjak A, Whelan T, Cancer Care Ontario Practice Guidelines Initiative Supportive Care Group. Meta-analysis of dose-fraction radiotherapy trias for the palliation of painful bone metastases. Int J Radiat Oncol Biol Phys. 2003;55(3):594–605.
23. Sze WM, Shelley MD, Held I, Wilt TJ, Mason MD. Palliation of metastatic bone pain; single fraction versus multifraction radiotherapy: a systemic review of randomized trials. Clin Oncol (R Coll Radiol). 2003;15(6):345–52.
24. Chow E, Harris K, Fan G, Tsao M, Sze WM. Palliative radiotherapy trials for bone metastases: systematic review. J Clin Oncol. 2007;25(11):1423–36.
25. Chow E, Zeng L, Salvo N, Dennis K, Tsao M, Lutz S. Update on the systematic review of palliative radiotherapy trials for bone metastases. Clin Oncol (R Coll Radiol). 2012;24(2):112–24. https://doi.org/10.1016/j.clon.2011.11.004.
26. Westhoff PG, de Graeff A, Monninkhof EM, Bollen L, Dijkstra SP, van der Steen-Banasik EM, et al. An easy tool to predict survival in patients receiving radiation therapy for painful bone metastases. Int J Radiat Oncol Biol Phys. 2014;90(4):739–47. https://doi.org/10.1016/j.ijrobp.2014.07.051.

27. Sim FH. Metastatic bone disease of the pelvis and femur. Instr Course Lect. 1992;41:317–27.
28. Bonarigo BC, Rubin P. Nonunion of pathologic fracture after radiation therapy. Radiology. 1967;88(5):889–98.
29. Frassica FJ, Frassica DA. Metastatic bone disease of the humerus. J Am Acad Orthop Surg. 2003;11(4):282–8.
30. Jacofsky DJ, Haidukewych GJ. Management of pathologic fractures of the proximal femur: state of the art. J Orthop Trauma. 2004;18(7):459–69.
31. Bickels J, Dadia S, Lidar Z. Surgical management of metastatic bone disease. J Bone Joint Surg Am. 2009;91(6):1503–16. https://doi.org/10.2106/JBJS.H.00175.
32. Biermann JS, Holt GE, Lewis VO, Schwartz HS, Yaszemski MJ. Metastatic bone disease: diagnosis, evaluation, and treatment. Instr Course Lect. 2010;59:593–606.
33. Ruggieri P, Mavrogenis AF, Casadei R, Errani C, Angelini A, Calabrò T, et al. Protocol of surgical treatment of long bone pathological fractures. Injury. 2010;41(11):1161–7. https://doi.org/10.1016/j.injury.2010.09.018.
34. Malviya A, Gerrand C. Evidence for orthopaedic surgery in the treatment of metastatic bone disease of the extremities: a review article. Palliat Med. 2012;26(6):788–96. https://doi.org/10.1177/0269216311419882.
35. Quinn RH, Randall RL, Benevenia J, Berven SH, Raskin KA. Contemporary management of metastatic bone disease: tips and tools of the trade for general practitioners. Instr Course Lect. 2014;63:431–41.
36. Willeumier JJ, van der Linden YM, Dijkstra PD. Lack of clinical evidence for postoperative radiotherapy after surgical fixation of impending or actual pathologic fractures in the long bones in patients with cancer; a systematic review. Radiother Oncol.
2016;121(1):138–42. https://doi.org/10.1016/j.radonc.2016.07.009.
37. Gunderson T. Clinical radiation oncology. 2nd ed. Philadelphia: Churchill Livingstone Elsevier; 2007.
38. Hoskin P, Goh V. Radiotherapy in practice—imaging. Oxford: Oxford University press; 2010. p. 260–1.
39. Taylor A, Powell ME. Intensity-modulated radiotherapy—what is it? Cancer Imaging. 2004;4(2):68–73. https://doi.org/10.1102/1470-7330.2004.0003.
40. Griffioen G, Dahele M, Jeulink M, Senan S, Slotman B, Verbakel WF. Bowel-sparing intensity-modulated radiotherapy (IMRT) for palliation of large-volume pelvic bone metastases: rationale, technique and clinical implementation. Acta Oncol. 2013;52(4):877–80. https://doi.org/10.3109/0284186X.2012.725943.
41. Bhattacharya IS, Hoskin PJ. Stereotactic body radiotherapy for spinal and bone metastases. Clin Oncol (R Coll Radiol). 2015;27(5):298–306. https://doi.org/10.1016/j.clon.2015.01.030.
42. Kim H, Rajagopalan MS, Beriwal S, Huq MS, Smith KJ. Cost-effectiveness analysis of single fraction of stereotactic body radiation therapy compared with single fraction of external beam radiation therapy for palliation of vertebral bone metastases. Int J Radiat Oncol Biol Phys. 2015;91(3):556–63.
43. Gomez-Iturriaga A, Cacicedo J, Navarro A, Morillo V, Willisch P, Carvajal C, et al. Incidence of pain flare following palliative radiotherapy for symptomatic bone metastases: multicenter prospective observational study. BMC Palliat Care. 2015;14:48. https://doi.org/10.1186/s12904-015-0045-8.
44. Chow E, Meyer RM, Ding K, Nabid A, Chabot P, Wong P. Dexamethasone in the prophylaxis of radiation-induced pain flare after palliative radiotherapy for bone metastases: a double-blind, randomised placebo-controlled, phase 3 trial. Lancet Oncol. 2015;16(15):1463–72. https://doi.org/10.1016/S1470-2045(15)00199-0.

The Role of Radiotherapy in Spinal Metastases

7

Francesca De Felice, Daniela Musio, and Vincenzo Tombolini

Abstract

Nowadays metastatic disease dominates the survival outcomes of cancer patients, due to modern combined modality therapies. The spine represents the most common site of bone metastases.

Treatment decisions primarily depend on clinical symptoms, spinal stability, extent of disease, and medical comorbidities. Radiation therapy (RT) plays a crucial role in the palliative management of spinal metastases (SM). The main objective is to provide pain relief and preserve neurological function.

Keywords

Spinal metastases · Palliative radiotherapy · External beam radiotherapy · Stereotactic body radiotherapy · Spinal cord compression Pain · Quality of life

7.1 Introduction

Spinal metastases (SM) constitute one of the major problems in oncology. The spine is involved in up to 40% of cancer patients that develop metastatic disease during the course of their illness [1]. SM are usually associated with a limited median survival (7 months), with an approximately 40% probability of survival up to 12 months, especially in case of oligometastatic breast or prostate cancer [2]. Most commonly seen tumor primary sites include prostate, breast, kidney, lung, thyroid, lymphoma, and myeloma. SM can determine important morbidity and negatively impact patient's quality of life (QoL), primarily due to spinal cord compression (SCC) risk. In fact, SCC exposes to a paralysis below the level of compression, prejudicing extremities movement, as well as bladder, bowel, and sexual function [2]. Thus, an early diagnosis and a prompt treatment of SM are a high priority, in order to prevent, reduce, or at least delay serious complications. Over the past 20 years, it has been estimated that the incidence of SM has increased due to improved survival of cancer patients, whereas, on the other hand, the incidence of SCC has decreased, primarily because magnetic resonance imaging (MRI) has become more widely available [3].

The thoracic spine is the most frequently involved region (60–80%), followed by lumbar (15–30%) and cervical vertebrae (10%). Breast and lung tumors metastasize usually to the thoracic spine, whereas prostate cancer metastasizes preferably in the lumbar-sacral region. It has been estimated that more than 50% of patients with SM have evidence of metastases at multiple

F. De Felice (✉) · D. Musio · V. Tombolini
Department of Radiological, Oncological and
Anatomo-Pathological Sciences, Policlinico Umberto
I "Sapienza" University of Rome, Rome, Italy
e-mail: francesca.defelice@uniroma1.it

© Springer International Publishing AG, part of Springer Nature 2019
V. Denaro et al. (eds.), *Management of Bone Metastases*, https://doi.org/10.1007/978-3-319-73485-9_7

levels of the spine [4]. The posterior portion of the vertebral body is the most common initial anatomic location and involvement of pedicles occurs thereafter.

Optimal management of SM encompasses a multidisciplinary approach, including radiology, spinal surgery, radiation therapy (RT), medical oncology, and rehabilitation medicine. We briefly examine the natural history of SM and focus on the clinical effectiveness and cost-effectiveness of subsequent RT treatment.

7.2   Natural History

Physiopathology The main method of tumor cells dissemination is through the venous plexus of Batson. Firstly described in 1940, this venous system is located in the epidural space between the spinal column bone and the dura mater. Its major characteristic is the lack of valves that control the blood flow received from other venous drainage, including the portal, caval, renal, pulmonary, intercostals, and azygous systems. Vertebral bodies represent one of the preferential tumor cell localization because of their rich vascularity that promotes adhesion of malignant cells to endothelial cells. The bone microenvironment is the most fertile soil for cellular implantation, due to its variety of growth factors, including cytokines, enzymes, and hormones. In pathological condition, the balance between bone resorption (osteoclast-mediated) and bone remodeling (osteoblast-mediated) is lost, resulting in osteolytic, osteoblastic, or mixed bone lesions formation [4].

SM can also occur as direct invasion or extension of primary tumor. For instance, prostate and colorectal lesions may become locally aggressive and invade the lumbar or sacral spine, leading to symptomatic SM, whereas lung cancers can extend posteriorly into the thoracic vertebral column.

Seeding of tumor cells in the cerebrospinal fluid represents other mechanism of SM spread, and it is usually secondary to a cerebral surgery approach [5].

Clinical Manifestation Structural failure of the vertebrae and pain, either local, referred, or radicular in nature, are common symptoms at diagnosis. However, sometimes SM can be asymptomatic [2].

Generally, the severity of symptoms depends on tumor growth, degree of bone involvement, and extent of systematic disease. SM can lead to severe complications, such as pathological fractures, motor dysfunction (causing myelopathy and radiculopathy), sensory dysfunction (including anesthesia, hyperesthesia, and paresthesia), and SCC with subsequent autonomic dysfunction [5].

7.3   Impact on Treatment Decision-Making

To optimize the treatment paradigms in SM patients, appropriate establishment of spinal stability and degree of SM occupancy of the vertebral body are crucial.

Spinal Instability Neoplastic Score The spine oncology study group (SOSG) developed the spinal instability neoplastic score (SINS) as a comprehensive classification system specific to SM [6]. SINS is an evidence-based medicine system able to predict stability of neoplastic lesions and identify those patients requiring surgical consultation. It is based on both patient symptoms and radiographic criteria of the spine. The final score includes the following factors: global spinal location of the tumor, type and presence of pain, bone lesion quality, radiographic spinal alignment, extent of vertebral body collapse, and posterolateral spinal element involvement. The greater is the extent of vertebra invasion, the more likely spinal fracture is to occur, and surgical assessment is important.

Bilsky Grading Scale To facilitate optimal patient care, a clear grading scheme to define epidural involvement is paramount. In fact, the degree of epidural disease can be essential to guide RT decision-making, due to constraints of spinal cord tolerance. Epidural disease is defined as grade 0 (bone only), grade 1 [epidural impingement, without (1a) or with (1b) deformation of thecal sac or spinal cord abutment (1c)], grade 2 (partial obliteration of cerebrospinal fluid space), and grade 3 (complete obliteration of cerebrospinal fluid space) [7]. Considering innovations in techniques, RT is utilized as primary treatment approach in patients with grade 0–1 epidural disease, whereas it can be used as adjuvant treatment after surgical management in grade 2 and 3 epidural disease.

7.4 Radiation Therapy

RT is a valuable therapy in SM management. The therapeutic objective is mainly to relieve pain and preserve neurological function. Beneficial effects on pain may necessitate several days to a few weeks, so analgesic medication must be optimized during that interval [8]. Pain relief ranges from 50 to 85% of cases—with up to one-third reporting complete response—and typically occurs within 4 weeks after RT to last approximately 19 weeks [9].

Imaging is essential to delineate target volume for radiation planning purposes. The major factors that should be taken into account when considering a patient for RT treatment are anatomic location and presence/absence of SCC. Current standard recommendations are listed in Table 7.1 [9, 10]. In case of SCC, definitive treatment, including surgical decompression followed by RT or RT alone in those patients unfit for surgical

approach, should be given as soon as possible [5, 11]. Adjuvant RT is indicated to achieve local tumor control and should be initiated as soon as possible.

External Beam Radiation Therapy External beam radiation therapy (EBRT) is the standard of care for the treatment of SM. Before EBRT, a computed tomography (CT) scan of the affected anatomic site is obtained, with the patient immobilized in a comfortable and reproducible treatment position. EBRT fields include the involved vertebral body (and if necessary the soft tissue mass), plus a vertebral body below and above. Single 8 Gy fraction, prescribed to the appropriate target volume, is nowadays the recommended dose to treat symptomatic and uncomplicated bone metastases [12].

There have been several randomized controlled trials comparing the effectiveness of pain control with various regimens of fractionated EBRT, including single 8 Gy dose and multiple fraction regimens, such as 30 Gy in ten fractions, 24 Gy in six fractions, and 20 Gy in five fractions [13–18]. Pain control rates were essentially similar regardless of the fractionation pattern, whereas re-treatment rates to the same anatomic site were significantly higher in those patients who received 8 Gy compared to fractionated courses (20% versus 8%, $p < 0.00001$) [19]. However, in daily practice, despite the proven 8 Gy clinical effectiveness and cost efficiency, the selection of the fractionation schemes is often influenced by patient characteristics (performance status, compliance to

Table 7.1 Radiation therapy in spinal metastases: indications

| Clinical circumstances | Treatment | Radiation therapy | | |
		Total dose	Fraction	Technique
Uncomplicated spinal metastases	Primary RT	8 Gy	1	EBRT
		15–24 Gy	1	SBRT
		18–36 Gy	3–6	
Spinal cord compression	Adjuvant RT			EBRT
Life expectancy >6 months		30 Gy	10	
Life expectancy ≤6 months		8 Gy; 20 Gy	1; 5	
Unfit for decompressive surgery	Primary RT	8 Gy	1	
Reirradiation	Primary RT	8 Gy	1	EBRT
		10–30 Gy	1–5	SBRT

RT radiation therapy, *Gy* gray, *EBRT* external beam radiation therapy, *SBRT* stereotactic body radiation therapy treatment, life expectancy), tumor-related factors (histology of the primary tumor, interval time from primary diagnosis to SM, time of developing pain or neurological deficits before RT), and logistic issues (treatment duration time, validity of family members assistance, hospital location, cost of therapy).

Stereotactic Body Radiation Therapy Nowadays, stereotactic body radiation therapy (SBRT) is gaining increasing popularity in SM treatment, due to its ability to overcome several EBRT dose limitations. SBRT is an emerging high-dose RT with tumor-ablative intent, while sparing surrounding tissues. Meticulous attention should be given to the accuracy of both target delineation and patient setup to maximize treatment effectiveness and safety. SBRT involves a multistep process, including patient immobilization, computer tomography (CT) image acquisition planning, target delineation, sophisticated treatment planning, and imaging guidance to detect and correct patient positional deviations [20]. The main advantage over EBRT is the higher biologically effective dose (BED) delivered to the SM. Typically, a total dose of 16–24 Gy in single fraction or 24 Gy in two fractions or 27 Gy in three fractions is delivered to the target volume, which is, respectively, normalized to a 34.7–68 Gy, 44 Gy, and 42.8 Gy equivalent BED ($\alpha/\beta = 10$). In addition, reducing target volume, more spinal cord is preserved compared to the large EBRT fields. On the other hand, treatment time is prolonged (45–90 min per fraction); if toxicity arises, it is more severe, and retreatment results are much more complicated.

Retrospective literature data highlight a great local control (up to 80%) in those series using SBRT as adjuvant or salvage postoperative treatment. However, due to the lack of randomized clinical trials comparing EBRT versus SBRT, nowadays it is still not possible to draw definitive conclusions. The Radiation Therapy Oncology Group (RTOG) 0631 study is currently recruiting participants (https://clinicaltrials.gov/NCT00922974). It randomizes patients with localized SM between 8 Gy in a single fraction EBRT and single 16 or 18 Gy SBRT dose to

determine whether SBRT could improve pain control and QoL as compared to conventional EBRT. Final results would be essential to better delineate SBRT clinical effectiveness, in this setting of patients.

Local failure in the epidural space adjacent to the spinal cord is the most common pattern reported in SBRT studies [21, 22]. It appears that recurrent disease is mainly related to radiation underdosing of the epidural space in order to meet spinal cord constraints and disease direct extension into the epidural space. Therefore, identifying the appropriate clinical target volume (CTV) is essential because the step dose gradients between target and adjacent normal tissues result in disease subdosage. The International Spine Radiosurgery Consortium (ISRC) generated recommendations for delineating the correct target volume when using SBRT [23]. Each vertebral body has been divided into six sectors: vertebral body (sector 1), left pedicle (sector 2), left transverse process and lamina (sector 3), spinous process (sector 4), right transverse process and lamina (sector 5), and right pedicle (sector 6). Detailed analysis of CTV delineation is beyond the aim of this chapter; thus we only briefly described it. As a general rule, the entire sector should be included in the CTV if any portion of any sector contained the lesion. For instance, if the SM involves part of vertebral body, pedicle, and base of transverse process, then the CTV should include all sectors 1, 2, and 3 (Fig. 7.1). In

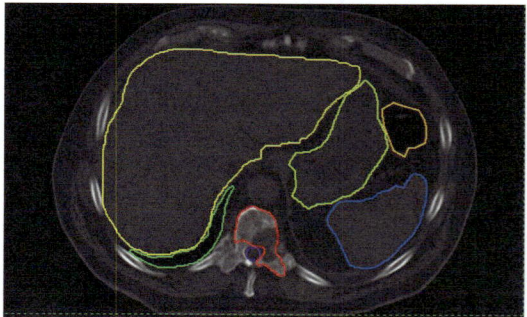

Fig. 7.1 Practical example of clinical target volume delineation. Spinal metastases involving lateral left vertebral body with extension to pedicle and base of transverse process, clinical target volume includes all sectors 1 (vertebral body), 2 (pedicle), and 3 (transverse process)

case of postoperative spine SBRT, the CTV should include the anatomic sectors involved based on both preoperative and postoperative diagnostic images [24]. However, the potential application of postoperative SBRT requires validation in prospective controlled studies.

7.5   Toxicity

Quantitative Analysis of Normal Tissue Effects in the Clinic (QUANTEC) Tissue radiation tolerance depends on its architecture and its reserve capacity, as well as the proportion of the organ included in the target, the fraction size and the dose received, the overall treatment time, and the length of follow-up [25]. Conventionally, it is assumed that each organ is composed of functional subunits (FSUs), and their spatial rapport is essential to maintain organ integrity [26]. The spinal cord is classified into serial organ, and the maximum absorbed dose is essential to predict tissue tolerance and, thus, tissue complication. The spinal cord extends from the base of the skull through the lumbar spine and consists of motor and sensory tracts. RT-induced injury can be severe and result in pain, paresthesias, sensory deficits, paralysis, Brown-Sequard syndrome, and bowel/bladder incontinence [27]. Portions of the spinal cord are always included in RT fields for SM treatment. In EBRT treatment plan, it is sufficient to identify the level of the involved spinal cord. In fact, considering that the radiation field encompasses the entire spinal cord circumference, the precise spinal cord definition is not critical. On the other hand, in SBRT technique, the delineation of the spinal cord is paramount, although there is not until now a consensus on the best approach to delineate it—the entire thecal sac or the spinal canal, or the spinal cord with/without a radial margin.

It is well established that the spinal cord can tolerate 45–50 Gy with conventional fractionation, resulting in an estimated radiation myelopathy (RM) risk of 0.03–0.2% [27]. Reirradiation

data suggested no RM cases for cumulative dose ≤60 Gy in 2 Gy equivalent doses, in at least 6 months interval between RT courses [27]. Using hypofractionated regimens, the recommended constraints are less accepted. It is well known that when the spinal cord is treated with large dose fractions, the biological effectiveness per unit of dose increases briskly [26]. RM incidence after SBRT to SM is less than 1% when the maximum spinal cord dose is limited to the equivalent of 13 Gy in a single fraction or 20 Gy in three fractions [27]. To reduce its local recurrence, it has been proposed a less strict spinal cord constraint of 9–10 Gy, but it is probably not appropriate for previously irradiated patients [21]. However, it should be noted that SBRT is a relatively recent technique; thus, reports of toxicity are rare, the follow-up time is short, and the patient numbers are small.

Radiation Therapy-Related Complications Potentially disabling serious adverse events include, mainly, vertebral compression fracture (VCF) and RM.

VCF arises secondary to bone tissue damage. It is a practically low-risk (<5%) adverse event after EBRT, whereas the crude risk of VCF after spinal SBRT ranges from 11 to 39% [28]. It is dependent on several clinical and dosimetric factors, including the evidence of kyphotic or scoliotic deformity, the presence of lytic tumor, and the SBRT dose per fraction [29]. The VCF incidence is alarming if the risk of subsequent surgical salvage interventions is considered [30]. However, the VCF incidence can potentially be minimized by performing careful RT and surgical planning.

According to the Common Terminology Criteria for Adverse Events (CTCAE), RM is defined as a grade ≥2 myelitis, with signs of sensory or motor deficits, loss of function, or pain (https://ctep.cancer.gov). RM occurs within 3 years the completion of RT, due to spinal cord necrosis. The risk of RM following RT depends on the maximum dose to the spinal cord, and, independently of RT technique, it has been estimated to be ≤5% if the recommended dose constraints are adhered to.

7.6 Reirradiation

According to the international consensus on palliative RT, reirradiation to a previously irradiated site is defined as a treatment given more than 4 weeks after the initial RT course [31]. Reirradiation might represent an option to control pain in those patients who have had no response after previous RT, in those other patients who have had partial response and thus there is the hope of additional benefit from repeat treatment, or in those patients who have had pain relapse after initial satisfactory response. At present no definitive recommendation can be given regarding dose and fractions. Actually, after initial multiple fractions schedule, the vast majority of patients are not referred to retreatment, primarily due to the limits of spinal cord radiation tolerance. Reirradiation with single 8 Gy fraction seems to be non-inferior and less toxic than 20 Gy in multiple fractions [32]. However, this conclusion needs a careful interpretation. In fact, it should be noticed that patients receiving retreatment to the spine were eligible if their previous treatment was with single fraction, 18 Gy in four fractions, or 20 Gy in five fractions. Previous treatment with 24 Gy in six fractions, 27 Gy in eight fractions, or 30 Gy in ten fractions was an exclusion criteria, as well as clinical or radiological evidence of SCC, a pathological fracture, or an impending fracture that needed to be fixed surgically. These criteria support the hypothesis that the misconception of high RM risk could interfere with potential retreatment indication.

The option to reirradiate SM using SBRT technique has been tested in several phase I/II clinical trials [33, 34]. Although it results in an effective and safe therapy, there is no evidence of SBRT superiority over conventional EBRT, especially in terms of pain control, and therefore further researches are mandatory in this field.

7.7 Spinal Cord Compression

SCC is an additional complication caused by SM. Considering that an immediate and aggressive treatment approach is essential to preserve the neurological function, SCC represents a medical emergency. Although corticosteroids and RT have routinely been considered the standard of care over the past decades, nowadays, due to improvements in spinal surgery techniques, new evidence suggests that direct decompressive surgery followed by adjuvant RT represents the best management in SCC in eligible patients [35]. Generally, a protracted hypofractionated schedule (30 Gy; 3 Gy/fraction) is reserved to those patients with expected longer survivals (>6 months), whereas shorter RT (20 Gy; 4 Gy/fraction, or single 8 Gy fraction) regimens are recommended for patient with SCC and life expectancy ≤6 months [36].

7.8 Summary

Improvement in survival rates of cancer patients has resulted in increased incidence of SM. Appropriate multidisciplinary management is essential in the evaluation and care of these complex patients. EBRT is considered the standard of care, and the single 8 Gy fraction should represent the first choice for uncomplicated SM treatment. Although rare, VCF and RM are the most significant RT-related adverse events, whereas SCC is the prevalent complication linked to SM and a prompt approach, including surgery plus RT, is paramount to preserve patient's neurological function.

Further advances are needed to routinely include SBRT technique in clinical practice.

References

1. Schmidt MH, Klimo P Jr, Vrionis FD. Metastatic spinal cord compression. J Natl Compr Cancer Netw. 2005;3(5):711–9.
2. Sutcliffe P, Connock M, Shyangdan D, Court R, Kandala NB, Clarke A. A systematic review of evidence on malignant spinal metastases: natural history and technologies for identifying patients at high risk of vertebral fracture and spinal cord compression. Health Technol Assess. 2013;17(42):1–274.
3. Jabehdar Maralani P, Lo SS, Redmond K, Soliman H, Myrehaug S, Husain ZA, Heyn C, Kapadia A, Chan A, Sahgal A. Spinal metastases: multimodality

imaging in diagnosis and stereotactic body radiation therapy planning. Future Oncol. 2017;13(1):77–91.

4. Maccauro G, Spinelli MS, Mauro S, Perisano C, Graci C, Rosa MA. Physiopathology of spine metastasis. Int J Surg Oncol. 2011;2011:107969.

5. Sciubba DM, Petteys RJ, Dekutoski MB, Fisher CG, Fehlings MG, Ondra SL, Rhines LD, Gokaslan ZL. Diagnosis and management of metastatic spine disease. A review. J Neurosurg Spine. 2010;13(1):94–108.

6. Fisher CG, DiPaola CP, Ryken TC, Bilsky MH, Shaffrey CI, Berven SH, Harrop JS, Fehlings MG, Boriani S, Chou D, Schmidt MH, Polly DW, Biagini R, Burch S, Dekutoski MB, Ganju A, Gerszten PC, Gokaslan ZL, Groff MW, Liebsch NJ, Mendel E, Okuno SH, Patel S, Rhines LD, Rose PS, Sciubba DM, Sundaresan N, Tomita K, Varga PP, Vialle LR, Vrionis FD, Yamada Y, Fourney DR. A novel classification system for spinal instability in neoplastic disease: an evidence-based approach and expert consensus from the Spine Oncology Study Group. Spine (Phila Pa 1976). 2010;35(22):E1221–9.

7. Bilsky MH, Laufer I, Fourney DR, Groff M, Schmidt MH, Varga PP, Vrionis FD, Yamada Y, Gerszten PC, Kuklo TR. Reliability analysis of the epidural spinal cord compression scale. J Neurosurg Spine. 2010;13(3):324–8.

8. Lutz S. The role of radiation therapy in controlling painful bone metastases. Curr Pain Headache Rep. 2012;16(4):300–6.

9. Lutz S, Berk L, Chang E, Chow E, Hahn C, Hoskin P, Howell D, Konski A, Kachnic L, Lo S, Sahgal A, Silverman L, von Gunten C, Mendel E, Vassil A, Bruner DW, Hartsell W, American Society for Radiation Oncology (ASTRO). Palliative radiotherapy for bone metastases: an ASTRO evidence-based guideline. Int J Radiat Oncol Biol Phys. 2011;79(4):965–76.

10. Bhattacharya IS, Hoskin PJ. Stereotactic body radiotherapy for spinal and bone metastases. Clin Oncol (R Coll Radiol). 2015;27(5):298–306.

11. Saarto T, Janes R, Tenhunen M, Kouri M. Palliative radiotherapy in the treatment of skeletal metastases. Eur J Pain. 2002;6(5):323–30.

12. Wu JS, Wong RK, Lloyd NS, Johnston M, Bezjak A, Whelan T, Supportive Care Guidelines Group of Cancer Care Ontario. Radiotherapy fractionation for the palliation of uncomplicated painful bone metastases—an evidence-based practice guideline. BMC Cancer. 2004;4:71.

13. No Authors. 8 Gy single fraction radiotherapy for the treatment of metastatic skeletal pain: randomised comparison with a multifraction schedule over 12 months of patient follow-up. Bone Pain Trial Working Party. Radiother Oncol. 1999;52(2):111–21.

14. Hartsell WF, Scott CB, Bruner DW, Scarantino CW, Ivker RA, Roach M 3rd, Suh JH, Demas WF, Movsas B, Petersen IA, Konski AA, Cleeland CS, Janjan NA, DeSilvio M. Randomized trial of short- versus long-

course radiotherapy for palliation of painful bone metastases. J Natl Cancer Inst. 2005;97(11):798–804.

15. Foro Arnalot P, Fontanals AV, Galcerán JC, Lynd F, Latiesas XS, de Dios NR, Castillejo AR, Bassols ML, Galán JL, Conejo IM, López MA. Randomized clinical trial with two palliative radiotherapy regimens in painful bone metastases: 30 Gy in 10 fractions compared with 8 Gy in single fraction. Radiother Oncol. 2008;89(2):150–5.

16. Steenland E, Leer JW, van Houwelingen H, Post WJ, van den Hout WB, Kievit J, de Haes H, Martijn H, Oei B, Vonk E, van der Steen-Banasik E, Wiggenraad RG, Hoogenhout J, Wárlám-Rodenhuis C, van Tienhoven G, Wanders R, Pomp J, van Reijn M, van Mierlo I, Rutten E. The effect of a single fraction compared to multiple fractions on painful bone metastases: a global analysis of the Dutch Bone Metastasis Study. Radiother Oncol. 1999;52(2):101–9.

17. Nielsen OS, Bentzen SM, Sandberg E, Gadeberg CC, Timothy AR. Randomized trial of single dose versus fractionated palliative radiotherapy of bone metastases. Radiother Oncol. 1998;47(3):233–40.

18. Gaze MN, Kelly CG, Kerr GR, Cull A, Cowie VJ, Gregor A, Howard GC, Rodger A. Pain relief and quality of life following radiotherapy for bone metastases: a randomised trial of two fractionation schedules. Radiother Oncol. 1997;45(2):109–16.

19. Chow E, Zeng L, Salvo N, Dennis K, Tsao M, Lutz S. Update on the systematic review of palliative radiotherapy trials for bone metastases. Clin Oncol (R Coll Radiol). 2012;24(2):112–24.

20. Sahgal A, Bilsky M, Chang EL, Ma L, Yamada Y, Rhines LD, Létourneau D, Foote M, Yu E, Larson DA, Fehlings MG. Stereotactic body radiotherapy for spinal metastases: current status, with a focus on its application in the postoperative patient. J Neurosurg Spine. 2011;14(2):151–66.

21. Chang EL, Shiu AS, Mendel E, Mathews LA, Mahajan A, Allen PK, Weinberg JS, Brown BW, Wang XS, Woo SY, Cleeland C, Maor MH, Rhines LD. Phase I/II study of stereotactic body radiotherapy for spinal metastasis and its pattern of failure. J Neurosurg Spine. 2007;7(2):151–60.

22. Koyfman SA, Djemil T, Burdick MJ, Woody N, Balagamwala EH, Reddy CA, Angelov L, Suh JH, Chao ST. Marginal recurrence requiring salvage radiotherapy after stereotactic body radiotherapy for spinal metastases. Int J Radiat Oncol Biol Phys. 2012;83(1):297–302.

23. Cox BW, Spratt DE, Lovelock M, Bilsky MH, Lis E, Ryu S, Sheehan J, Gerszten PC, Chang E, Gibbs I, Soltys S, Sahgal A, Deasy J, Flickinger J, Quader M, Mindea S, Yamada Y. International Spine Radiosurgery Consortium consensus guidelines for target volume definition in spinal stereotactic radiosurgery. Int J Radiat Oncol Biol Phys. 2012;83(5):e597–605.

24. Redmond KJ, Robertson S, Lo SS, Soltys SG, Ryu S, McNutt T, Chao ST, Yamada Y, Ghia A, Chang EL, Sheehan J, Sahgal A. Consensus contouring guidelines for postoperative stereotactic body

radiation therapy for metastatic solid tumor malignancies to the spine. Int J Radiat Oncol Biol Phys. 2017;97:64–74.

25. De Felice F, Musio D, Tombolini V. Osteoradionecrosis and intensity modulated radiation therapy: an overview. Crit Rev Oncol Hematol. 2016;107:39–43.

26. Withers HR, Taylor JM, Maciejewski B. Treatment volume and tissue tolerance. Int J Radiat Oncol Biol Phys. 1988;14(4):751–9.

27. Kirkpatrick JP, van der Kogel AJ, Schultheiss TE. Radiation dose-volume effects in the spinal cord. Int J Radiat Oncol Biol Phys. 2010;76(3 Suppl):S42–9.

28. Chang JH, Shin JH, Yamada YJ, Mesfin A, Fehlings MG, Rhines LD, Sahgal A. Stereotactic body radiotherapy for spinal metastases: what are the risks and how do we minimize them? Spine (Phila Pa 1976). 2016;41(Suppl 20):S238–45.

29. Cunha MV, Al-Omair A, Atenafu EG, Masucci GL, Letourneau D, Korol R, Yu E, Howard P, Lochray F, da Costa LB, Fehlings MG, Sahgal A. Vertebral compression fracture (VCF) after spine stereotactic body radiation therapy (SBRT): analysis of predictive factors. Int J Radiat Oncol Biol Phys. 2012;84(3):e343–9.

30. Sahgal A, Whyne CM, Ma L, Larson DA, Fehlings MG. Vertebral compression fracture after stereotactic body radiotherapy for spinal metastases. Lancet Oncol. 2013;14(8):e310–20.

31. Chow E, Hoskin P, Mitera G, Zeng L, Lutz S, Roos D, Hahn C, van der Linden Y, Hartsell W, Kumar E, International Bone Metastases Consensus Working Party. Update of the international consensus on palliative radiotherapy endpoints for future clinical trials in bone metastases. Int J Radiat Oncol Biol Phys. 2012;82(5):1730–7.

32. Chow E, van der Linden YM, Roos D, Hartsell WF, Hoskin P, Wu JS, Brundage MD, Nabid A, Tissing-Tan CJ, Oei B, Babington S, Demas WF, Wilson CF, Meyer RM, Chen BE, Wong RK. Single versus multiple fractions of repeat radiation for painful bone metastases: a randomised, controlled, non-inferiority trial. Lancet Oncol. 2014;15(2):164–71.

33. Sahgal A, Ames C, Chou D, Ma L, Huang K, Xu W, Chin C, Weinberg V, Chuang C, Weinstein P, Larson DA. Stereotactic body radiotherapy is effective salvage therapy for patients with prior radiation of spinal metastases. Int J Radiat Oncol Biol Phys. 2009;74(3):723–31.

34. Choi CY, Adler JR, Gibbs IC, Chang SD, Jackson PS, Minn AY, Lieberson RE, Soltys SG. Stereotactic radiosurgery for treatment of spinal metastases recurring in close proximity to previously irradiated spinal cord. Int J Radiat Oncol Biol Phys. 2010;78(2):499–506.

35. Patchell RA, Tibbs PA, Regine WF, Payne R, Saris S, Kryscio RJ, Mohiuddin M, Young B. Direct decompressive surgical resection in the treatment of spinal cord compression caused by metastatic cancer: a randomised trial. Lancet. 2005;366(9486):643–8.

36. Maranzano E, Trippa F, Casale M, Costantini S, Lupattelli M, Bellavita R, Marafioti L, Pergolizzi S, Santacaterina A, Mignogna M, Silvano G, Fusco V. 8Gy single-dose radiotherapy is effective in metastatic spinal cord compression: results of a phase III randomized multicentre Italian trial. Radiother Oncol. 2009;93(2):174–9.

Management of Metastases to the Spine and Sacrum

8

Riccardo Ghermandi, Gisberto Evangelisti,
Marco Girolami, Valerio Pipola, Stefano Bandiera,
Giovanni Barbanti-Bròdano, Cristiana Griffoni,
Giuseppe Tedesco, Silvia Terzi, and Alessandro Gasbarrini

Abstract

The incidence of bone metastatic deposit from carcinoma is second only to pulmonary and hepatic metastases. The most frequently affected segment of the skeleton is the vertebral column. Refinement of the protocols for treating tumour patients has led to a progressive improvement in the prognosis for many tumour histotypes in terms of increase of life expectancy. The choice of the most appropriate treatment is of crucial importance for the patient who may be severely disabled by the presence of untreated spinal metastases. It is commonly accepted that bone metastases are an expression of a systemic disease, and therefore require multi-disciplinary treatment, integrating radiotherapy (RT), chemotherapy (CHT) and surgery. The most appropriate treatment for patients with metastatic disease of the vertebral column is controversial. Appropriate surgical treatment of bone metastases and tumours in general has now become an integral part of the correct approach to the tumour patient. The evolution of anaesthetic techniques now allows more aggressive treatment of some patients with spinal and sacral metastases. These procedures can dramatically improve the patient's quality of life and may prolong the patient's life expectancy by preventing complications related to paralysis.

8.1 Introduction

The incidence of bone metastatic deposit from carcinoma is second only to pulmonary and hepatic metastases. The most frequently affected segment of the skeleton is the vertebral column. It is estimated that more than 10% of tumour patients develop symptomatic spinal metastases [1–5].

The vertebral bodies are reached largely via the bloodstream. Neoplastic substitution of the bone tissue causes progressive structural destruction leading to loss of stability and/or compression of the intracanal nerve structures.

Refinement of the protocols for treating tumour patients has led to a progressive improvement in the prognosis for many tumour histotypes in terms of increase of life expectancy. As a consequence, symptomatic spinal metastases in patients without other evidence of disease are increasing and severely affect the quality of life of the patients [5].

The choice of the most appropriate treatment is of crucial importance for the patient who may be severely disabled by the presence of untreated spinal metastases. These spinal metastases may not only be the cause of severe deterioration in

R. Ghermandi · G. Evangelisti · M. Girolami
V. Pipola · S. Bandiera · G. Barbanti-Bròdano
C. Griffoni · G. Tedesco · S. Terzi
A. Gasbarrini (✉)
Department of Oncologic and Degenerative
Spine Surgery, IRCCS Istituto Ortopedico Rizzoli,
Bologna, Italy
e-mail: gasbarrini@me.com

© Springer International Publishing AG, part of Springer Nature 2019
V. Denaro et al. (eds.), *Management of Bone Metastases*, https://doi.org/10.1007/978-3-319-73485-9_8

the quality of life, but also the direct or indirect cause of death. Therefore the correct treatment of spine metastasis affects the life expectancy. Although there is widespread agreement in literature regarding the need to treat symptomatic metastases, the best treatment protocol to adopt is still a matter of discussion.

Spinal metastases have different patterns and behaviour related to the large varieties of histotypes and spread modality of the primary tumour. These metastases may develop early and must be considered severe complications requiring multidisciplinary approach by collaboration of oncologists, radiotherapists and surgeons.

It is commonly accepted that bone metastases are an expression of a systemic disease, and therefore require multi-disciplinary treatment, integrating radiotherapy (RT), chemotherapy (CHT) and surgery [6].

The most common presenting symptom in patients with spinal tumour is pain [7, 8].

This is extremely frequent and often intractable, not even sensitive even to major analgesic drugs. Although spinal tumours might be asymptomatic for relatively long periods, pain can be caused by:

- tumour expansion beyond the cortex of vertebral body, stretching the periosteum and stimulating pain receptors, and eventually breaking it invading into the paravertebral tissues,
- tumour compression of the spinal cord and/or nerve roots,
- instability caused by progressive replacement of bone with tumour tissue, which does not have the same mechanical properties, thus increasing risk of fracture of the vertebral body (impending fracture) (Table 8.1),
- pathological fracture in the vertebra weakened by tumour erosion. It causes acute onset of pain and usually patients do not report history of trauma or, if any, this is low energy.

Neurological deficits may be caused by either direct compression of the tumour on the myeloradicular structures or by sudden retropulsion into

Table 8.1 Spinal instability neoplastic score

Location	
Junctional (occiput-C2, C7-T2, T11-L1, L5-S1)	*3 pt*
Mobile spine (C3–C6, L2–L4)	2 pt
Semi-rigid (T3–T10)	1 pt
Rigid (S2–S5)	0 pt
Pain relief with recumbency and/or pain with movement/loading of the spine	
Yes	3 pt
No (occasional pain but not mechanic)	*1 pt*
Pain free lesion	0 pt
Bone lesion	
Lytic	*2 pt*
Mixed (lytic/blastic)	1 pt
Blastic	0 pt
Radiographic spinal alignment	
Subluxation/translation present	4 pt
De novo deformity (kyphosis/scoliosis)	2 pt
Normal alignment	*0 pt*
Vertebral body collapse	
>50%	3 pt
<50%	2 pt
No collapse with >50% body involved	1 pt
None of the above	*0 pt*
Posterolateral involvement of the spinal elements (facet, pedicle or CV joint fracture or replacement with tumour)	
Bilateral	3 pt
Unilateral	*1 pt*
None of the above	0 pt

Score: 0–6, stability; 7–12, indeterminate instability; 13–18, instability

the canal of tumour and bone debris caused by pathological fracture [9, 10].

8.1.1 Role of Spine Surgery in Metastasis Treatment

Controversy exists over the most appropriate treatment for patients with metastatic disease of the vertebral column. The evolution of anaesthesiological techniques allowed surgical treatments that few years ago were considered prohibitive. The problem is to know which is the best sequential process to arrive at the most appropriate treatment considering the individual general conditions of the patient and the parameters of the metastasis [11–16].

The aim of surgery might be one, or an association, of the following:

- pain relief,
- neurological function preservation, or recovery from a neurological deficit,
- spinal stability restoration,
- local control of the tumour.

Even though local control of the tumour is a target for the treatment of metastases, it is not always achieved surgically. In fact, the wide variety of histotypes which may deposit in the spine differ in their sensitivity to non-surgical treatments (such as RT, hormonal therapy, immunotherapy) [11, 13, 14].

Moreover, it is intuitive that the longer the expected survival of the patient, the greater the possibility that the disease might relapse (with eventual compression of the spinal cord and/or pathological fracture), thus the differential importance of achieving a durable local control.

It is important for the surgeon to be aware of the various options available to achieve local control of the various different histotypes, whether surgical or not.

From our perspective the surgical techniques in spine metastasis can be summarized into (1) decompression and stabilization, (2) intralesional excision (curettage, debulking) and (3) en bloc resection, these latter two followed by reconstructive procedures (with various techniques). All these operations can be performed by either the anterior, posterior or combined approaches.

1. *Decompression and stabilization*: this is the quickest and less aggressive surgical procedure and even though it might involve a direct approach to the tumour, it is aimed to just circumferentially decompress the spinal cord without aiming at complete removal of the mass. It is mandatory to stabilize the spinal column at the same time. It is indicated for patients with short-term prognosis, in cases of neurological damage and/or pathological fracture, making this the procedure of choice in case of emergency, but also for tumours highly sensitive to radiotherapy or hormonal treatment. Preoperative selective arterial embolization makes this procedure easier and safer. The surgical approach used for this purpose is posterior only.

2. *Intralesional excision* "debulking". The tumour is directly approached and managed as far as possible by piecemeal removal, not only to achieve circumferential decompression of the spinal cord, but also to extensively reduce the mass. This procedure is often performed as part of a multi-disciplinary approach and is preceded by selective preoperative arterial embolization. This operation is indicated for metastases not sensitive to radiotherapy, with pathological fracture and/or signs of cord compression, or when a tumour debulking is required to enhance the oncological treatments. Surgical approach for this purpose can be posterior, anterior or combined anterior and posterior.

3. *En bloc resection*: this procedure, mostly indicated for primary tumours, is sometimes the correct solution for solitary metastases of radioresistant tumours with middle or long-term favourable prognosis. The operation can be performed by a posterior approach alone or by double approach. En bloc resection is associated with the lower local recurrence rate but the cost to benefit ratio is very high due to the morbidity of these long operations (8–16 h). This kind of procedure should be considered in patients with a long life expectancy. Another point to be considered is the lower morbidity of en bloc resection versus intralesional excision in highly vascularized tumours. En bloc resection is the surgical technique which showed the best results in terms of local control (local recurrence of the disease is less likely to occur).

Supplemental application of adjuvant treatments (i.e. RT, hormonal therapy) may increase the effectiveness of the surgical treatment. The surgical reduction of the tumour mass (debulking) is another important target finalized to the local control of the disease mostly in combination with other treatments. As the number of treatment options for metastatic spinal disease has grown, it has become clear that effective implementation of these treatments can only be achieved by multi-disciplinary approach [13].

8.1.2 The Role of Minimally Invasive (MI) Techniques in Vertebral Metastasis

Various new minimally invasive techniques are emerging for the treatment of spinal metastases. For a technique to be considered minimally invasive there must be less collateral tissue damage but same exact intended surgical goal as traditional open procedure. These techniques aim at decreased morbidity, allow a quicker functional recovery but without compromising postoperative results.

Stabilization can be achieved using percutaneous cannulated screws and, if histotypes of the tumour allow to, local control can be subsequently achieved using adjuvant therapies, thus limiting the extent of the surgery just to restore stability. Pedicle screws rod constructs act as an internal brace allowing quick functional recovery [17].

MI decompression can be performed using endoscopic tubular retractors; usually final decompression is not always comparable to that achieved by open techniques, thus systematic use should be limited to the lower grades of neurologic compression (Bilsky score grade 1).

Some authors suggested to combine posterior procedures with MI anterior approaches, such as extreme lateral (XLIF or LLIF) and mini-thoraco or thoracoscopic approaches, in order to relieve anterior compression and reconstruct the anterior column.

Extreme care must be taken in patient selection when these challenging techniques for anterior column exposure are taken into consideration in this patient population, since the general conditions often preclude their use (i.e. single lung ventilation), or equal results could be achieved by multi-disciplinary treatment plans (i.e. surgery + RT/CHT/hormonal/immunotherapy). In our experience, indications are so uncommon that their use should be considered anecdotal [10].

Local control of the disease can be achieved using various energy sources—i.e. high-frequency alternating current, argon gas and plasma fields, that have been applied directly on the tumour through probes in order to produce tissue necrosis [18–22].

These techniques—radiofrequency ablation, cryoablation, cavity coblation, respectively—can be combined with stabilization techniques in order to restore segmental stability and achieve local control of the disease with the least tissue exposure possible.

Radiofrequency ablation not only produces the thermal destruction of the tumour (even if not completely histologically shown), but also thrombosis of the perivertebral venous plexus. The most severe complication of this technique is the thermal cytolysis of the neural structures, even it seems that the integrity of the back cortical wall may be a protective barrier for the neural structures, as the presence of cortical bone can significantly reduce the temperature. Indeed, the authors think that the presence of cerebrospinal fluid between the tumour mass and the spinal cord is enough to avoid some thermal damages, even if they dissuade the use of thermoablation in the case of wide vertebral osteolysis with invasion of the back vertebral wall [21, 23].

Electrochemotherapy combines systemic bleomycin use with electric pulses delivered locally. These electric pulses permeabilize cell membranes (electroporation) in the tissue, allowing bleomycin delivery diffusion inside the cell and its cytotoxicity. The applied electrical field is generated using stainless steel electrodes that are placed around the tumour tissue [20, 24].

The authors include selective arterial embolization in this group even if it cannot be considered a real minimally invasive technique but rather a minimal treatment that can be used as a palliative procedure (and eventually repeated) in nonoperable patients or in case of inoperable lesions. More often it is performed as adjuvant preoperative procedure, in order to decrease intra-operative blood loss in case of any procedure that implies violation of the tumour pseudocapsule (decompression and stabilization with or without tumour debulking) [25–27].

Percutaneous vertebral body augmentation techniques (vertebro- or kyphoplasty) can be done in order to restore the strength of the affected verte-bra. Several authors reported good results in terms of pain control after PMMA injection [28–33].

However, its use in spinal metastases differs from what is performed in osteoporotic vertebral compression fractures.

In fact, while osteoporosis decreases bone mass, the tumour occupying the vertebra has predomi-nantly solid consistency and when the cement is injected inside the vertebra without having first removed it, this can go inside the spinal canal, causing compression, or anyway outside of the ver-tebra, causing further dissemination of the disease.

An interesting experimental study by Reidy and collaborators [34] showed that the presence of tumour causes an increase of pressure of about eight times inside the vertebral body and this can determine the uncontrolled migration of tumour material or cement. This would be justified by the different hydraulic permeability of the neoplastic tissue so that its smaller "porosity" prevents and hinders diffusion of the PMMA within it. This also could explain the dishomogeneous distribu-tion of cement inside the vertebral body.

Vertebroplasty does not determine a local con-trol of the disease, even though an anti-neoplastic role of PMMA has been hypothesized so far; if the tumour does not respond to adjuvant thera-pies and continues to grow, PMMA can be fur-therly displaced into the epidural space [35].

Some authors, trying to get a local control of the disease and reduce the migration of the cement inside the perivertebral vessels, pro-pose the combined use of techniques such as radiofrequency ablation with vertebroplasty. Some changes of the physical properties of the tumour mass and the hydraulic permeability can reduce the intravertebral pressure follow-ing vertebroplasty and therefore the risk of PMMA spillage (the most common complica-tion) [28, 36–38].

8.2   Decision-Making Process in Vertebral Metastases

The first element to be considered in the decision-making process for treatment of spine metastases is the diagnosis. Excluding a number of lesions easily diagnosed with instrumental and technical-laboratory examinations (i.e. osteoid osteoma), the majority of tumours require a pathological evaluation. In the spine, a CT-guided trocar biopsy performed through the pedicle without invading the epidural space seems to be the best way to reduce the spread of the tumour cells [39].

While for the treatment of primary tumours a systematic approach has been accepted, there are no accepted guidelines for the treatment of spinal metastases.

Protocols of chemotherapy (CHT), hormone therapy, immunotherapy and radiotherapy exist and are progressively increasing survival for the majority of solid and hematologic tumours.

However, drugs cannot effectively control pain and functional impairment from vertebral body collapse and cord compression from epi-dural space invasion [6, 10, 40].

Moreover, the erroneous certainty that patients with secondary skeletal localisations should be considered terminal, and therefore not of ortho-paedic interest, makes often surgery urgent and essential (if feasible), with increased operative risks for the patient, difficulties to its relatives/caregivers/beloved and to the healthcare facility taking in charge of these problems.

Many factors must be taken into account when choosing the most appropriate surgical tech-nique: the general conditions of the patient, the histotype of the primary tumour and its sensitivity to adjuvant treatments, the spread of the disease and the current neurological conditions [10].

Briefly, it can be stated that a patient with dif-fuse neoplastic disease, generally impaired con-ditions and incipient neurological deficit should be treated with palliative decompression and sta-bilization followed by radiotherapy which may noticeably improve the quality of life.

On the other hand, in a patient in good general conditions suffering from a primary tumour with a relatively positive prognosis and a symptomatic isolated spinal metastasis, more aggressive treat-ment similar to that for a primary tumour is justified.

Sioutos et al. [5] statistically analysed the fac-tors influencing the incidence of complications and length of survival after surgical treatment of spinal metastases and showed that this is influenced by preoperative neurological conditions, the histotype of the primary tumour and the number of vertebrae involved, but not by the degree of diffusion of the disease or the age of the patient.

On the basis of these observations, the authors recommend careful selection of both patients candidates for surgical treatment and the kind of surgical treatment itself.

The literature proposes many preoperative scoring systems to classify patients by creating repeatable treatment protocols [10, 13, 14, 41–43].

These systems are characterized by the fact that each parameter is attributed a score and the sum of these scores suggests the most appropriate treatment. Equal importance is therefore attached to the various parameters considered in individual cases. For example, the histotype of the primary tumour and the general conditions of the patient have the same influence on the final score and therefore the choice of type of treatment.

On the basis of the personal experience, the authors have built up an algorithm [13, 44] for treating spinal metastases in which the importance of the parameters varies according to when they are considered.

Each patient follows his or her "personal" sequential process which does not necessarily consider all the parameters every time as some may be irrelevant for the purposes of choosing the type of treatment. For example, a patient in poor general conditions with a high "ASA" score is usually not a candidate for surgery, irrespective of the histotype of the primary tumour or the number of secondary localisations. For this patient, the most important parameter will therefore be the sensitivity of the tumour histotype to adjuvant treatment. In the same way, a patient with acute and progressive spinal cord damage will undergo emergency palliative decompression and stabilization surgery without considering a more demanding operation.

Finally, the patient is not considered just in terms of the disease, reducing the choice of treatment to an overly simplistic mathematical score. Instead, the case is analysed holistically, firstly considering the individual and his or her general conditions, and only subsequently the parameters of the metastases.

8.3 Flow-chart for Multi-disciplinary Management of Metastases in the Mobile Spine

Without considering all the clinical and instrumental examinations which the patient undergoes on admission and forming part of preoperative staging, our treatment algorithm begins with the diagnosis of spinal metastases [13].

The first assessment must be performed by the anaesthetist who must determine whether the patient is operable or not.

If the patient is not operable due to a high American Society of Anesthesiologists (ASA) score, non-surgical options are considered. Next, the sensitivity of the tumour histotype to adjuvant therapies (CHT, RT, hormonal) is taken into account. If the tumour does not respond to any form of treatment, the only option for the patient is pain therapy.

If the patient is operable, the severity of the spinal cord compression and neurological damage is evaluated by means of the Frankel score. If there is neurological deficit or paralysis, the possibility of recovery is evaluated on the basis of time from the onset of symptoms.

Finally, if in our opinion neurological recovery of the patient is not possible, sensitivity to adjuvant treatments is re-evaluated. If, on the other hand, the patient has acute and progressive spinal cord damage, emergency surgery is performed.

If there is no deficit or the damage is recoverable and stable, sensitivity to adjuvant treatments is evaluated. If the tumour histotype is not sensitive and there is a single metastasis only, resection of the lesion is chosen. On the other hand, decompression and stabilization is indicated if there are multiple metastases and they are treatable. If they are not treatable, pain therapy alone is administered.

When there is no deficit or the damage is recoverable and not progressive, and the tumour is sensitive to some form of adjuvant treatment, pathological fracture (actual or impending) is evaluated. This parameter is, in fact, decisive in orienting the choice towards either surgical treatment with compression and stabilization or adjuvant treatment only.

Resection of the tumour may be performed en bloc with a wide margin or through debulking. Generally speaking en bloc removal is suggested by the authors for hypervascularised tumours, metastases from renal cell carcinoma and from sarcoma, and the cases in which this type of operation is easy to perform (Fig. 8.1).

8.4   Experience at Our Institution

8.4.1   Materials and Methods

Since 1972, 1070 cases of spinal metastases from a solid tumour have been treated at the Rizzoli Orthopedic Institute in Bologna. For the purpose of this paper, we retrospectively reviewed all the patients suffering from spinal metastases from January 2000 and June 2015 and treated at the Oncologic and Degenerative Spine Unit at

Rizzoli Orthopedic Institute. Patients suffering from plasmacytoma and lymphoma were excluded from the study as the therapeutic approach and prognostic evaluation are, in our experience, different.

In the analysed period 546 patients have been treated (286 males and 260 female) with a mean age of 59.4 years (±12.1 SD; range 15–86 years). We identified 50 metastases located in the cervical section, 309 in the thoracic section and 187 in the lumbar section. The most frequently affected metameres were L1 and L2 affected respectively 45 and 50 times (Fig. 8.2).

The anatomical location of the primary tumour is reported in (Fig. 8.3). The most frequent locations were kidney, lung, breast and colon. In 4.2% of the cases the original tumour was not known at the onset of the vertebral symptoms.

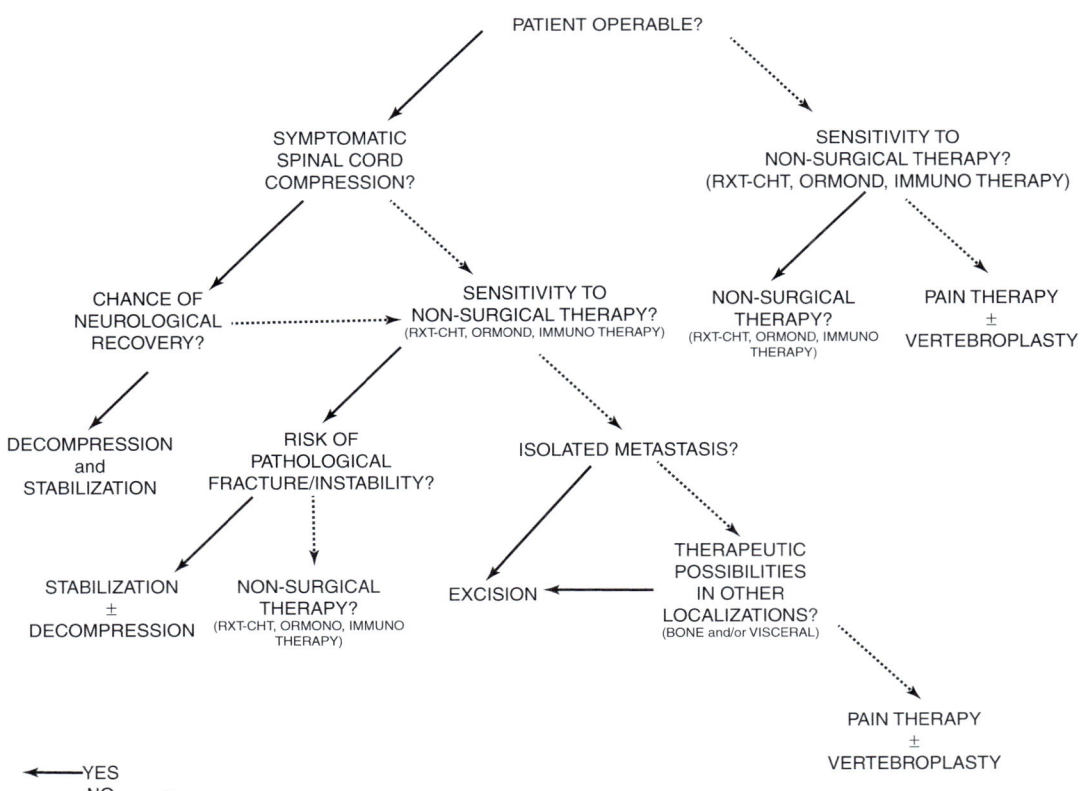

Fig. 8.1 Flow-chart for the treatment of spinal metastases

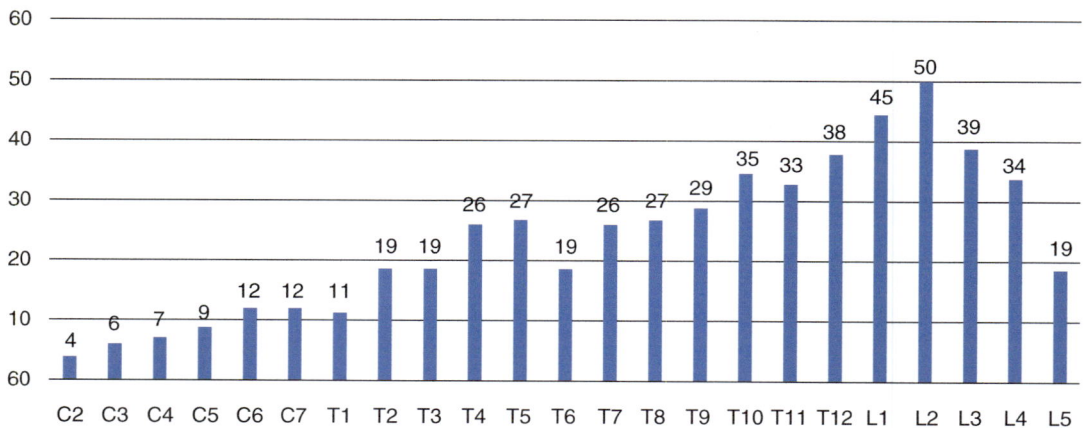

Fig. 8.2 Affected metamers

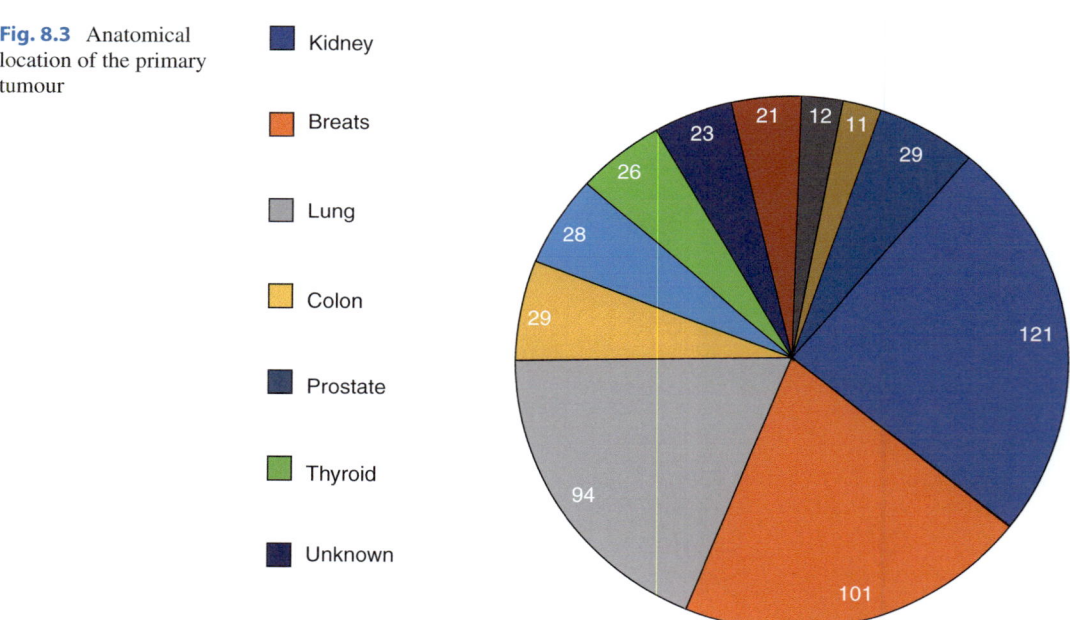

Fig. 8.3 Anatomical location of the primary tumour

The Frankel score was used to assess neurological impairment; 367 patients had no neurological impairment (Frankel E), 39 patients were Frankel D3, 33 cases were D2, 38 cases were D1, 50 cases were C, 18 cases were B and 1 cases A.

On admission, there was pathological fracture of the vertebra concerned in 172 cases (31.5%). Before surgery all the patients underwent an anaesthesiological evaluation in order to assess comorbidities and the risks of surgery: 30 patients were considered inoperable due to their poor general conditions and therefore they were directed to palliative care. It should be kept in mind that the patients referred at the authors institution had already been selected by the oncologists, and this explains the high number of surgical operations.

The remaining 516 patients have undergone one of the following surgical treatments.

1. Vertebroplasty or Kyphoplasty in 14 cases (2.7%): this is the quickest and less aggressive procedure. The aim is to stabilize the anterior column and reduce the pain. It was chosen for patients with short-term prognosis as palliative treatment to combine with both chemo and radiotherapy (Fig. 8.4).

2. Decompression and stabilization in 169 cases (32.8%): this surgical procedure does not necessarily involve a direct approach to the tumour. The aim is to circumferentially decompress the spinal cord and stabilize the spinal column. It was chosen for patients with short-term prognosis in cases of neurological damage as a result of pathological fracture, but also in conditions of very high sensitivity to radiotherapy or hormonal treatment. In the majority of these patients, a preoperative embolisation of the tumour mass was performed to reduce intra-operative bleeding (Fig. 8.5).

3. Intralesional resection "debulking" in 290 cases (56.2%): the tumour was attacked directly and removed as far as possible not only in order to achieve circumferential decompression of the spinal cord but also to reduce the mass of the tumour. This procedure was performed as part of a multi-disciplinary approach to treating the metastases and was preceded by appropriate surgical planning including selective preoperative arterial embolisation (performed in the majority of the cases). We chose this operation in presence of metastases not sensitive to radiotherapy, with pathological fracture and/or signs of spinal cord compression, or when the oncologist considered it necessary to remove the tumour to enable adjuvant treatments to act more effectively on the remaining cells. Surgical access was posterior in 235 cases, anterior in 39 cases and combined anterior plus posterior in the remaining 16 cases (Figs 8.6 and 8.7).

4. En bloc resection in 43 cases (8.3%): this was performed on patients suffering from a single spinal metastasis deriving from the primary tumour, with a long life expectancy and already treated. The operation was performed with a double approach in 21 cases, a posterior approach alone in 21 cases and an anterior approach alone in 1 case. The criteria making

this operation possible include: tumour size, volume, location. Three possible en bloc resections have been described according to the WBB system: resection of the vertebral body (37 cases), sagittal resection (2 cases) and posterior resection (4 cases) (Fig. 8.8).

8.4.2 Results

All patients underwent periodic outpatient visits in which a clinical examination was combined with X-ray examination of the spinal column, CT and/or MRI of the operated segment and any other examinations indicated in the individual case. The main elements recorded for each patient were functional assessment of the neurological conditions according to the Frankel scale, complications associated with the operation, local recurrence or local progression of the disease and general clinical status.

The 546 patients included in our study were followed up for a mean of 19 months (±21.8 SD; range 5 days–142 months). At the longest available follow-up 160 patients had died (a mean distance of 16.7 months after admission to hospital (±17.7 SD; range 5 days–96 months)).

In total, there were 34 (6.5%) intra-operative complications: 11 cases of excessive bleeding, 11 cases of dural lesion that has been sutured, 5 cases of pleural lesion, 2 cases of peritoneum lesion, 1 case of lesion of inferior vena cava, 1 case of chylothorax, 1 fracture of the seventh rib, 1 case of lesion of L3 nerve root and 1 case of unstable blood pressure with bradycardia. We had 50 (9.7%) early complications: early infection with wound dehiscence (25), cerebrospinal fluid fistula (3), screw mal-placement (3), paraplegia (3), postoperative bleeding (2), pleural effusion (2), pseudomeningoceles (1), hematoma (1), bowel obstruction (1), pulmonary embolism and cardiac arrest (1), paroxysmal supraventricular tachycardia (1), bronchopneumonia (1), pericardial tamponade (1), seizures (1), acute pulmonary edema (1), acute kidney failure (1), massive hemothorax (1), subcutaneous emphysema (1). We had 29 (5.6%) late complication: deep infection (18), breakage of fixation devices (5), aseptic loosening (5), junctional syndrome (1).

Fig. 8.4 R.G., female, 38 years, multiple metastases from breast carcinoma previously submitted to radiotherapy and currently under hormone therapy. She experienced sudden onset of intractable back pain, increasing with standing and refractory to any combination of painkillers. (**a**) MRI revealing a pathological fracture of L3 without epidural space involvement (Bilsky grade 0), confirmed by the CT scan analysis (**b**). According to the proposed algorithm (**c**), she underwent a percutaneous vertebroplasty by a biportal approach (**d**), after the performance of a transpedicular biopsy to confirm the diagnosis. The postoperative CT scan (**e**) shows the correct position of the cement inside the vertebrae

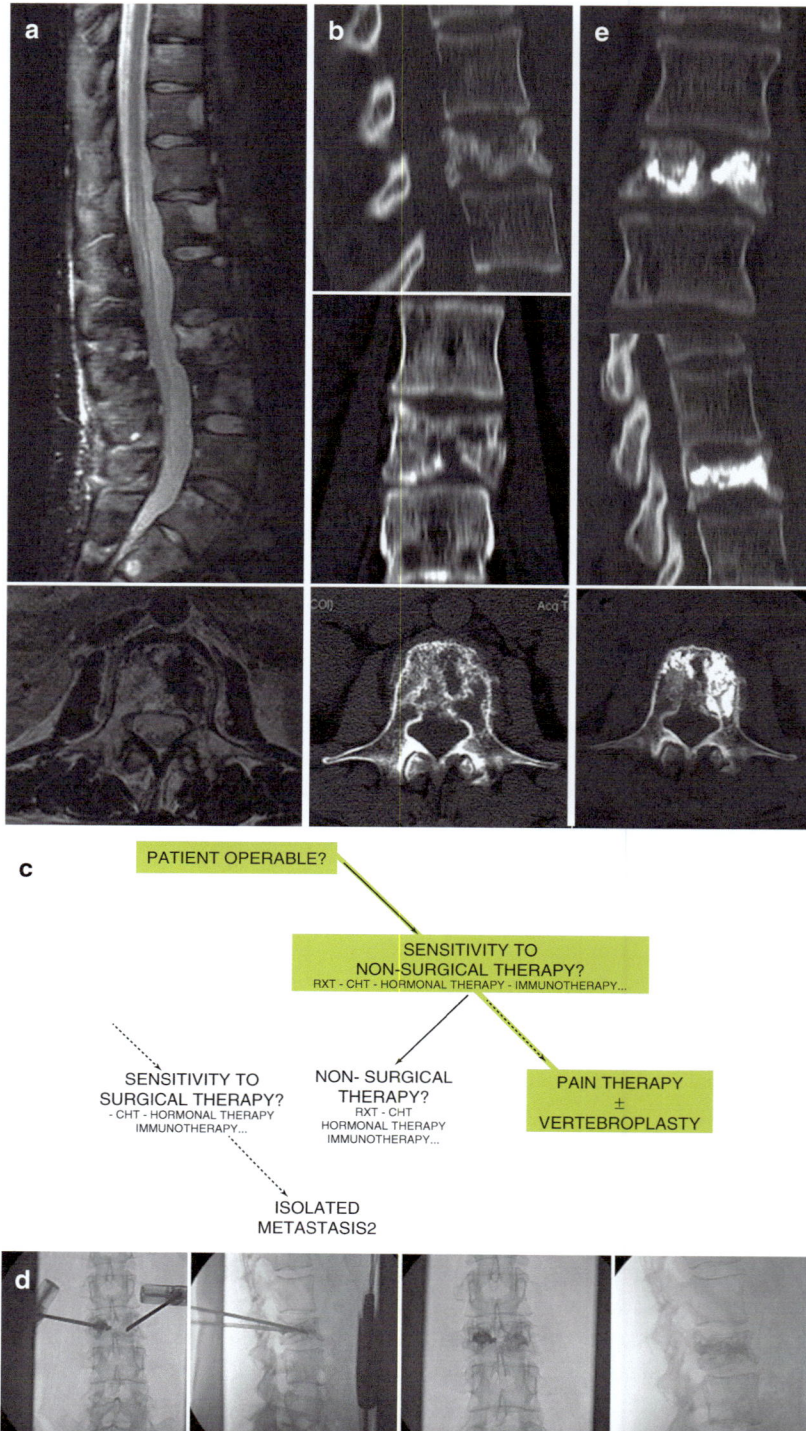

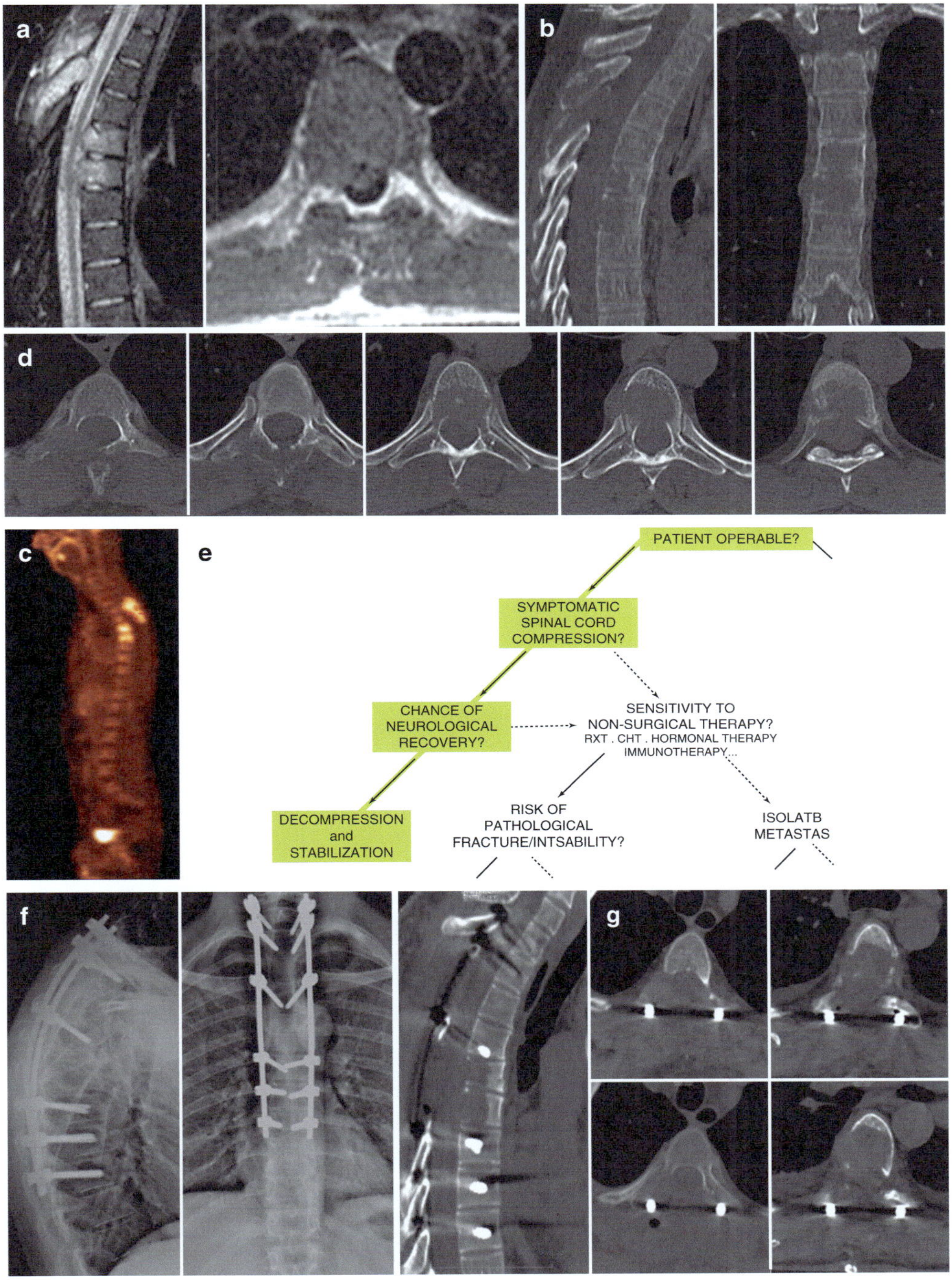

Fig. 8.5 D.T., male, 34 years, history of parathyroid tumour. He presented sudden onset of back pain and motor deficits, progressively increasing up to Frankel C paraplegia. Sagittal and axial MRI (**a**) showed multiple lesions to posterior arch of T2–T3 and vertebral bodies of T5–T6 with spinal cord compression (Bilsky grade 2). Osteolysis and vertebral involvement were assessed by CT scan in either sagittal or coronal (**b**) and axial images (**c**), and by PET-scan (**d**). According to the proposed algorithm (**e**), he was submitted to decompression and stabilization, with immediate regression of deficits (**f**). Post-operative CT scan shows hardware position and extent of decompression (**g**). After healing of the surgical wound, lesions were submitted to radiotherapy and patient started specific chemotherapy protocol

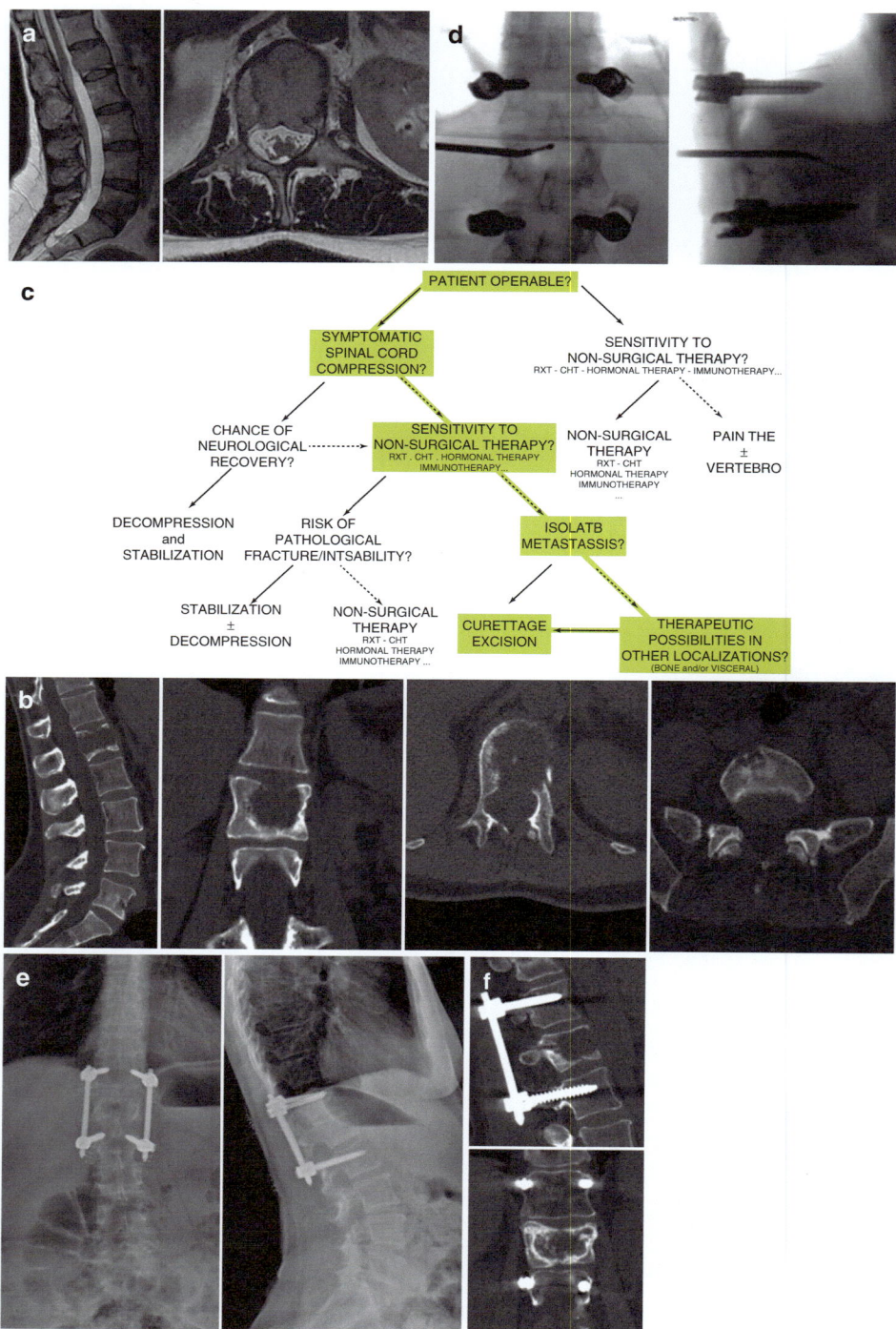

Fig. 8.6 M.P., female, 55 years, metastases from melanoma (Δt = 1 year). She experienced progressive onset of back pain, progressively irresponsive to painkillers. MRI (**a**) and CT scan (**b**) showed a metastasis in L1 with mild epidural space invasion (Bilsky grade 1a). SINS score for the lesion in L1 results 9 pts. (impending instability), with a synchronous asymptomatic lesion in L5. According to the proposed algorithm (**c**), she was submitted to percutaneous stabilization and local control of the disease by radiofrequency thermo-ablation (**d**), with good pain relief. Postoperative radiographic control showed the stabilization of the affected segment (**e**). Both lesions were later submitted to stereotactic radiosurgery (SRS), with partial consolidation of the lesions (**f**)

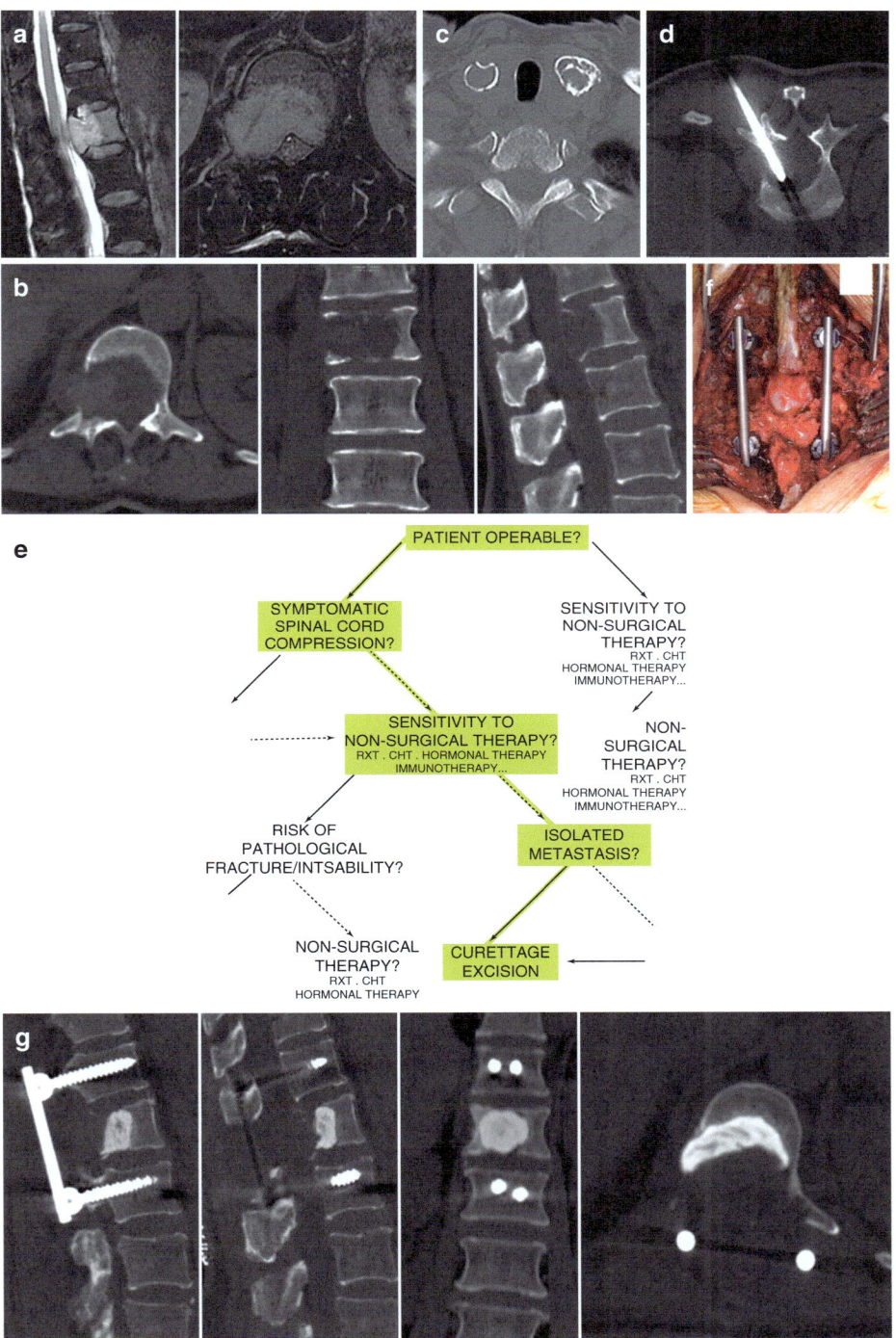

Fig. 8.7 R.T., female, 68 years, progressive back pain radiating in the right thigh and leg with L5 dermatome distribution. MRI (**a**) and CT scan (**b**) revealed a lesion in L1 with severe epidural space invasion causing compression of the neurostructures (Bilsky grade 3). A CT scan showed enlarged thyroid lobes with round calcium deposits (**c**). The lesion was submitted to CT-guided transpedicular biopsy which resulted diagnostic for metastases from follicular thyroid cancer (**d**). According to the proposed algorithm (**e**), the patient underwent contextual thyroidectomy and debulking of the L1 metastases (**f**), decompression and stabilization, and the lesion was filled with bone cement (**g**)

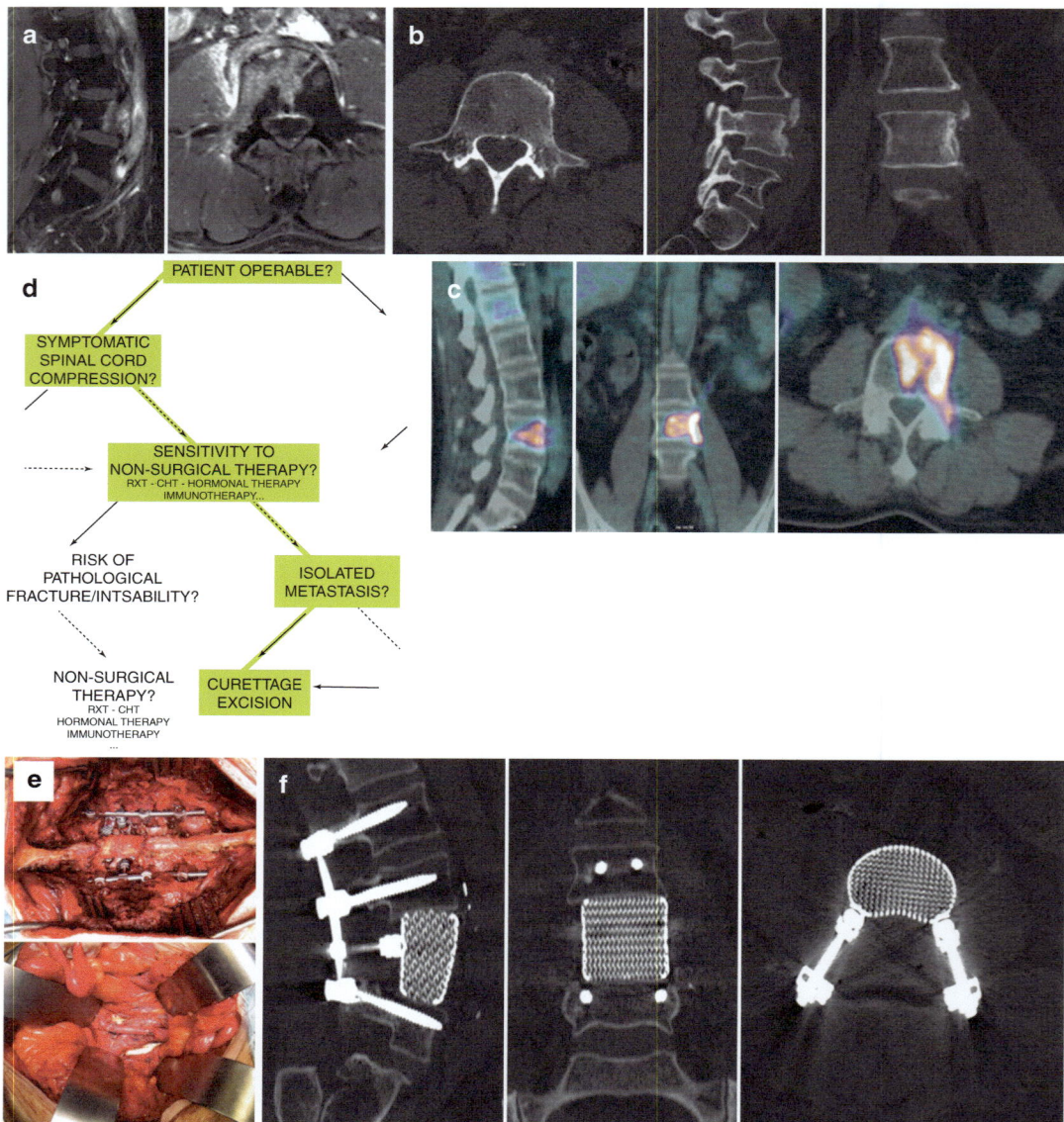

Fig. 8.8 R.B., male, 55 years, presenting for local progression of disease at an L4 lesion which was diagnosed as metastasis from adenocarcinoma. He already had a debulking done (with intralesional margin) by general surgeons through a transperitoneal approach 18 months before. Past medical history included a seminoma that was treated with orchiectomy 27 years before. He complained of non-mechanical severe back pain, particularly during the night. MRI (**a**) and CT (**b**) imaging revealed the lesion extending into the prevertebral layer (WBB layer A) without evidence of epidural disease (Bilsky grade 0). PET-CT scan (**c**) did not show other lesions. According to the proposed algorithm (**d**), he was submitted to en bloc vertebrectomy by a combined anterior and posterior approach (**e**), and reconstruction by a 3D printed custom-made titanium prosthesis. The pathologist indicated wide margin on surgical specimen

Seventy-four patients (14.3%) have been operated more than one time due to local recurrence: 54 patients required a second surgery, 16 patients required third surgery and 4 patients required fourth surgery.

As regards variations in the neurological profile, at the longest available follow-up 70.6% had no neurological impairment (Frankel E), 6% were Frankel D3, 4.8% were D2, 6.5% were D1, 6.8% were C, 5% were B and 0.3% were A. It appears that it was not a neurological worsening. However, a limitation of this assessment is that it takes into account different types of treatment and different types of tumour. Obviously, the longer the follow-up, the greater the possibility that the disease will relapse with possible compression of the spinal cord and/or pathological fracture which could worsen the neurological conditions. In the same way, the best results have been obtained in cases of en bloc resection where local recurrence of the disease is less likely.

8.5 Management of Sacral Metastases

The goals of the treatment of sacral metastases are the same of those previously presented for the mobile spine: control of symptoms and recovery, as far as possible, of neurological functions [36, 45–49].

Being it not a curative treatment, this must be aggressive just enough to achieve a durable local control of the disease with the lowest possible surgical trauma to minimize the complications, which can be potentially fatal in this population of patients. There are many different treatment options and the most appropriate should be chosen considering multiple factors related to both the disease and the patient.

A flow-chart was proposed to condense the shared decision-making process (Fig. 8.9). This was obtained by a consensus of spinal surgeons, oncologists, radiologists and pathologists involved in the treatment of these complex lesions. Treatment options are divided into three

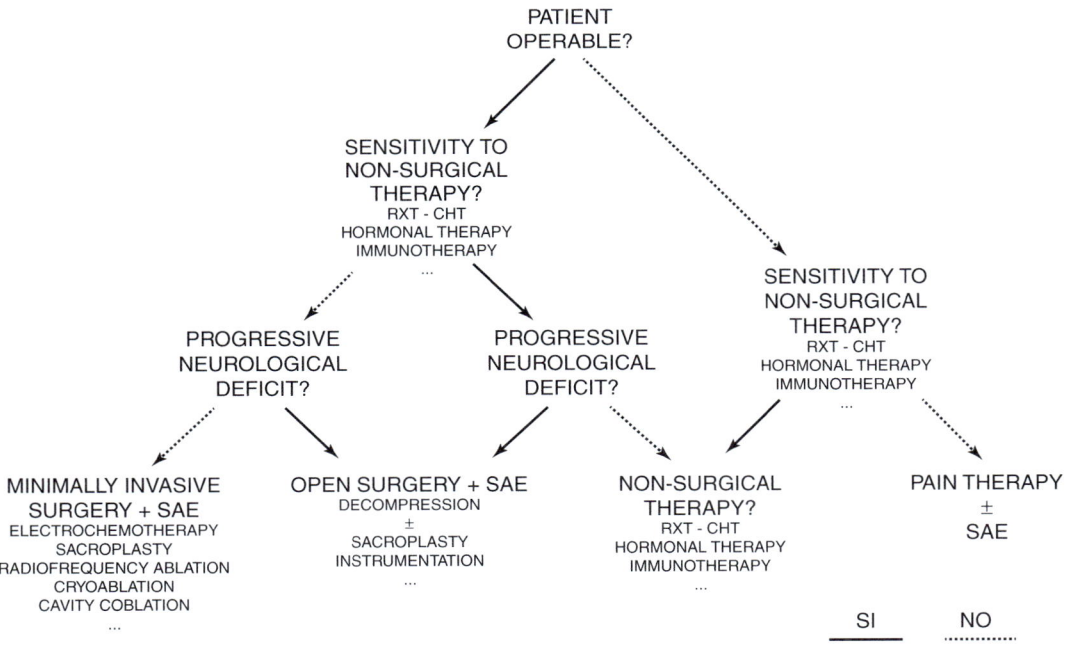

Fig. 8.9 Flow-chart for the treatment of sacral metastases

major groups: conservative treatment, which includes chemo-, immuno-, radiation, hormonal and pain therapies, alone or in association, open and minimally invasive surgical treatments [46].

Radiation therapy is the most frequently used local treatment for patients affected by sacral metastases. It was proven to be successful in achieving local control of sacral metastases, but it is not indicated in case of pathological fractures (or impending) and severe compression on the neurological structures. Moreover it is most effective in case of radiosensitive tumours, such as lymphoma, or prostate and breast cancer. On the contrary, gastrointestinal and renal cell tumours are considered radioresistant [50].

Spinal stereotactic radiosurgery (SRS) is emerging as the recommended technique of radiation therapy for metastatic lesions. It allows the delivery of a more focused radiation beam to the tumour, while sparing the healthy surrounding tissues; therefore, higher doses can be given with hypofractionated schedules (even single-fraction). According to a recent prospective study on 500 patients affected by spinal metastases (including 103 sacral metastases), this technique

has been proven to be safe and effective, showing increased rates of local control and low rate of complications when compared with conventional external beam radiotherapy (CEBRT) [50].

Despite the availability of techniques to resect en bloc the sacrum with wide or marginal margins which could offer the lowest recurrence rates, these are burdened by particularly disabling sequelae, such as rectal and bladder incontinence, loss of sexual functions, sensory and motor deficits in the lower limbs (Tables 8.2 and 8.3), as well as a high rate of complications. Therefore, indications for en bloc resection for sacral metastases are almost absent and, if any, reserved for highly selected patients [46, 51–54].

Despite these considerations, surgery still has a strong and defined role in the treatment of sacral metastases, which most frequently include decompression (Fig. 8.10) through a posterior approach. In this way, it is possible to decompress the nerve roots and cauda equina from neoplastic tissue invading the epidural space, and also to access the sacral wings and the vertebral body of the sacral vertebrae through the pedicles to excise the tumour (with intralesional margins) [48, 55].

Subsequently, the remaining cavity can be filled with poly-methyl-methacrylate (PMMA), restoring the weight-bearing anterior column of the sacrum. Occasionally, it is necessary to sacrifice sacral roots infiltrated by the tumour; however, these isolated roots sacrifices result in less disabling functional losses that can be treated with an external orthoses [53, 54, 56].

Table 8.2 Motor function after sacrectomy

Preserved levels	Unilateral	Bilateral
L5	Normal 0% Minor deficit 25% Major deficit 75%	
S1	Normal 56% Minor deficit 6% Major deficit 38%	
S2	Minor deficit	100% preserved

Table 8.3 Bladder and bowel functions after sacrectomy.

Preserved levels	Bladder function		Bowel function	
S1	100% impaired		100% impaired	
S2	*Unilat.*	*Bilat.*	*Unilat.*	*Bilat.*
	Impaired 75%	Preserved 39.6% Min. disf. 22.9% Maj. disf. 37.5%	Preserved 12.5% Min. disf. 50% Maj. disf. 37.5%	Preserved 50% Min. disf. 25% Maj. disf. 25%
S3	*Unilat.*	*Bilat.*	*Unilat.*	*Bilat.*
	Preserved 72.7% Min. disf. 18.2% Maj. disf. 9.1%	Preserved 83% Min. disf. 14.8% Maj. disf. 1.8%	Preserved 70% Min. disf. 20% Maj. disf. 10%	Preserved 93% Min. disf. 4.4% Maj. disf. 2.2%
S4	100% preserved		100% preserved	

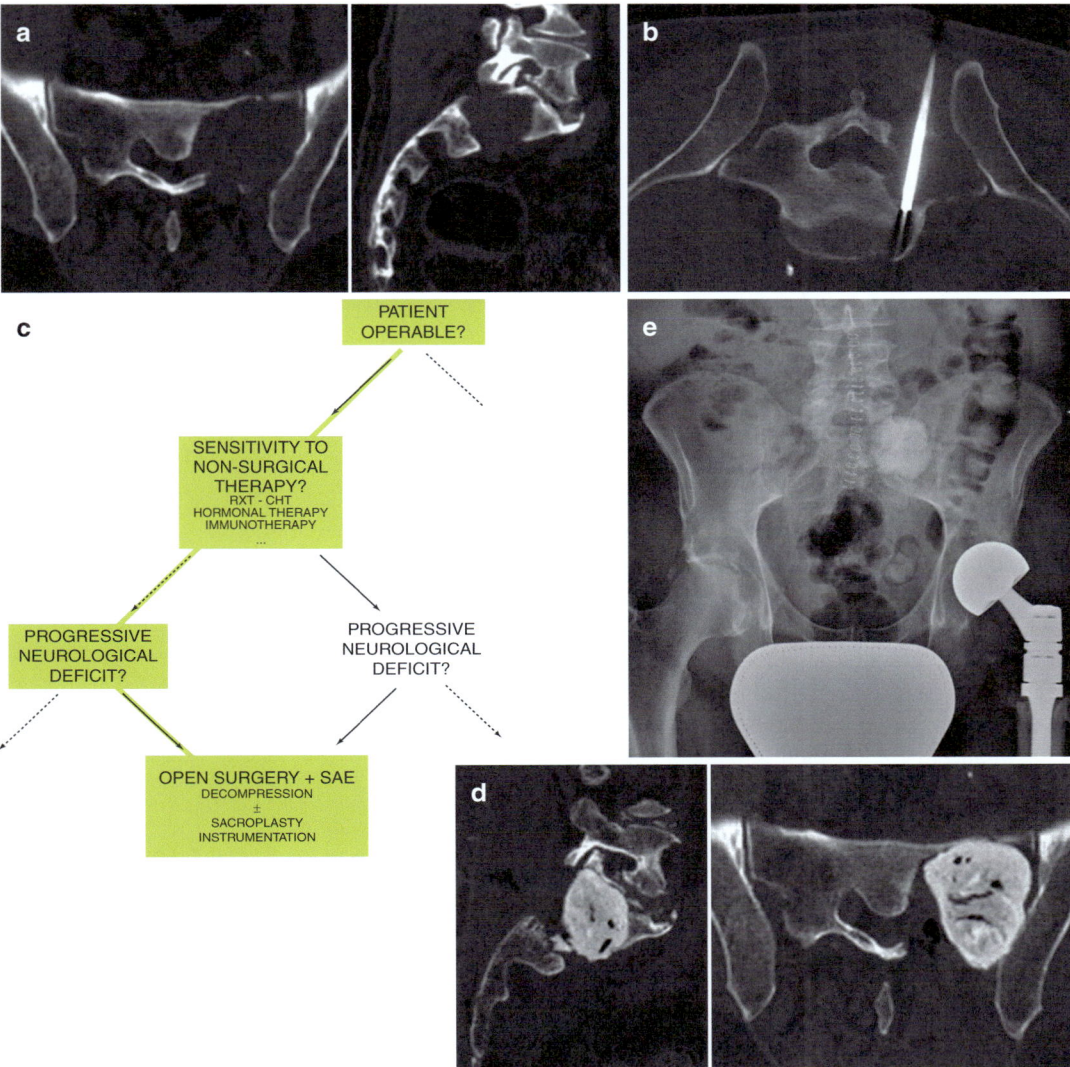

Fig. 8.10 E.M., male, 57 years, progressive onset of low-back pain and left sciatica. Past medical history revealed a liver transplant 2 years before, and early post-operative detection of a metastasis in the left proximal femur that was treated by resection with wide margins and prosthetic reconstruction. CT imaging of the sacrum (**a**) revealed an osteolytic lesion of the left wing with dislocation of the nerve roots. CT-guided trocar biopsy (**b**) was performed which was diagnostic for metastasis from hepatic carcinoma. According to the proposed algorithm (**c**), he was subjected to selective arterial embolization, followed by decompression and excision of the tumour, as evidenced by CT scan (**d**) and postoperative X-rays (**e**)

Recent studies have shown that combining surgery and radiotherapy further increases local control, compared to radiotherapy alone, as performed in the past. In the rare cases in which radiotherapy is performed before surgery, there are significantly higher rates of complications.

Several minimally invasive techniques for the treatment of metastases are emerging in recent years, including radiofrequency thermo-ablation, cryoablation, cavity coblation, sacroplasty, and electrochemotherapy [18–20, 24, 36, 49, 57, 58, 59].

The first three techniques use different energy sources (long waves of electromagnetic radiation, argon gas and ionized gas, respectively), which are applied directly on the tumour through percutaneous probes and induce necrosis limited to the neoplastic tissue, thus preserving the surrounding healthy tissues. To stabilize the treated segment, reducing the risk of a pathologic fracture, it is possible to complete these procedures by injecting PMMA into the residual cavity. However, the isolated percutaneous injection of PMMA in the sacrum (sacroplasty) is an option in case of pathological fractures, allowing a good pain control [49].

Electrochemotherapy (ECT) is a technique based on the application of pulsed electric fields at the tumour level that increase the cell membrane permeability to chemotherapy drugs contextually administered systemically (Bleomycin). The local electric field is produced by electrodes positioned percutaneously directly into the tumour tissue under fluoroscopy or CT guide [20, 24].

Selective arterial embolization must be mentioned as a percutaneous technique that may be used, and eventually repeated, to stop the tumour growth and to control pain in patients with poor general condition, or in case of inoperable lesions. Moreover it is used pre-operatively (within 72 h) in order to reduce bleeding during surgery [25–27].

Conclusions

Appropriate surgical treatment of bone metastases and tumours in general has now become an integral part of the correct approach to the neoplastic patient.

The evolution of anaesthetic techniques now allows correct treatment of spinal metastases, both dramatically improving the quality of life and prolonging the patient's life expectancy, protecting him or her from the complications of these lesions, often either directly or indirectly fatal.

In the majority of cases, it is therefore possible to restore or maintain movement, sensitivity, dignity and hope, as well as controlling pain, reducing the use of adjuvant and analgesic treatments.

The surgical indication for spinal metastases must consider:

- life expectancy of the patient;
- need to improve function and to limit pain;
- need for complete local control, to prevent recurrence;
- possibility of associating adjuvant treatments to improve the efficacy of the treatment, thereby reducing morbidity.

Acknowledgements The authors thank Mr. Carlo Piovani for his helpful collaboration in patients' images storage and editing.

References

1. Wise JJ, Fischgrund JS, Herkowitz HN, Montgomery D, Kurtz LT. Complication, survival rates and risk factors of surgery for metastatic disease of the spine. Spine. 1999;24(18):1943–51.
2. Ryken TC, Eichholz KM, Gerszten PC, Welch WC, Gokaslan ZL, Resnick DK. Evidence-based review of the surgical management of vertebral column metastatic disease. Neurosurg Focus. 2003;15(5):11.
3. Sundaresan N, Rothman A, Manhart K, Kelliher K. Surgery for solitary metastases of the spine. Rationale and results of the treatment. Spine. 2002;27:1802–6.
4. Hosono N, Yonenobu K, Fuji T, Ebara S, Yamashita K, Ono K. Orthopaedic management of spinal metastases. Clin Orthop. 1995;312:148–59.
5. Sioutos PJ, Arbit E, Meshulam CF, Galicich JH. Spinal metastases from solid tumors. Analysis of factors affecting survival. Cancer. 1995;76(8):1453–9.
6. Schuster JM, Grady MS. Medical management and adjuvant therapies in spinal metastatic disease. Neurosurg Focus. 2001;11(6):1–3.
7. Helweg-Larsen S, Sørenson PS. Symptoms and signs in metastatic spinal cord compression: a study from first symptom until diagnosis in 153 patients. Eur J Cancer. 1994;30:396–8.
8. Livingstone KE, Perrin RG. The neurosurgical management of spinal metastases causing cord and cauda equina compression. J Neurosurg. 1978;49:839–43.
9. Loblaw DA, Laperriere NJ, Mackillop WJ. A population-based study of malignant spinal cord compression in Ontario. Clin Oncol (R Coll Radiol). 2003;15:211–7.
10. Quraishi NA, Gokaslan ZL, Boriani S. The surgical management of metastatic epidural compression of the spinal cord. J Bone Joint Surg. 2010;92-B(8):1054–60.
11. Bradley Jacobs W, Perrin RG. Evaluation and treatment of spinal metastases: an overview. Neurosurg Focus. 2001;11(6):e10.

12. Greenberg HS, Kim JH, Posner JB. Epidural spinal cord compression from metastatic tumor: results with a new treatment protocol. Ann Neurol. 1980;8:361–6.
13. Gasbarrini A, Cappuccio M, Mirabile L, Bandiera S, Terzi S, Barbanti Bròdano G, Boriani S. Spinal metastases: treatment evaluation algorithm. Eur Rev Med Pharmacol Sci. 2004;8:265–74.
14. Harrington kDa. Orthopedic surgical management of skeletal complications of malignancy. Cancer. 1997;15(80):1614–27.
15. Young RF, Post EM, King GA. Treatment of spinal epidural metastases. Randomized prospective comparison of laminectomy and radiotherapy. J Neurosurg. 1980;53:741–8.
16. Klimo P, Schmidt MH. Surgical management of spinal metastases. Oncologist. 2004;9:188–96.
17. Holly LT, Foley KT. Three-dimensional fluouroscopy-guided percutaneous thoracolumbar pedicle screw placement: technical note. J Neurosurg. 2003; 99(Suppl):324–9.
18. Callstrom MR, Dupuy DE, Solomon SB, Beres RA, Littrup PJ, Davis KW, Paz-Fumagalli R, Hoffman C, Atwell TD, Charboneau JW, Schmit GD, Goetz MP, Rubin J, Brown KJ, Novotny PJ, Sloan JA. Percutaneous image-guided cryoablation of painful metastases involving bone: multicenter trial. Cancer. 2013;119(5):1033–41.
19. Dabravolski D, Esser J, Lahm A, et al. Treatment of tumors and metastases of the spine by minimally invasive cavity-coblation method (plasma field therapy). J Neurosurg Sci. 2016;61:565–78.
20. Gasbarrini A, Campos WK, Campanacci L, et al. Electrochemotherapy to metastatic spinal melanoma: a novel treatment of spinal metastasis? Spine (Phila Pa 1976). 2015;40:E1340–6.
21. Goetz MP, Callstrom MR, Charboneau JW, Farrel MA, Maus TP, Welch TJ, Wong GY, Sloan JA, Novotny PJ, Petersen IA, Beres RA, Regge D, Capanna R, Saker MB, Groenenmeyer D, Gevargez A, Ahrar K, Choti MA, de Baere TJ, Rubin J. Percutaneous image-guided radiofrequency ablation of painful metastases involving bone: a multicenter study. J Clin Oncol. 2004;22:300–6.
22. Halpin RJ, Bendok BR, Liu JC. Minimally invasive treatments for spinal metastases: vertebroplasty, kyphoplasty and radiofrequency ablation. J Support Oncol. 2004;2:339–55.
23. Dupuy DE, Hong R, Oliver B, Nahum Goldberg S. Radiofrequency ablation of spinal tumors: temperature distribution in the spinal canal. AJR. 2000;175: 1263–6.
24. Bianchi G, Campanacci L, Ronchetti M, et al. Electrochemotherapy in the treatment of bone metastases: a phase II trial. World J Surg. 2016;40: 3088–94.
25. Gellad FE, Sadato N, Numaguchi Y, et al. Vascular metastatic lesions of the spine: preoperative embolization. Radiology. 1990;176:683–6.
26. Sundaresan N, Choi IS, Hughes JE, et al. Treatment of spinal metastases from kidney cancer by pre-surgical embolization and resection. J Neurosurg. 1990;73:548–54.
27. Prabhu VC, Bilsky MH, Jambhekar K, et al. Results of preoperative embolization for metastatic spinal neoplasms. J Neurosurg. 2003;98(Spine 2):156–64.
28. Hoffmann RT, Jakobs TF, Trumm C, Weber C, Helmberger TK, Reiser MF. Radiofrequency ablation in combination with osteoplasty in the treatment of painful metastatic bone disease. J Vasc Interv Radiol. 2008;19(3):419–25.
29. Alvarez L, Pérez-Higueras A, Quinones D, Calvo E, Rossi RE. Vertebroplasty in the treatment of vertebral tumors: postprocedural outcome and quality of life. Eur Spine J. 2003;12:356–60.
30. Fourney DR, Schomer DF, Nader R, Chlan J, Suki D, Ahrar K, Rhines LD, Gokaslan ZL. Percutaneous vertebroplasty and kyphoplasty for painful vertebral body fractures in cancer patients. J Neurosurg Spine. 2003;98:21–30.
31. Groenemeyer D, Schirp S, Gevargez A. Image-guided radiofrequency ablation of spinal tumors: preliminary experience with expandable array electrode. Cancer J. 2002;8(1):33–9.
32. Pilitsis JG, Rengachary SS. The role of vertebroplasty in metastatic spinal disease. Neurosurg Focus. 2001;11:E9.
33. Shimony JS, Gilula LA, Zeller AJ, Brown DB. Percutaneous vertebroplasty for malignant compression fractures with epidural involvement. Radiology. 2004;232:846–53.
34. Reidy D, Ahn H, Mousavi P, Finkelstein J, Whine CM. A biomechanical analysis of intravertebral pressures during vertebroplasty of cadaveric spines with and without simulated metastases. Spine. 2003;28:1534–9.
35. Hide IG, Gangi A. Percutaneus vertebroplasty: history, technique and current perspectives. Clin Radiol. 2004;59:461–7.
36. Madaelil TP, Wallace AN, Jennings JW. Radiofrequency ablation alone or in combination with cementoplasty for local control and pain palliation of sacral metastases: preliminary results in 11 patients. Skelet Radiol. 2016;45:1213–9.
37. Nakatsuka A, Yamakado K, Maeda M, Yasuda M, Akeboshi M, Takaki H, Hamada A, Takeda K. Radiofrequency ablation combined with bone cement injection for the treatment of bone malignancies. J Vasc Interv Radiol. 2004;15(7):707–12.
38. Schaefer O, Lohrmann C, Markmiller M, Uhrmeister P, Langer M. Combined treatment of a spinal metastases with radiofrequency heat ablation and vertebroplasty. AJR. 2003;180:1075–7.
39. Babu NV, Titus VT, Chittaranjan S, Abraham G, Prem H, Korula RJ. Computed guided biopsy of the spine. Spine. 1994;19:2436–42.
40. Yu MK, Buys SS. Medical management of skeletal metastasis. Neurosurg Clin N Am. 2004;15:529–3.
41. Tokuhashi Y, Matsuzaki Y, Toriyama S, Kawano H, Ohsaka S. Scoring system for the preoperative evalu-

ation of metastatic spine tumor prognosis. Spine. 1990;15:1110–3.

42. Tomita K, Kawahara N, Kobayashi T, et al. Surgical strategy for spinal metastases. Spine. 2001;26: 298–306.

43. Fisher CG, DiPaola CP, Ryken TC, Bilsky MH, Shaffrey CI, Berven SH, Harrop JS, Fehlings MG, Boriani S, Chou D, Schmidt MH, Polly DW, Biagini R, Burch S, Dekutoski MB, Ganju A, Gerszten PC, Gokaslan ZL, Groff MW, Liebsch NJ, Mendel E, Okuno SH, Patel S, Rhines LD, Rose PS, Sciubba DM, Sundaresan N, Tomita K, Varga PP, Vialle LR, Vrionis FD, Yamada Y, Fourney DR. A novel classification system for spinal instability in neoplastic disease: an evidence-based approach and expert consensus from the Spine Oncology Study Group. Spine (Phila Pa 1976). 2010;35(22):E1221–9.

44. Boriani S, Gasbarrini A. Point of view. Spine. 2005;30:2227–9.

45. Fourney DR, Gokaslan ZL. Sacral tumors: primary and metastatic. In: Dickman CA, Fehlings MG, Gokaslan ZL, editors. Spinal cord and spinal column tumors: principles and practice. New York: Thieme; 2006. p. 404–19.

46. Gasbarrini A, Di Martino A, Biagini R, et al. Therapeutic flow-chart for the treatment of sacral metastases: recommendations from the Italian Orthopaedic Society bone metastasis study group. Ital J Orthop Traumatol. 2016;42:242–50.

47. Quraishi NA, Giannoulis KE, Edwards KL, et al. Surgical treatment of cauda equina compression as a result of metastatic tumours of the lumbo-sacral junction and sacrum. Eur Spine J. 2013;22:S33–7.

48. Varga PP, Bors I, Lazary A. Sacral tumors and management. Orthop Clin North Am. 2009;40:105–23.

49. Nebreda C, Vallejo R, Aliaga L, Benyamin R. Percutaneous sacroplasty and sacroiliac joint cementation under fluoroscopic guidance for lower back pain related to sacral metastatic tumors with sacroiliac joint invasion. Pain Pract. 2011;11(6):564–9.

50. Gerszten PC, Ozhasoglu C, Burton SA, et al. CyberKnife frameless single-fraction stereotactic radiosurgery for tumors of the sacrum. Neurosurg Focus. 2003;15:E7.

51. Fujimura Y, Maruiwa H, Takahata T, et al. Neurological evaluation after radical resection of sacral neoplasms. Paraplegia. 1994;32:396–406.

52. Guo W, Tang X, Zang J. One-stage total en bloc sacrectomy: a novel technique and report of 9 cases. Spine (Phila Pa 1976). 2013;38:E626–31.

53. Nakai S, Yoshizawa H, Kobayashi S, et al. Anorectal andbladder function after sacrifice of the sacral nerves. Spine (Phila Pa 1976). 2000;25:2234–9.

54. Salehi SA, McCafferty RR, Karahalios D. Neural function preservation and early mobilization after resection of metastatic sacral tumors and lumbosacro-pelvic junction re- construction. Report of three cases. J Neurosurg. 2002;97:88–93.

55. Uemura A, Matsusako M, Numaguchi Y, Oka M, Kobayashi N, Niinami C, Kawasaki T, Suzuki K. Percutaneous sacroplasty for hemorrhagic metastases from hepatocellular carcinoma. AJNR Am J Neuroradiol. 2005;26(3):493–5.

56. Li D, Guo W, Tang X, et al. Preservation of the contra-lateral sacral nerves during hemisacrectomy for sacral malignancies. Eur Spine J. 2014;23:1933–9.

57. Masala S, Konda D, Massari F, Simonetti G. Sacroplasty and iliac osteoplasty under combined CT and fluoroscopic guidance. Spine. 2006;31(18): E667–9.

58. Tomasian A, Wallace A, Northrup B, Hillen TJ, Jennings JW. Spine cryoablation: pain palliation and local tumor control for vertebral metastases. AJNR Am J Neuroradiol. 2016;37(1):189–95.

59. Damron TA, Sim FH. Surgical treatment for metastatic disease of the pelvis and the proximal end of the femur. Instr Course Lect. 2000;49:461–70.

Metastases to the Long Bones: Algorithm of Treatment

Maurizio Scorianz, Franco Gherlinzoni, and Domenico A. Campanacci

Abstract

Metastases of the long bones represent a frequent clinical condition.

Multiple treatment options are available, ranging from the more aggressive resections and arthroplasty to palliative care and from long-lasting reconstruction to minimally invasive therapies.

When selecting a treatment, it is paramount to consider not only the mechanical characteristics of the lesions but also the tumoral behavior, medical state, and expected survival of the patient. In addition, other factors should be taken into account: the presence of a single metastatic lesion, the site in the long bone (diaphysis or metaepiphysis), mechanical stability (impending or pathological fracture), and the effectiveness of nonsurgical therapies.

Several prognostic criteria were assessed in the last 20 years and, being familiar with them may help in treatment selection.

An algorithm of treatment has been the objective to guide the decision-making process in a multidisciplinary approach to metastasis of the long bones.

A collaboration between the orthopedic surgeon, the oncologist, and the radiotherapist leads to the best choice of treatment for the different scenarios.

Keywords

Metastases · Long bones · Algorithm · Metastases resection · Osteosynthesis · Palliative therapy

9.1 Introduction

Correctly treating metastases of the long bones can be challenging. Furthermore, due to the increasing incidence of long bone metastases, a larger number of orthopedic surgeons will have to face this pathological condition [1, 2].

Several treatment options are available, ranging from resection to palliative care.

Patient selection is critical, and life expectancy of the patient and their operability must be evaluated carefully to choose the best treatment.

M. Scorianz
Orthopaedic Oncology and Reconstructive Unit, Careggi University Hospital, Florence, Italy

F. Gherlinzoni
Orthopedic and Traumatology Unit, Gorizia General Hospital, Gorizia, Italy

D. A. Campanacci (✉)
Orthopaedic Oncology and Reconstructive Unit, Careggi University Hospital, Florence, Italy

Department of Surgery and Translational Medicine, University of Florence, Florence, Italy
e-mail: domenico.campanacci@unifi.it

The occurrence of skeletal metastases is a negative prognostic factor for the oncological patient, especially when the lesion requires a surgical treatment [3].

A multicentric study from the Scandinavian Sarcoma Group on 460 nonvertebral bone metastatic lesions treated surgically reported that 44% of the patients died within 6 months from surgery; the survival rates at 1 year and 3 years were 39% and 18%, respectively [4]. Two other studies on secondary lesions of the skeleton, including spine, found 1-year survival rate of 48 and 54% and 3-year survival rate of 23 and 27% [5, 6].

During the last two decades, interest has increased to assess prognostic factors for patients with metastatic carcinoma.

A multivariate analysis from a multicentric study of the Scandinavian Sarcoma Group [4] identified the following risk factors: histology of primary tumor, the presence of pathological fracture, visceral metastases, preoperative hemoglobin level ≤ 7 g/dL, and Karnofsky performance status [7].

Bohm et al. established the following prognostic criteria: histology of primary tumor, the presence of pathological fracture, visceral metastases, and the time from tumor diagnosis to metastases >3 years [5]. The study was carried out on 94 patients.

A prospective study by Nathan et al. identified the following prognostic factors: histology of primary tumor, Eastern Cooperative Oncology Group (ECOG) performance status, visceral metastases, number of bone metastases, hemoglobin count, and surgeon survival estimate. The study was conducted on 191 patients that had been previously treated for a pathological fracture [8].

Katagiri et al. assessed five prognostic factors in a study on 350 patients. These were histology of primary tumor, ECOG performance status [9, 10], visceral/brain metastases, isolated or multiple bone lesions, and previous chemotherapy.

These authors also developed a prognostic scoring system. A score ≤ 2 indicated that the likelihood of 1-year survival was 89%. On the contrary, a score ≥ 6 implied that the probability of 1-year survival was at 11% [6].

A Bayesian classification to estimate survival of patients undergoing surgery was proposed in 2011 by Forsberg et al. [11]. They developed two different Bayesian networks, called the "Bayesian Estimated Tools for Survival (BETS) models." These networks could estimate the expected survival at 3 and 12 months for patients that were eligible for bone metastases surgery.

The authors validated these criteria on a sample of 815 patients from the Scandinavian Skeletal Metastasis Registry. These patients were affected by bone metastases of the limbs, and they were treated in eight Scandinavian centers between 1999 and 2008. BETS models at 3 and 12 months were also effective when data was incomplete or missing. At 4 months, four preoperative criteria were found to be significant: surgeon survival estimate, hemoglobin level, number of bone metastases, and histology of the primary tumor [12, 13].

9.2   Histology

The histology of the primary tumor is the most important prognostic factor because it is determinant of its biological behavior.

A relatively good prognosis is usually expected for carcinomas of the breast, prostate, and thyroid.

Multiple myelomas and lymphomas, although not carcinomas, are included in the treatment protocols of bone metastases due to their similar behavior.

Renal carcinomas have a different prognosis based on their histotype. Clear cell carcinoma, the most common histotype, has a favorable prognosis if treated promptly and correctly. On the contrary, the transitional cell cancer of the renal pelvis, being more aggressive, implies a worse prognosis [14]. Another factor that leads to poor prognosis of clear cell carcinomas is the development of synchronous metastases. On the other hand, the development of metachronous metastases is considered a positive prognosis factor.

Lung tumors and cancer of unknown origin (tumors where a full body CT scan cannot identify the primary tumor) are always associated to a poor prognosis [4, 5, 15].

Katagiri et al. divided tumors into slow growth tumors (breast, prostate, myeloma, lymphoma), moderate growth tumors (other carcinomas and sarcomas), rapid growth tumors (liver, pancreas, stomach, and lung) [6].

Forsberg et al. developed this classification further by adding some modifications: slow growth tumors (breast, prostate, kidney, thyroid, myeloma and lymphoma), moderate growth tumors (other carcinoma and sarcomas), and rapid growth tumors (lung, stomach, liver and melanoma). A statistically significant difference in 3- and 12-month survivals was found between these three groups [12].

Potential responses that follow nonsurgical treatments are ossification and repair of the lesion. These therapies can be either a local (radiotherapy) or systemic treatment (chemotherapy, molecular therapy, hormonal therapy, bisphosphonates, denosumab, radioreceptorial therapy).

A positive response of the skeletal metastatic lesions can be expected in the following: breast, prostate, and thyroid cancer, myeloma, and lymphoma. On the contrary, kidney and lung carcinomas usually respond poorly [14].

When a positive response is not expected and life expectancy is >1 year, excisional surgery is considered appropriate.

If a good response from nonsurgical treatment is anticipated, the orthopedic surgery should be limited to prevent an impending fracture or treating a pathological fracture. An excision of the lesion in this clinical scenario is usually not needed.

9.3 Solitary Metastases

When approaching a solitary bone metastasis, performing an excision has proven to improve prognoses for secondary lesions of the kidney [7, 16–21] and thyroid (favorable prognosis histotypes) [22–27]. There is no evidence of a prognostic improvement for breast [28–31] and prostate metastases [32, 33]. Additionally, there is no prognostic difference between wide and marginal margins or an intralesional curettage [16, 21, 26, 27].

Patients of this group can become long-term survivors, so the surgical treatment must include the excision of the metastatic lesion and a long-lasting reconstruction.

The development of solitary metastases after a long time from the removal of the primary tumor can be considered a favorable prognostic factor. In this clinical situation, adequate surgical margins should be considered.

9.4 Pathological Fracture

A pathological fracture is a dramatic event for the metastatic patient.

The main objective of treatment in these cases is not the consolidation of the fracture, although that can sometimes occur, but rather the intent should be restoring the resistance to flexion and torsion of the bone segment, allowing for immediate weight-bearing and ambulation [34].

Occasionally the fracture will consolidate, but literature data are lacking on this topic because most of the studies report the survival data of patients or implants and consolidation of the fracture is generally not taken into consideration. Poitout et al. [35] reported the healing of pathological fractures in 5–20% of the patients. Gainor and Buchert [36] found a 35% chance of fracture consolidation. They found a different rate of fracture healing in different histotypes: 67% for myeloma, 44% for kidney carcinoma, 37% for breast cancer, and 0% for lung cancer. Radiation therapy, up to a total dose of 30 Gy, did not seem to influence the healing of the fracture. One of the conclusions of this study was that at 6–9 months from surgery, there is a high risk of failure of the osteosynthesis.

In another study, Sim indicates that breast cancer and myeloma are the histotypes with the best chances of pathological fracture healing [37].

9.5 Impending Fracture

The femur is the skeletal segment with the highest risk of pathological fracture due to the considerable flexion and torsion mechanical stresses at this level. The high-risk sites are the femoral neck, the subtrochanteric region, and the supracondylar area.

A pathological fracture is a severe complication for the oncological patient with negative effects on quality of life and psychological status. Moreover, pathological fracture was seen to represent a negative prognostic factor, and it was observed that such an event increases the cost of care for the health system. A prophylactic surgical treatment of impending fractures was seen to be effective in improving survival and the quality of life of the patient [4, 38].

Harrington's criteria predict the risk of a pathological fracture in the following scenarios: when the lesion of the peritrochanteric area is >25 mm, when the lesion involves more than 50% of the cortical bone, when the lesion is osteolytic, and when there is an increasing pain [39], particularly following irradiation.

Mirels in 1989 [40] developed the most commonly used scoring system to evaluate the risk of a pathological fracture. The system considers the anatomical region, the pain level, the radiological characteristics of the lesion (blastic, mixed, lytic), and the size of the lesion compared to the diameter of the bone segment [41].

Other authors suggest to consider the following as indicators of increased risk: lesions located above the lesser trochanter or at the proximal half of the humerus, breast histotype, the patient not being in treatment with bisphosphonates, and primary or secondary osteoporosis [42].

In 2004, van der Linden et al. evaluated the correlation between pathological fractures and the risk factors previously described by different authors. Their conclusion was that the Mirels criteria overestimated the risk of a pathological fracture [43]. Notably, the only statistically significant criteria they observed were an axial cortical involvement >30 mm and a circumferential cortical involvement >50%.

Future developments in predicting a pathological fracture might include the use of quantitative computed tomography and case-specific finite element analyses based on 3D CT [44–47].

9.6   General Considerations

The life expectancy of the patient is one of the most important criteria when selecting the appropriate treatment for metastases of the long bones.

If the prognosis of the patient is poor in relation to tumor histotype, staging, and medical state, then palliative treatment should be considered. The objective should be to improve quality of life of the patient through pain management and prevention or treatment of complications.

On the other hand, when the prognosis is favorable, the treatment of the metastases should be more aggressive, and long-lasting reconstructions should be considered (i.e., excisional surgery) [48, 49].

Before surgery, careful attention must be given to the biological and mechanical characteristics of the metastatic lesion. Each of the following parameters should be considered in order to choose the appropriate surgical solution: the presence of solitary metastasis, site of the lesion (metaepiphysis or diaphysis), mechanical stability (presence or risk of pathological fracture), and sensitivity to nonsurgical treatments [50].

A surgical resection of the metastases and replacement with a prosthetic implant are the recommended treatment for impending or pathological fractures of the metaepiphysis, solitary metastases of renal cell and thyroid carcinomas of the metaepiphysis, and metastatic lesions of the metaepiphysis with a poor expected response from nonsurgical treatment, especially when these lesions are located in the proximal femur (Fig. 9.1).

Prosthetic replacement allows an earlier functional recovery with a low risk of reoperation due to progression of the disease or failure of reconstruction [51–53].

Steensma et al. observed that prosthetic reconstruction leads to fewer complications and longer survival when compared to osteosynthesis in metastatic patients with pathological or impending fractures of the proximal femur [54].

In metaphyseal fractures of the proximal humerus, prosthetic replacements last longer than other solutions because they are more resistant to torsional forces. Moreover, prosthetic

Fig. 9.1 Impending fracture of the proximal femoral metaphysis due to metastatic renal cell carcinoma. (**a**, **b**) Preoperative radiographic images of the metastatic lesion. (**c**) Surgical resection specimen and proximal femur prosthetic implant. (**d**) Postoperative radiographic control after modular prosthesis replacement with cemented stem and bipolar cup

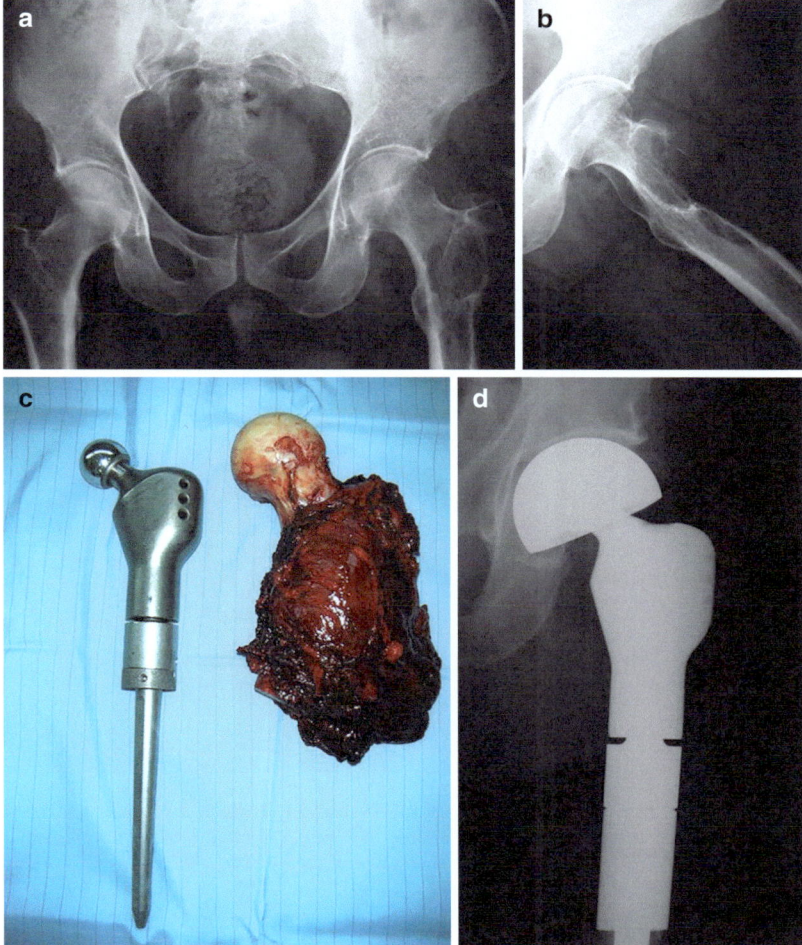

replacement is considered the treatment of choice for metastases of the distal humerus, since mechanically stable osteosynthesis with plate and cement in this area is very difficult to obtain.

In diaphyseal metastatic lesions, when the patient has a favorable prognosis and response to nonsurgical treatments is not expected, osteosynthesis reinforced with polymethyl methacrylate (PMMA) cement can be performed (Fig. 9.2). Tumoral tissue can be removed either through intralesional curettage or intercalary resection, and local adjuvants may be used to improve surgical margins [55–60]. Then the defect is filled with PMMA cement that can be injected into the medullary canal to improve the mechanical strength of the osteosynthesis [61].

Locked nails have proven to be more durable implants than plates for metastatic lesions of the femur and tibia, because of their better mechanical stability and resistance in case of local progression of the disease [54]. Plate and screw fixation, however, must be considered for humeral lesions and for long bones of the forearm.

In diaphyseal metastatic lesions, when the prognosis of the patient is favorable and the expected response to nonsurgical therapy is good, simple osteosynthesis obtained through a locked nail may be performed (Fig. 9.3). This must be considered especially when facing mixed or osteoblastic lesions (breast, prostate) and lesions responding to medical therapy, radiotherapy, bisphosphonate, and denosumab.

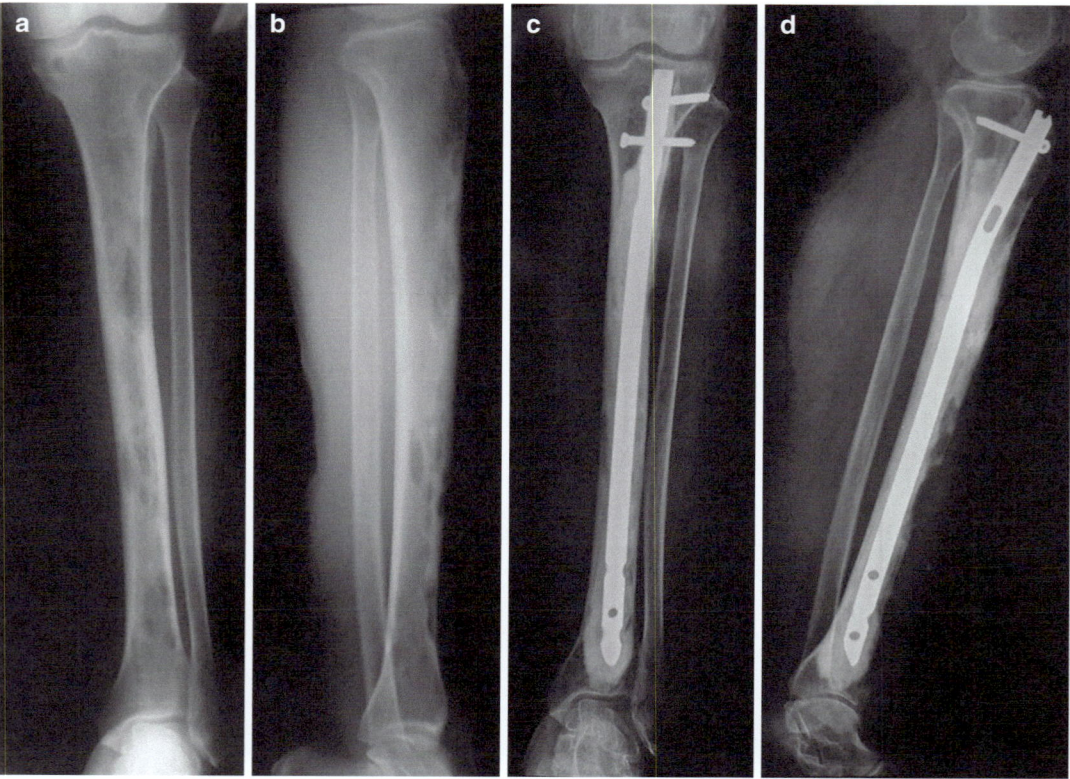

Fig. 9.2 Multifocal diaphyseal metastatic lesions of the tibia from breast cancer with progression despite of radiation therapy. (**a, b**) Radiographic view of diaphyseal mul- tifocal metastatic lesions of the tibia. (**c, d**) Postoperative images of the intramedullary nail reinforced with PMMA cement

If the prognosis is poor, the diaphyseal metastasis should be treated with simple osteosynthesis: locked nail for lesions of the femur, tibia, and humerus and plate and screws for lesions of the forearm [14].

In patients with poor prognosis and poor general conditions, in case of persistent pain notwithstanding nonsurgical treatments, minimally invasive therapies should be considered. When surgery is not indicated, pain control may be achieved by tumoral tissue ablation through percutaneous minimally invasive techniques [62]. Originally developed as treatment for benign lesions, minimally invasive therapies, like cryoablation, thermoablation, embolization, and others, represent an effective option for this patient group [63–66].

9.7 Algorithm of Treatment

Several studies have attempted to standardize the treatment of bone metastases.

Capanna and Campanacci divided bone metastases into four different classes [14, 67]. This classification selected patients who needed a surgical treatment providing guidelines for the indication to simple osteosynthesis, osteosynthesis with cement, and prosthetic replacement. The selection between the surgical options was done basing on a score obtained from the following parameters: life expectancy, according to the type of tumor, site/location of the lesion (epiphyseal, metaphyseal, or diaphyseal), extension of the lesion, and sensitivity to nonsurgical therapies.

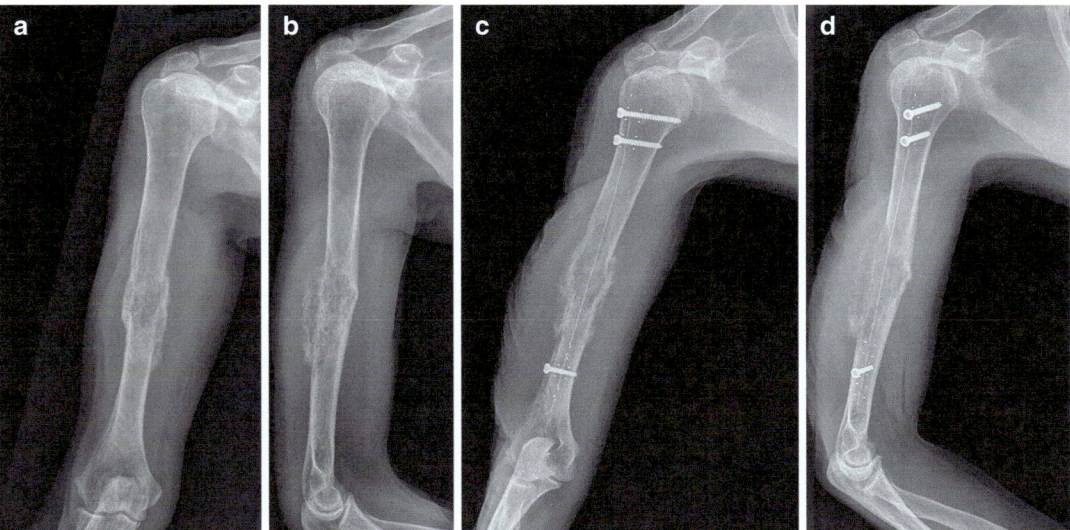

Fig. 9.3 Impending fracture of the humeral diaphysis in metastatic lesions from breast cancer. (**a**, **b**) Preoperative radiographic images of the lesion. (**c**, **d**) Postoperative images after intramedullary nail fixation using a carbon fiber device

In 2014, the Italian Orthopaedic and Traumatology Society (SIOT) Bone Metastasis Study Group developed a new algorithm for the treatment of metastases of the long bones (Fig. 9.4). The algorithm was based on the protocol of Capanna and Campanacci, integrated with the most recent evidence from literature [14, 69–77].

The following parameters were considered:

– The presence of a pathological fracture or impending fracture
– The presence of a solitary metastasis from a carcinoma of the kidney or thyroid
– The localization of the metastases (meta-epiphysis or diaphysis)
– The expected response to nonsurgical therapies
– The survival estimate for the patient

The eligibility of the patient to surgical treatment is determinant, and the evaluation is made by the anesthesiologist according to the ASA score. The surgical procedure can be performed if the ASA score is lower or equal to 3 (on a scale from 1 to 5).

The final treatment options of the algorithm are the following: excisional surgery (resection and prosthesis, resection/intralesional excision, and osteosynthesis with cement augmentation), simple osteosynthesis, nonsurgical therapies, and palliative care (minimally invasive treatments, pain management).

The steps of this algorithm are designed mostly for lytic or mixed pattern metastatic lesions of weight-bearing long bones. For this reason, this algorithm cannot be applied in some circumstances: a pathological fracture or impending fracture due to osteolytic metastases of a non-weight-bearing long bone or osteoblastic metastases, regardless of their location. If those lesions are painful, then surgery should be considered when nonsurgical treatment is unsuccessful.

The SIOT algorithm assumes the integration of the orthopedic surgeon with a medical oncologist and a radiation oncologist in a multidisciplinary team [77].

Although the steps of this algorithm can seem an excessive simplification of high-complexity concepts, the aim of the SIOT algorithm is to

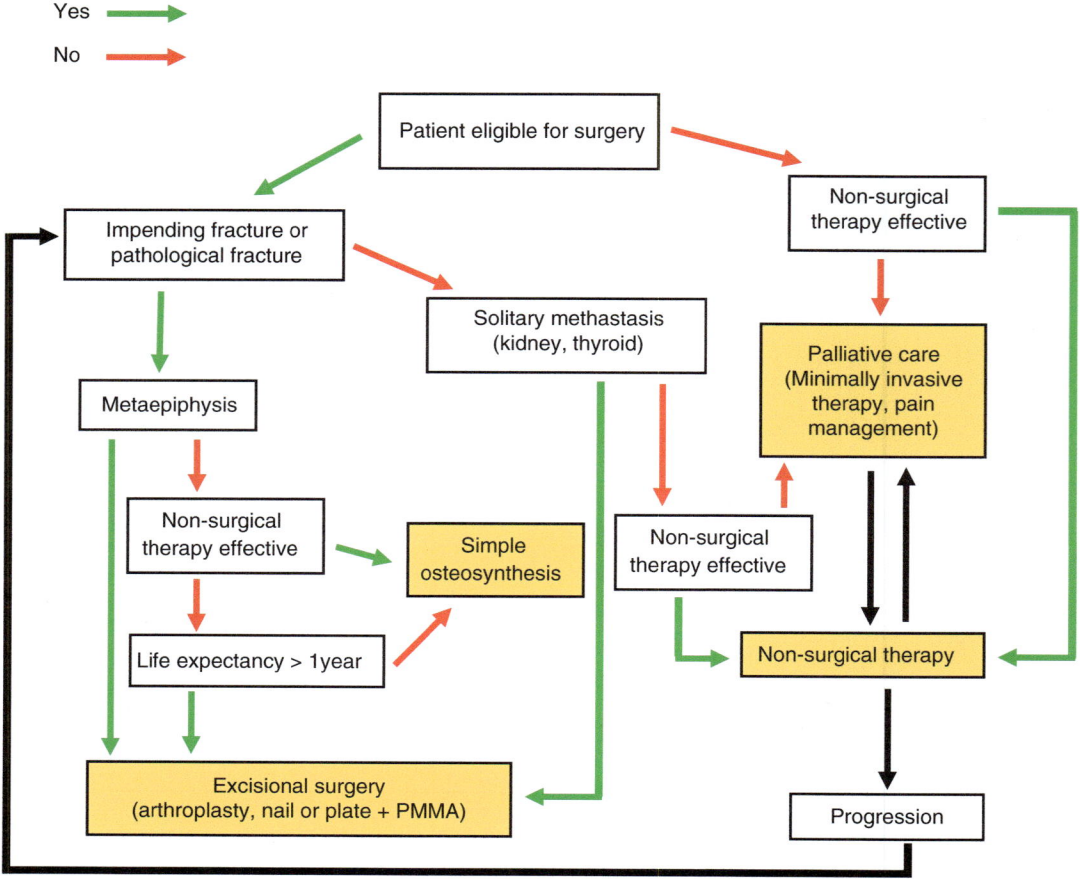

Fig. 9.4 Flowchart for the treatment of long bone metastases. Modified with permission from [68]

guide the orthopedic surgeon in the decision-making process when approaching a patient affected by long bone metastases.

References

1. Li S, Peng Y, Weinhandl ED, et al. Estimated number of prevalent cases of metastatic bone disease in the US adult population. Clin Epidemiol. 2012;4:87–93.
2. Ibrahim T, Farolfi A, Mercatali L, et al. Metastatic bone disease in the era of bone-targeted therapy: clinical impact. Tumori. 2013;99:1–9.
3. Saad F, Lipton A, Cook R, et al. Pathologic fractures correlate with reduced survival in patients with malignant bone disease. Cancer. 2007;110:1860–7.
4. Hansen BH, Keller J, Laitinen M, et al. The Scandinavian Sarcoma Group skeletal metastasis register. Survival after surgery for bone metastases in the pelvis and extremities. Acta Orthop Scand. 2004;75:11–5.
5. Bohm P, Huber J. The surgical treatment of bony metastases of the spine and limb. J Bone Joint Surg Br. 2002;84B:521–9.
6. Katagiri H, Takahashi M, Wakai K, et al. Prognostic factors and scoring system for patients with skeletal metastasis. J Bone Joint Surg Br. 2005;87-B:698–703.
7. Karnofsky DA, Burchenal JH. The clinical evaluation of chemotherapeutic agents. In: MacLeod CM, editor. Evaluation of chemotherapeutic agents. New York: Columbia University Press; 1949. p. 191–205.
8. Nathan SS, Healey JH, Mellano D, et al. Survival in patients operated on for pathologic fracture: implications for end-of-life orthopedic care. J Clin Oncol. 2005;23:6072–82.
9. Conill C, Verger E, Salamero M. Performance status assessment in cancer patients. Cancer. 1990;65:1864–6.
10. Oken MM, Creech RH, Tormey DC, et al. Toxicity and response criteria of the Eastern Cooperative Oncology Group. Am J Clin Oncol. 1982;5:649–55.
11. Forsberg JA, Eberhardt J, Boland PJ, et al. Estimating survival in patients with operable skeletal metastases:

an application of a Bayesian belief network. PLoS One. 2011;6:e19956.

12. Forsberg JA, Wedin R, Bauer H, et al. External validation of the Bayesian Estimated Tools for Survival (BETS) models in patients with surgically treated skeletal metastases. BMC Cancer. 2012;12:493.

13. Forsberg JA, Sjoberg D, Chen QR, et al. Treating metastatic disease: which survival model is best suited for the clinic? Clin Orthop Relat Res. 2013;471:843–50.

14. Capanna R, Campanacci DA. The treatment of metastasis in appendicular skeleton. J Bone Joint Surg Br. 2001;83:471–81.

15. Rougraff BT. Diagnosis of bone metastases evaluation of the patient with carcinoma of unknown origin metastatic to bone. Clin Orthop Relat Res. 2003;415S:S105–9.

16. Fuchs B, Trousdale RT, Rock MG. Solitary bony metastasis from renal cell carcinoma. Significance of surgical treatment. Clin Orthop Rel Res. 2005;431:187–92.

17. Althausen P, Althausen A, Jennings LC, et al. Prognostic factors and surgical treatment of osseous metastases secondary to renal cell carcinoma. Cancer. 1997;80:1103–9.

18. Durr HR, Maier M, Pfahler M, et al. Surgical treatment of osseous metastases in patients with renal cell carcinoma. Clin Orthop Rel Res. 1999;367:283–90.

19. Jung ST, Ghert MA, Harrelson JM, et al. Treatment of osseous metastases in patients with renal cell carcinoma. Clin Orthop Rel Res. 2003;409:223–31.

20. Balock KG, Grimer RJ, Carter SR, et al. Radical surgery for the solitary bony metastasis from renal-cell carcinoma. J Bone Joint Surg Br. 2000;82-B:62–7.

21. Lin PP, Mirza AN, Lewis VO, et al. Patient survival after surgery for osseous metastases from renal cell carcinoma. J Bone Joint Surg Am. 2007;89:1794–801.

22. Casara D, Rubello D, Saladini G, et al. Distant metastases in differentiated thyroid cancer: long-term results of radioiodine treatment and statistical analysis of prognostic factors in 214 patients. Tumori. 1991;77:432–6.

23. Sampson E, Brierley JD, Le LW, et al. Clinical management and outcome of papillary and follicular (differentiated) thyroid cancer presenting with distant metastasis at diagnosis. Cancer. 2007;110:1451–6.

24. Proye CA, Dromer DH, Carnaille BM, et al. Is it still worthwhile to treat bone metastases from differentiated thyroid carcinoma with radioactive iodine? World J Surg. 1992;16:640–5.

25. Schlumberger M, Challeton C, De Vathaire F, et al. Radioactive iodine treatment and external radiotherapy for lung and bone metastases from thyroid carcinoma. J Nucl Med. 1996;37:598–605.

26. Niederle B, Roka R, Schemper M, et al. Surgical treatment of distant metastases in differentiated thyroid cancer: indication and results. Surgery. 1986;100:1088–97.

27. Boyle MJ, Hornicek FJ, Robinson DS, et al. Internal hemipelvectomy for solitary pelvic thyroid cancer metastases. J Surg Oncol. 2000;75:3–10.

28. Durr HR, Muller PE, Lenz T, et al. Surgical treatment of bone metastases in patients with breast cancer. Clin Orthop Rel Res. 2002;396:191–6.

29. Jimeno A, Amador ML, Gonzalez-Cortijo L, et al. Initially metastatic breast carcinoma has a distinct disease pattern but an equivalent outcome compared with recurrent metastatic breast carcinoma. Cancer. 2004;100:1833–42.

30. Oka H, Kondoh T, Seichi A, et al. Incidence and prognostic factors of Japanese breast cancer patients with bone metastasis. J Orthop Sci. 2006;11:13–9.

31. Koizumi M, Yoshimoto M, Kasumi F, et al. Comparison between solitary and multiple skeletal metastatic lesions of breast cancer patients. Ann Oncol. 2003;14:1234–40.

32. Weiss RJ, Forsberg JA, Wedin R. Surgery of skeletal metastases in 306 patients with prostate cancer. Indications, complications, and survival. Acta Orthop. 2012;83:74–9.

33. Cheville JC, Tindall D, Boelter C, et al. Metastatic prostate carcinoma to bone. Clinical and pathologic features associated with cancer-specific survival. Cancer. 2002;95:1028–36.

34. Healey JH, Brown HK. Complications of bone metastases - surgical management. Cancer. 2000;88:2940–51.

35. Poitout DG, Tropiano P, Clouet D'Orval B, et al. Surgery for bone metastasis of the limbs. In: Poitout DG, editor. Bone metastases medical, surgical and radiological treatment. London: Springer; 2002. p. 97–100.

36. Gainor BJ, Buchert P. Fracture healing in metastatic bone disease. Clin Orthop. 1983;178:297–302.

37. Sim FH. Operative treatment—general considerations. In: Sim FH, editor. Diagnosis and management of metastatic bone disease—a multidisciplinary approach. New York: Raven Press; 1987. p. 161–70.

38. Ward WG, Holsenbeck S, Dorey FJ, et al. Metastatic disease of the femur: surgical treatment. Clin Orthop Relat Res. 2003;415(Suppl):S230–44.

39. Harrington KD. The role of surgery in the management of pathologic fractures. Orthop Clin North Am. 1977;8:841.

40. Mirels M. Metastatic disease in long bones: a proposed scoring system for diagnosis impending pathologic fractures. Clin Orthop. 1989;249:256–64.

41. Damron TA, Morgan H, Prakash D, et al. Critical evaluation of Mirels' rating system for impending pathological fractures. Clin Orthop Rel Res. 2003;415(Suppl):S201–7.

42. Patel B, DeGroot H. Evaluation of the risk of pathologic fractures secondary to metastatic bone disease. Orthopedics. 2001;24:612–7.

43. Van der Linden YM, Dijkstra PDS, Kroon HM, et al. Comparative analysis of risk factors for pathological fracture with femoral metastases. Results based on a randomized trial of radiotherapy. J Bone Joint Surg Br. 2004;86B:566–73.

44. Tanck E, van Aken JB, van der Linden YM, et al. Pathological fracture prediction in patients with

metastatic lesions can be improved with quantitative computed tomography based computer models. Bone. 2009;45:777–83.

45. Keyak JH, Kaneko TS, Rossi SA, et al. Predicting the strength of femoral shafts with and without metastatic lesions. Clin Orthop Rel Res. 2005;439:161–70.

46. Keyak JH, Kaneko TS, Tehranzadeh J, et al. Predicting proximal femoral strength using structural engineering models. Clin Orthop Relat Res. 2005;437:219–28.

47. Derikx LC, van Aken JB, Janssen D, et al. The assessment of the risk of fracture in femora with metastatic lesions: comparing case-specific finite element analyses with predictions by clinical experts. J Bone Joint Surg Br. 2012;94:1135–42.

48. Piccioli A, Maccauro G, Rossi B, et al. Surgical treatment of pathologic fractures of humerus. Injury. 2010;41:1112–6.

49. Piccioli A, Maccauro G, Scaramuzzo L, et al. Surgical treatment of impending and pathological fractures of tibia. Injury. 2013;44:1092–6.

50. Piccioli A, Ventura A, Maccauro G, et al. Local adjuvants in surgical management of bone metastases. Int J Immunopathol Pharmacol. 2011;24:129–32.

51. Jacofsky DJ, Haidukewych JH. Management of pathologic fractures of the proximal femur state of the art. J Orthop Trauma. 2004;18:459–69.

52. Capanna R, Scoccianti G, Campanacci DA, et al. Surgical technique: extraarticular knee resection with prosthesis-proximal tibia-extensor apparatus allograft for tumors invading the knee. Clin Orthop Relat Res. 2011;469:2905–14.

53. Harvey N, Ahlmann ER, Allison DC, et al. Endoprostheses last longer than intramedullary devices in proximal femur metastases. Clin Orthop Rel Res. 2012;470:684–91.

54. Steensma M, Boland PJ, Morris CD, et al. Endoprosthetic treatment is more durable for pathologic proximal femur fractures. Clin Orthop Relat Res. 2012;470:920–6.

55. Lackman RD, Hosalkar HS, Ogilvie CM, et al. Intralesional curettage for graves II and III Giant cell tumors of bone. Clin Orthop. 2005;438:123–7.

56. Quint U, Muller RT, Muller G. Characteristics of phenol. Arch Orthop Trauma Surg. 1998;117:43–6.

57. Gage AA, Baust JG. Mechanisms of tissue injury in cryosurgery. Cryobiology. 1998;37:171–86.

58. Marcove RC, Lyden JP, Huvos AG, et al. Giant cell tumors treated by cryosurgery. A report of twenty-five cases. J Bone Joint Surg Am. 1973;55A:1633.

59. Baust JG, Gage AA. The molecular basis of cryosurgery. BJU Int. 2005;95:1187–91.

60. Robinson D, Halperin N, Nevo Z. Two freezing cycles ensure interface sterilization by cryosurgery during bone tumor resection. Cryobiology. 2001;43:4–10.

61. Dijkstra S, Wiggers T, Van Geel BN, et al. Impending and actual pathological fractures in patients with bone metastases of the long bones—a retrospective study of 233 surgically treated fractures. Eur J Surg. 1994;160:535–42.

62. Capanna R, De Biase P, Sensi L. Minimally invasive techniques for treatment of metastatic cancer. Orthopade. 2009;38:343–7.

63. Carrafiello G, Laganà D, Pellegrino C, et al. Ablation of painful metastatic bone tumors: a systematic review. Int J Surg. 2008;6:S47–52.

64. Choi J, Raghavan M. Diagnostic imaging and image-guided therapy of skeletal metastases. Cancer Control. 2012;19:10212.

65. Callstrom MR, Charboneau JW, Goetz MP, et al. Image-guided ablation of painful metastatic bone tumors: a new and effective approach to a difficult problem. Skelet Radiol. 2006;35:1–15.

66. Lee JH, Stein M, Roychowdhury S. Percutaneous treatment of a sacral metastasis with combined embolization, cryoablation, alcohol ablation and sacroplasty for local tumor and pain control. Interv Neuroradiol. 2013;19:250–3.

67. Capanna R. A new system for classification and treatment of long bone metastases. In: Instructional course lecture – EFORT, 1998.

68. Piccioli A, Campanacci DA, Daolio P, et al. Linee Guida SIOT. Gruppo di Studio SIOT sulle metastasi ossee. Trattamento delle metastasi ossee nello scheletro appendicolare. GIOT. 2014;40:1–15.

69. Gruppo di Studio SIOT sulle Metastasi Ossee. Linee Guida SIOT. Il trattamento dell metastasi ossee. 2008.

70. Attar S, Steffner RJ, Avedian R, et al. Surgical intervention of nonvertebral osseous metastasis. Cancer Control. 2012;19:113–21.

71. Theriault RL, Theriault RL. Biology of bone metastases. Cancer Control. 2012;19:92101.

72. Zou X, Zou L, He Y, et al. Molecular treatment strategies and surgical reconstruction for metastatic bone diseases. Cancer Treat Rev. 2008;34:527–38.

73. Eastley N, Newey M, Ashford RU. Skeletal metastases and the role of the orthopaedic and spinal surgeon. Surg Oncol. 2012;21:216–22.

74. Malvija A, Gerrand C. Evidence for orthopaedic surgery in the treatment of metastatic bone disease of the extremities. A review article. Palliat Med. 2012;26:788–96.

75. Yu HM, Tsai Y, Hoffe SE. Overview of diagnosis and management of metastatic disease to bone. Cancer Control. 2012;19:84–91.

76. Capanna R, De Biase P, Campanacci DA. A new protocol of surgical treatment of long bone metastases. Ortop Traumatol Rehabil. 2003;5:271–5.

77. Ibrahim T, Flamini E, Fabbri L, et al. Multidisciplinary approach to the treatment of bone metastases: osteo-oncology center, a new organizational model. Tumori. 2009;95:291–7.

Metastases to the Pelvis: Algorithm of Treatment

10

Andrea Angelini, Giulia Trovarelli,
and Pietro Ruggieri

Abstract

Introduction. Patients with pelvic bone metastasis present a wide range of symptoms, and therapeutic strategies should be individualized in order to obtain the best possible quality of life despite the advanced stage of disease. A multidisciplinary approach among the oncologist, radiation therapist, and orthopedic surgeon is mandatory. The goals of treatment in these patients are pain control, maintenance of independence and prevention of tumor progression, and improvement of the quality of remaining life. We propose a treatment algorithm for patients with bone metastasis in the pelvis. This algorithm aims to simplify the choices of the team from diagnosis to treatment and to avoid under- or overtreatment of pelvic bone metastases.

Material and Methods. We conducted a comprehensive review of the literature for clinical studies that reported diagnosis, modalities of treatment, pain relief and function outcomes, as well as perioperative complications and mortality, in patients with bone metastasis to the pelvis and/or acetabulum. Multiple databases from the experienced centers involved were searched up to June 2016. Data have been analyzed in order to prepare an algorithm of treatment based simply on questions with yes/no answers, from diagnosis to follow-up.

Results. The algorithm consists of 11 questions that guide physicians since the discovery of a pelvic bone lesion. Treatments are reported in squares and included biopsy, nonsurgical treatment group, radiotherapy, minimally invasive palliative procedures (MIPPs), noninvasive MR-guided FUS (focused ultrasound), surgery, and embolization. In acetabular involvement, the amount of the periacetabular bone loss was classified according to Harrington classification (ranging from groups I to IV) and metastatic acetabular classification (MAC, ranging from types 1 to 4).

Conclusion. The treatment of cancer patients with bone metastases is multidisciplinary. Currently, modern treatments are available for the palliative management of patients with metastatic bone disease. These include modern radiation therapy, chemotherapy, embolization, electrochemotherapy, radiofrequency ablation, MIPPs, and MR-guided FUS. Special attention should be directed to osteolytic lesions in the periacetabular region, as they can provoke pathologic fractures and subsequent functional impairment. Different reconstruction techniques for the pelvis are available; the choice depends on the patient's prognosis, size of the bone defect,

A. Angelini · G. Trovarelli · P. Ruggieri (✉)
Department of Orthopaedics and Orthopedic
Oncology, University of Padova, Padova, Italy
e-mail: pietro.ruggieri@unipd.it

and response of the tumor to adjuvant treatment. If all the conservative treatments are exhausted and the patient is not eligible for surgery, one of the various MIPPs can be considered.

Keywords

Pelvis · Palliative treatments · Pain · Cancer Flowchart · Metastatic disease · Surgery Multidisciplinary approach · Pathologic fracture · Bone tumors

10.1 Introduction

Primary malignant cancer can spread to distant organs forming a metastasis via the blood or lymphatic circulation. Theoretically any organ can be affected from metastases, but the lung, liver, and bone are the most frequent sites. Carcinomas with the greatest tendency to metastasize to the bone include prostate, breast, kidney, lung, and thyroid histotypes [1, 2]. In fact, these primary carcinomas account for 80% of all the metastases to the bone [2–4]. Bone metastases are associated with relevant skeletal morbidity including bone pain (usually severe), pathologic fractures, spinal cord or nerve root compression, and general symptoms such as malignant hypercalcemia [2, 5]. These events greatly compromise the quality of life of the patients. In the past decades, the life expectancy of these patients has improved considerably because of advances in diagnostic work-up, chemotherapy, immunotherapy, hormonal treatment, and radiotherapy [6]. However, this has resulted in an increased number of patients at risk of developing bone metastases or experiencing a pathologic fracture [7]. These patients demand a more reliable and stable reconstructive technique. The clinical presentation is varied between patients with bone metastases of the spine, pelvis, or long bones, but the impact on quality of life is often significant. In the archive of the Rizzoli Institute [8], 833 (18.8%) of all

4431 metastatic lesions registered were found to occur in the pelvis: ilium 559 cases (12.6%), ischium 80 cases (1.8%), and pubis 53 cases (1.2%).

Current treatment options for metastatic bone disease of the pelvis are usually performed without a curative purpose but are often palliative in nature. The therapeutic approach is based on a combination of local and systemic treatments. Chemotherapy, medical treatments (including bisphosphonates), radiotherapy, surgery, and minimally invasive palliative procedures are included in the armamentarium [2, 5, 9–11]. In this contest, it is important to define which patients need a surgical treatment, with which technique, the reconstruction modality, and the correct timing. Most of the techniques can help alleviate pain and control tumor growth, but sometimes surgical interventions help to achieve an adequate pain control by preventing or stabilizing pathologic fractures. In selected cases, a complete resection with adequate margins may improve the survival rate of the patients [10, 12].

To our knowledge, there are no universally accepted treatment algorithms for pelvic bone metastasis, even if the topic is highly debated in the recent literature [10, 13, 14]. Patients with bone metastases are treated today by a multidisciplinary team (composed of orthopedic surgeons, oncologists, radiologists, radiotherapists, etc.) without guidelines that consider a possible surgical treatment. In the present study we report a treatment algorithm for patients with pelvic metastasis, easily accessible for all specialists involved in the teamwork, in order to guide the therapeutic approach and to define the surgical indications.

10.2 Actual Guidelines in the Treatment of Pelvic Metastases

In 2001, Capanna and Campanacci [15] analyzed metastatic disease of the long bones, dividing the patients into four classes: (1) solitary lesion with good prognosis, (2) pathologic fracture, (3) impending fracture, and (4) other lesions not otherwise classified. This classification has been used as an algorithm of treatment of patients with long bone metastases and is based on a multidisciplinary approach. Important parameters such as expected survival, oncologic histotype, stage, presence of visceral metastases, and sensitivity to radio-/chemotherapy are considered. The same classification has been adapted in 2015 for metastatic disease of the pelvis [10]: class 1, solitary lesion of a primary tumor with a good prognosis (papillary or follicular thyroid, renal and hormone-sensitive breast carcinomas) or with an interval of more than 3 years from the diagnosis to the development of bone metastasis; class 2, pathologic fracture of the periacetabular area; class 3, periacetabular osteolytic lesions; and class 4, multiple osteoblastic diffuse lesions, osteolytic or mixed lesions in the ilium or ischiopubis branches, or small osteolytic periacetabular lesions. The authors [10] analyzed the surgical and nonsurgical indications based on the combination of three data: prognostic class (classes 1–4), anatomic area involved using Enneking classification (zones 1–4, Fig. 10.1) [16], and periacetabular bone loss. Periacetabular bone destruction was analyzed according to the Harrington classification [17]: minimal involvement of the acetabulum in subchondral bone (group I); the medial wall of the acetabulum is destroyed, but the roof and the lateral wall are still preserved (group II); extensive osteolysis affects not only the medial wall but also the roof

and the lateral rim of the acetabulum (group III); and complete acetabular collapse (group IV).

10.3 Algorithm of Treatment

The algorithm (Fig. 10.2) has been realized as a flowchart with positive/negative consecutive questions based on the principal prognostic factors on metastatic disease: (1) biologic characteristics such as life expectancy (histotype of primary tumor), extension of the disease (solitary or multiple lesions), general patient's health (performance status), and free interval of disease from excision of primary tumor, (2) biomechanic characteristics as pathologic or impending fracture (site and volume of the lesion, lytic or osteoblastic lesion), and (3) sensitivity to nonsurgical therapies (chemotherapy, radiation therapy, hormonotherapy, etc.).

The algorithm starts from the discovery of a bone lesion localized in the pelvis. The lesion should be initially evaluated on a standard AP pelvic radiograph to determine the extent of tumor involvement. Radiographs are useful for surgical planning and are helpful to evaluate the integrity of anterior and posterior columns, the roof and quadrilateral lamina of the acetabular area. The entire femur should also be imaged to identify additional disease. CT scan of the pelvis and acetabular area is useful in assessing the degree of bony destruction, the consistency of the tumor (osteolytic, osteoblastic, or mixed), and the quality of the bone for fixation of further eventual reconstruction [18, 19]. Pelvic MRI is useful to determine the soft tissue extension of permeative lesions [20]. A complete staging with total-body CT scan and bone scan or FDG-PET-CT can help to determine the exact extension of the disease [21].

10.3.1 Solitary Lesion?

The rationale of the first question should be found in the fact that a patient with a metastatic lesion of the pelvis usually presents multiple bone lesions [2, 22, 23]. If the patient has multiple

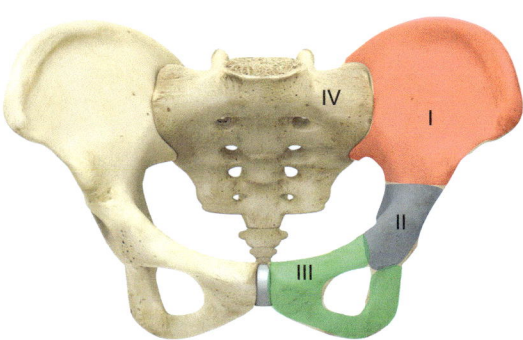

Fig. 10.1 Anatomic areas of the pelvis according to Enneking classification [16]: the iliac wing (zone 1), the periacetabular area (zone 2), anterior branches (zone 3), and the sacrum (zone 4)

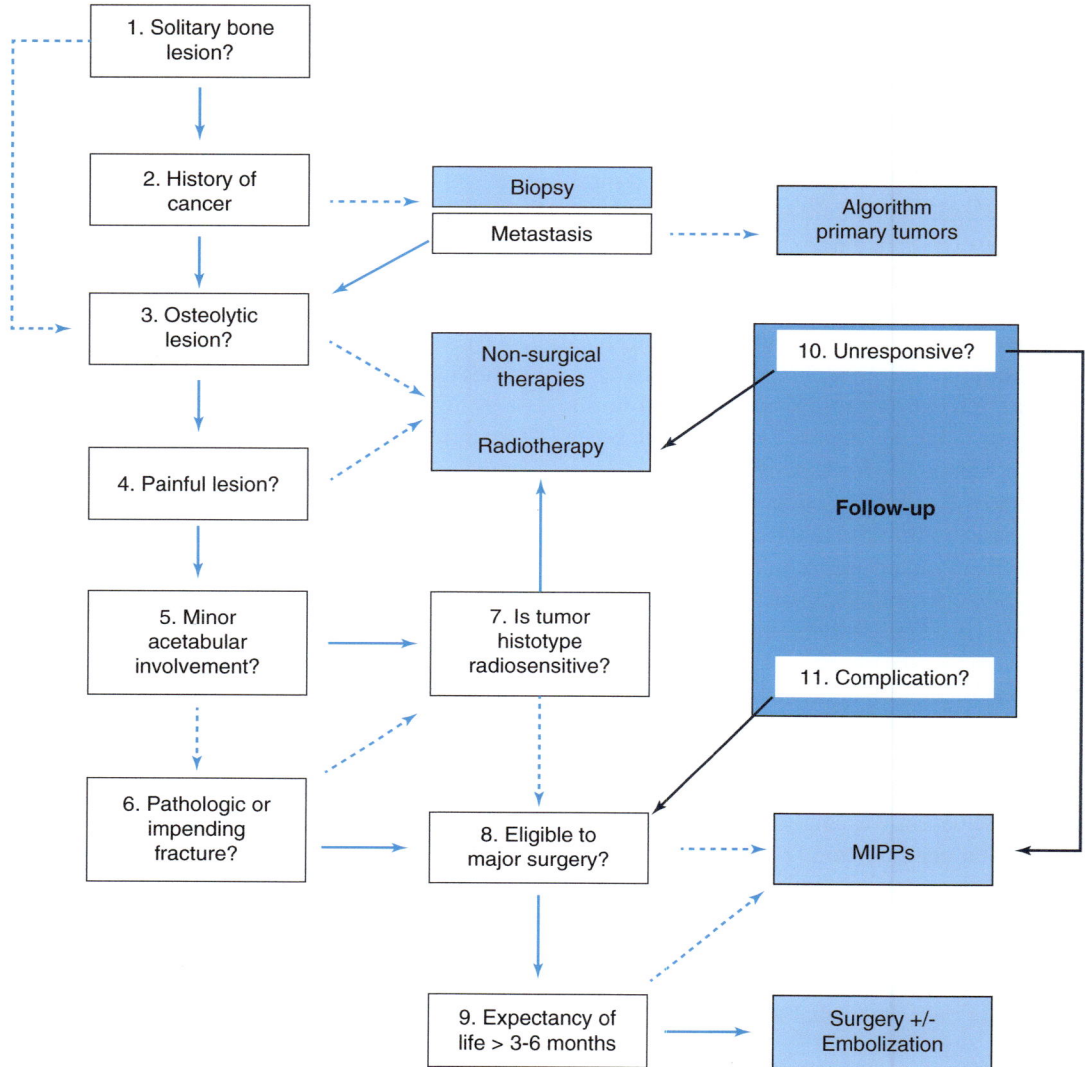

Fig. 10.2 Algorithm of treatment for metastatic lesion of the pelvis. Arrows with solid line indicate affirmative answer, whereas those with dashed line indicate negative answer

bone lesions, the algorithm guides the therapeutic strategy toward nonsurgical treatments, except for osteolytic painful lesions or unresponsive to nonsurgical therapies [24, 25]. The discovery of metastatic periacetabular solitary lesion in a patient with negative oncologic history is reported as the primary symptom in only 5% of the cases [23]. In this case, the possible differential diagnosis with primary bone tumors should be considered.

10.3.2 History of Cancer?

In a patient with a history of cancer, the probability that a solitary acetabular lesion could be a metastasis is high [26], and sometimes a biopsy is not required before treatment. It has been reported that the probability for a solitary acetabular lesion to be a metastatic lesion in patients aged >40 years is high, even in the absence of a history of cancer [27]. Biopsy should always be performed to confirm that the solitary acetabular lesion is a metastatic tumor in patients with a negative history of cancer [26, 28]. If the histologic examination reveals a primary bone tumor, the patient should be referred to the relative algorithm of treatment. In case of solitary lesion diagnosed as metastasis from a primary tumor with a good prognosis (thyroid, prostate, breast, clear cell renal, or colorectal carcinoma) or a disease-free interval of more than 3 years from the detection of the primary tumor to the development of bone metastasis, the patient should be considered for surgical treatment [10, 15].

10.3.3 Osteolytic Lesion?

Bone remodeling is a physiologic phenomenon that involves the interaction between different cell types, including osteoclasts and osteoblasts, and an array of cytokines and hormones. During the normal bone remodeling, there is a dynamic equilibrium between osteoclast-mediated bone resorption and osteoblast-mediated bone formation [29]. Both types of cells could be activated in bone metastases, causing osteolytic, osteoblastic, or mixed lesions [30, 31]. There is a key role of interaction between RANK receptor and RANK-ligand in osteoclast activation, and this fact is one of the reasons of osteolytic aspects of most carcinomas. Moreover, expression of RANK has been detected in a large percentage of bone metastases deriving from several histotypes including the breast and prostate [32]. It has been described that the RANK expression status of cancer cells directs tumor migration to bone, where the RANK-ligand is abundantly expressed [33].

In the presence of osteoblastic lesions (commonly observed in breast and prostate carcinomas), the gold standard of treatment is nonsurgical and includes chemotherapy, narcotic analgesics, radiation therapy, and often hormonal therapy. Bisphosphonates are an important advance in supportive care of patients with bone metastases. They inhibit normal and pathologic osteoclast-mediated bone resorption by direct inhibition of cellular mechanisms such as osteoclast attach-

ment, differentiation, and survival [5, 34]. In a recent meta-analysis including nine randomized controlled trials (2806 patients with bone metastases from breast cancer), it has been observed that intravenous zoledronic acid 4 mg and intravenous pamidronate 90 mg reduced the risk of skeletal-related events by 15% [35]. In the presence of an osteolytic lesion, we suggest to move to the following question.

10.3.4 Painful Lesion?

About 90% of patients with advanced cancer or metastatic disease can have a significant pain cancer-related. Pain related to bone is a common and debilitating symptom in half or more of the patients with a diagnosis of malignant tumor [22]. Pain is usually severe, progressive, and caused by different pathogenic mechanisms; therefore, a multimodal analgesic strategy should include systemic pharmacological approach (NSAIDS, opioid and adjuvant drugs), supplemented on demand with additional multidisciplinary forms of treatment. Whereas the treatment of asymptomatic multiple osteolytic lesions is substantially the same of that for bone-forming lesions, the strategy of treatment of painful lesions is different. Most of the palliative treatments for metastatic bone disease used to treat cancer-related pain may be used also to improve quality of life and maintenance of independence, to reduce skeletal morbidity, and to prevent (or treat) pathologic fracture, spinal cord compression, and other "skeletal-related events." Treatments for pain control include systemic analgesics, intrathecal analgesics, radiation (external beam radiation, radiopharmaceuticals), glucocorticoids, mini-invasive ablative techniques, bisphosphonates, inhibitors of RANK-RANKL interaction, chemotherapeutic agents, hormonal therapies, interventional techniques, and surgery [22]. Approximately 85–90% of patients with advanced disease may control cancer-related pain with oral analgesic drugs [36, 37]. In the case of refractory pain despite an adequate analgesic therapy, we suggest to move to the following question.

10.3.5 Minor Acetabular Involvement?

Metastatic lesions affect the strength of bone improving the risk of pathologic fracture, especially in osteolytic patterns. Highly stressed anatomical sites such as periacetabular area are particularly predisposed to pathologic fractures. The amount of acetabular involvement dictates the type of surgical treatment and reconstruction. There are two good tools to evaluate the acetabular destruction: the Harrington classification [17], ranging from groups I to IV, and the "metastatic acetabular classification" (MAC), ranging from types 1 to 4 [26]. The MAC classifications describes lesion involvement of the acetabular dome (type 1), of the medial wall (type 2), of a single posterior or anterior column (type 3), and of the two columns (type 4). For both classifications, when the acetabular destruction is minor (Harrington I or MAC 1), the patients should be guided to chemo-/radiotherapy, or it may be managed by curettage, cementation of the lesion, followed by total hip arthroplasty with conventional cemented components. In the case of major acetabular destruction, we should move to the next question.

10.3.6 Is There a Pathologic or Impending Fracture?

The evaluation of risk of occurrence of a pathologic fracture depends on the imaging appearance of the lesion and the site. Osteolytic lesions are at higher risk of fracture compared to osteoblastic or mixed lesions, as well as lesions with permeative pattern despite the reassuring radiographic aspect. In the presence of pathologic or impending fracture, the patient should be considered a candidate for surgical stabilization because of the low potential of fracture healing itself [5, 15, 38]. Even when healing is possible, it is often delayed [39].

10.3.7 Is Tumor Histotype Radiosensitive?

Radiation therapy is effective in providing pain relief correlate to bone metastases, up to a complete resolution of symptoms in about 20–50% of the treated patients [40–43]. Radiotherapy is therefore considered the standard of care in terms of palliation for patients with localized bone pain. It is indicated for radiosensitive tumors with a low risk of pathologic fracture, even if it may be used for any metastatic bone lesion (even less radiosensitive such as thyroid, prostatic, or renal carcinomas), to minimize the need of a surgical treatment [26, 44, 45]. Commonly used radiation therapy schemes include 8 Gy in a single fraction, 20 Gy in 5 fractions, and 30 Gy in 10 fractions [42, 46, 47].

10.3.8 Is the Patient Eligible to Major Surgery?

Summarizing, surgery is indicated in large, osteolytic, painful, periacetabular lesions with pathologic/impending fractures, in patients unresponsive (inadequate pain relief and limited quality of life) to conservative treatments. Criteria for successful procedure include proper patient's selection with precise clinical exam of eligible patients and careful evaluation of the general health status.

10.3.9 Expectancy of Life >3–6 Months?

The surgical treatment of pelvic metastases is often dictated by the systemic burden and life expectancy. The surgical indication should be discussed in a multidisciplinary team coordinated by the oncologist, balancing the quod vitam prognosis and surgical risks. Most of the studies in literature advocate a life expectancy greater than 3–6 months as a cutoff for surgical intervention due to the long rehabilitation and high incidence of early complications [10, 15, 26, 48–50]. For patients with poor prognosis, treatments such as MIPPs should be considered.

10.3.9.1 Surgical and Mini-invasive Treatments

Nowadays, the indication to major surgical procedures in patients with metastatic disease of the pelvis is increasing, even if in selected cases. Lesions eligible to surgery are:

1. Lesions located in periacetabular area (zone 2 according to Enneking [16]) characterized by functional inability and pain refractory to pharmacological therapy, protected weight bearing, and radiotherapy
2. Periacetabular lesions with pathological or impending fractures
3. Lesions that involve the highly stressed anatomical sites in the pelvis, affecting the pelvic girdle
4. Solitary lesions in class 1 according to Muller and Capanna [10] or solitary lesions from primary tumor with good prognosis [3, 13, 17, 51–56]

Surgical options include resection with/without reconstruction, intralesional curettage associated with local adjuvants (phenol and/or cement and/or cryotherapy), and filling of the defect. Internal fixation or prosthetic reconstruction may be used [3, 13, 17, 53, 55, 56]. In patients with a solitary metastatic lesion, a survival benefit of en bloc resection has been reported [57]. Considering the complex anatomy of the pelvis, surgical excision is usually preferred to resection techniques when it is difficult to achieve wide margins at the preoperative planning [13]. Preoperative angiography with selective embolization provides devascularization, size reduction, and pain relief [58–60] and reduces intraoperative blood loss, needs of transfusions, and surgical time [35, 61, 62]. Since all metastatic bone lesions are hypervascular [58, 60], all the patients may be indicated for embolization. In our experience [61, 63–65], a selective arterial embolization of feeding vessels is always suggested in the case of hypervascular lesions (such as clear cell renal carcinoma or thyroid carcinoma) and in the presence of large extraosseous lesions. The main limitation is represented by the renal toxicity in high-risk patients with poor kidney compensation and a vascularization of the lesion conjunct to relevant non-targeted vessel [61, 65].

In the presence of minimal acetabular bone loss (Harrington I or MAC 1), a simple curettage of the lesion may be performed with cement filling. This procedure may be sufficient for local control of the disease and may be carried out percutaneously [66, 67]. In other cases, a conventional total hip replacement with cemented components may be performed. In the presence of extensive acetabular osteolysis (Harrington II/III or MAC 2/3), the reconstruction typically involves the use of implants or internal fixation devices that extend to uninvolved portions of the pelvis [3, 68, 69]. Harrington described a technique with large threaded pins placed through the remaining hemipelvis, to support the cementation of acetabular lesions [70]. In other cases, more challenging reconstructive procedures should be performed, using flanged cups or cages [17, 71, 72], cemented acetabular components with total retention or dual-mobility cups [48], modular prostheses [16, 54], massive allograft-prosthesis composite [14, 68], saddle prosthesis (rarely used nowadays) [3, 52], or iliofemoral coarctation [73].

Nowadays, a wide range of minimally invasive palliative procedures (MIPPs) are available for patients with advanced cancer not eligible for open surgery [5, 74]. In literature, described procedures are [5, 75–82] radiofrequency ablation (RFA) with/without cementoplasty, microwave ablation (MWA) with/without cementoplasty, percutaneous cementoplasty, local application of ethanol, laser-induced interstitial thermotherapy (LITT), cryoablation, electrochemotherapy (ECT), and electroporation. Each procedure presents specific indications and limitations; therefore, the use should be customized to the patient [74]. Recently, a noninvasive technique named "magnetic resonance-guided focused ultrasound" (MRgFUS) is available for selected patients with painful metastatic bone disease [83–85].

10.3.10 Is Patient Unresponsive to Therapies?

In some cases, a progressive increase of number/volume of bone lesions occurs despite surgical and nonsurgical therapies, whereas other patients report inadequate pain palliation. Palliative radiation therapy can be administered (if it has not been used before), whereas previously irradiated patients could be treated only if the administered dose was lower for dose-limiting organs. MIPPs should be considered as alternative treatments.

10.3.11 Is This a Complication of Previous Treatment?

The therapeutic procedures of pelvic metastases are technically demanding and require a thorough knowledge of the pelvic anatomy and proximity of vital structures to minimize complications. Wood et al. [9] recently published a systematic review on the surgical management of bone metastases, finding that the complication rate following acetabular/pelvis replacement surgery for metastatic bone disease was 19.5%. However, in reality, complication rates may be higher considering all the MIPPs and nonsurgical treatments (mainly radiation therapy) applied to this patient population. In our experience and for the purpose of the algorithm, all patients admitted to a surgical ward for complications should be reevaluated as eligible for major surgical treatments.

Conclusions

The treatment of cancer patients with bone metastases is multidisciplinary, and pelvic involvement is a growing concern in the field of orthopedic surgery. Currently, modern treatments are available for the palliative management of patients with metastatic bone disease. These include modern radiation therapy, chemotherapy, embolization, electrochemotherapy, radiofrequency ablation, MIPPs, and MR-guided FUS. Special attention should be directed to the osteolytic lesions in the periacetabular region, as these can lead to pathologic fractures and subsequent functional impairment. Different reconstruction techniques for the pelvis are available; the choice depends on the patient's prognosis, size of the bone defect, and response of the tumor to adjuvant treatment. If all the conservative treatments are exhausted and the patient is not eligible for surgery, one of the various MIPPs should be considered. This algorithm has been realized to simplify the choices of the multidisciplinary team from diagnosis to treatment and to avoid under- or overtreatments of patients affected by pelvic bone metastases.

Conflict-of-Interest Statement No benefits have been or will be received from a commercial party related directed or indirectly to the subject matter of this article.

References

1. Weinstein RS, Pauli BU. Cell junctions and the biological behaviour of cancer. Ciba Found Symp. 1987;125:240–60.
2. Coleman RE. Metastatic bone disease: clinical features, pathophysiology and treatment strategies. Cancer Treat Rev. 2001;27(3):165–76.
3. Aboulafia AJ, Levine AM, Schmidt D, Aboulafia D. Surgical therapy of bone metastases. Semin Oncol. 2007;34(3):206–14. Review.
4. Bauer HC. Controversies in the surgical management of skeletal metastases. J Bone Joint Surg Br. 2005;87(5):608–17.
5. Mavrogenis AF, Angelini A, Vottis C, Pala E, Calabrò T, Papagelopoulos PJ, Ruggieri P. Modern palliative treatments for metastatic bone disease: awareness of advantages, disadvantages, and guidance. Clin J Pain. 2016;32(4):337–50.
6. Hage WD, Aboulafia AJ, Aboulafia DM. Incidence, location, and diagnostic evaluation of metastatic bone disease. Orthop Clin N Am. 2000;31(4):515–28.
7. Li S, Peng Y, Weinhandl ED, et al. Estimated number of prevalent cases of metastatic bone disease in the US adult population. Clin Epidemiol. 2012;4(1):87–93.
8. Picci P, Manfrini M, Fabbri N, Gambarotti M, Vanel D. Atlas of musculoskeletal tumors and tumorlike lesions. Berlin: Springer; 2014.
9. Wood SL, Pernemalm M, Crosbie PA, Whetton AD. The role of the tumor-microenvironment in lung cancer-metastasis and its relationship to potential therapeutic targets. Cancer Treat Rev. 2014;40(4):558–66.
10. Muller DA, Capanna R. The surgical treatment of pelvic bone metastases. Adv Orthop. 2015;2015:525363.
11. Nathan SS, Chan L, Tan WL, Tan I, Go M, Chuah B, et al. The need for a system of prognostication in skeletal metastasis to decide best end-of-life care: a call to arms. Ann Acad Med Singap. 2010;39(6):476–81.
12. Wedin R. Surgical treatment for pathologic fracture. Acta Orthop Scand. 2001;72(302):21–9.
13. Enneking WF. Metastatic carcinoma (418 cases). In: Enneking WF, editor. Musculoskeletal tumor surgery. New York: Churchill Livingstone; 1983.
14. Angelini A, Calabrò T, Pala E, Trovarelli G, Maraldi M, Ruggieri P. Resection and reconstruction of pelvic bone tumors. Orthopedics. 2015;38(2):87–93.
15. Capanna R, Campanacci DA. The treatment of metastasis in appendicular skeleton. J Bone Joint Surg Br. 2001;83(4):471–81.
16. Enneking WF, Dunham WK. Resection and reconstruction for primary neoplasms involving the innominate bone. J Bone Joint Surg. 1978;60A:734–46.

17. Harrington KD. The management of acetabular insufficiency secondary to metastatic malignant disease. J Bone Joint Surg Am. 1981;4:653–64.
18. Cimerman M, Kristan A. Preoperative planning in pelvic and acetabular surgery: the value of advanced computerised planning modules. Injury. 2007;38(4):442–9.
19. Hsieh MS, Tsai MD, Yeh YD. Three-dimensional hip morphology analysis using CT transverse sections to automate diagnoses and surgery managements. Comput Biol Med. 2005;35(4):347–71.
20. Schwab JH, Boland PJ. Metastatic disease about the hip. In: Callaghan JJ, Rosenberg AG, Rubash HE, editors. The adult hip, vol. 1. Philadelphia: Lippincott Williams and Wilkins; 2007. p. 559–71.
21. Rougraff BT, Kneisl JS, Simon MA. Skeletal metastases of unknown origin: a prospective study of a diagnostic strategy. J Bone Joint Surg Am. 1993;75(9):1276–81.
22. Smith HS. Painful osseous metastases. Pain Physician. 2011;14(4):E373–403.
23. Böhm P, Huber J. The surgical treatment of bony metastases of the spine and limbs. J Bone Joint Surg Br. 2002;84(4):521–9.
24. Rechl H, Mittelmeier W, Plotz W, Gradinger R. Surgical management of pelvic metastases. Orthopade. 1998;27:287–93.
25. Rhodes ML, Yu Ming K, RSLG. An application of computer graphics and networks to anatomic model and prosthesis manufacturing. IEEE CG&A. 1987;7:12–25.
26. Issack PS, Kotwal SY, Lane JM. Management of metastatic bone disease of the acetabulum. J Am Acad Orthop Surg. 2013;21(11):685–95.
27. Weber KL. Evaluation of the adult patient (aged >40 years) with a destructive bone lesion. J Am Acad Orthop Surg. 2010;18(3):169–79.
28. Mavrogenis AF, Angelini A, Errani C, Rimondi E. How should musculoskeletal biopsies be performed? Orthopedics. 2014;37(9):585–8.
29. Bussard KM, Gay CV, Mastro AM. The bone microenvironment in metastasis: what is special about bone? Cancer Metastasis Rev. 2008;27:41–55.
30. Yoneda T, Sasaki A, Mundy GR. Osteolytic bone metastasis in breast cancer. Breast Cancer Res Treat. 1994;32:73–84.
31. Papachristou DJ, Basdra EK, Papavassiliou AG. Bone metastases: molecular mechanisms and novel therapeutic interventions. Med Res Rev. 2012;32(3):611–36.
32. Santini D, Perrone G, Roato I, et al. Expression pattern of receptor activator of NFjB (RANK) in a series of primary solid tumors and related bone metastases. J Cell Physiol. 2011;226:780–4.
33. Jones DH, Nakashima T, Sanchez OH, et al. Regulation of cancer cell migration and bone metastasis by RANKL. Nature. 2006;440:692–6.
34. Hultborn R, Gundersen S, Ryden S, Holmberg E, Carstensen J, Wallgren UB, Killany S, Andreassen L, Carlsson G, Fahl N, Hatschek T, Sommer HH, Hessman Y, Hornmark-Stenstam B, Johnsborg S, Klepp R, Laino R, Niklasson LG, Rudenstam CM, Sundbeck A, Söderberg M, Tejler G. Efficacy of pamidronate in breast cancer with bone metastases: a randomized, double-blind placebo-controlled multicenter study. Anticancer Res. 1999;19(4C):3383–92.
35. Wong MH, Stockler MR, Pavlakis N. Bisphosphonates and other bone agents for breast cancer. Cochrane Database Syst Rev. 2012;2:CD003474.
36. Chambers WA. Nerve blocks in palliative care. Br J Anaesth. 2008;101(1):95–100.
37. Zech DF, Grond S, Lynch J, Hertel D, Lehmann KA. Validation of World Health Organization Guidelines for cancer pain relief: a 10-year prospective study. Pain. 1995;63(1):65–76.
38. Bickels J, Dadia S, Lidar Z. Surgical management of metastatic bone disease. J Bone Joint Surg Am. 2009;91(6):1503–16.
39. Ruggieri P, Mavrogenis AF, Casadei R, et al. Protocol of surgical treatment of long bone pathological fractures. Injury. 2010;41:1161–7.
40. Bates T. A review of local radiotherapy in the treatment of bone metastases and cord compression. Int J Radiat Oncol Biol Phys. 1992;23(1):217–21.
41. Maher EJ. The use of palliative radiotherapy in the management of breast cancer. Eur J Cancer. 1992;28(2–3):706–10.
42. Culleton S, Kwok S, Chow E. Radiotherapy for pain. Clin Oncol. 2010;23:399–406.
43. Sze WM, Shelley M, Held I, et al. Palliation of metastatic bone pain: single fraction versus multifraction radiotherapy—a systemic review of randomized trials. Clin Oncol. 2003;15:345–52.
44. Coleman RE. Clinical features of metastatic bone disease and risk of skeletal morbidity. Clin Cancer Res. 2006;12(20 Pt 2):6243s–9s. Review.
45. Selvaggi G, Scagliotti GV. Management of bone metastases in cancer: a review. Crit Rev Oncol Hematol. 2005;56(3):365–78.
46. Ben-Josef E, Shamsa F, Williams AO, Porter AT. Radiotherapeutic management of osseous metastases: a survey of current patterns of care. Int J Radiat Oncol Biol Phys. 1998;40(4):915–21.
47. Hartsell WF, Scott CB, Bruner DW, Scarantino CW, Ivker RA, Roach M 3rd, Suh JH, Demas WF, Movsas B, Petersen IA, Konski AA, Cleeland CS, Janjan NA, DeSilvio M. Randomized trial of short- versus long-course radiotherapy for palliation of painful bone metastases. J Natl Cancer Inst. 2005;97(11):798–804.
48. Brown HK, Healey JH. Pathologic pelvis fractures and acetabular reconstruction in metastatic disease. In: Tile M, Helfet DL, Kellam JF, editors. Fractures of the pelvis and acetabulum. Philadelphia: Lippincott Williams and Wilkins; 2003. p. 795–806.
49. Jacofsky DJ, Papagelopoulos PJ, Sim FH. Advances and challenges in the surgical treatment of metastatic bone disease. Clin Orthop Relat Res. 2003;415(Suppl):S14–8.
50. Marco RA, Sheth DS, Boland PJ, Wunder JS, Siegel JA, Healey JH. Functional and oncological

outcome of acetabular reconstruction for the treatment of metastatic disease. J Bone Joint Surg Am. 2000;82(5):642–51.

51. Healey JH, Brown HK. Complications of bone metastases: surgical management. Cancer. 2000;88:2940–51.

52. Lackman RD, Torbert JT, Hosalkar HS, et al. Treatment of metastases to the extremities and pelvis. Oper Tech Orthop. 2005;14:288–95.

53. Ogilvie CM, Fox EJ, Lackman RD. Current surgical management of bone metastases in the extremities and pelvis. Semin Oncol. 2008;35:118–28.

54. Ruggieri P, Mavrogenis AF, Angelini A, Mercuri M. Metastases of the pelvis: does resection improve survival? Orthopedics. 2011;34(7):e236–44.

55. Satcher RL Jr, O'Donnell RJ, Johnston JO. Reconstruction of the pelvis after resection of tumors about the acetabulum. Clin Orthop. 2003;409:209–17.

56. Vena V, Hsu J, Rosier RN, O'Keefe RJ. Pelvic reconstruction for severe periacetabular metastatic disease. Clin Orthop. 1999;362:171–80.

57. Giurea A, Ritschl P, Windhager R, Kaider A, Helwig U, Kotz R. The benefits of surgery in the treatment of pelvic metastases. Int Orthop. 1997;21(5):343–8.

58. Forauer AR, Kent E, Cwikiel WH, et al. Selective palliative transcatheter embolization of bony metastases from renal cell carcinoma. Acta Oncol. 2007;46:1012–8.

59. Barton PP, Waneck RE, Karnel FJ, et al. Embolization of bone metastases. J Vasc Interv Radiol. 1996;7:81–8.

60. Hansch A, Neumann R, Pfeil A, et al. Embolization of an unusual metastatic site of hepatocellular carcinoma in the humerus. World J Gastroenterol. 2009;15:2280–2.

61. Rossi G, Mavrogenis AF, Casadei R, Bianchi G, Romagnoli C, Rimondi E, Ruggieri P. Embolisation of bone metastases from renal cancer. Radiol Med. 2013;118(2):291–302.

62. Sun S, Lang EV. Bone metastases from renal cell carcinoma: preoperative embolization. J Vasc Interv Radiol. 1998;9(2):263–9.

63. Facchini G, Di Tullio P, Battaglia M, Bartalena T, Tetta C, Errani C, Mavrogenis AF, Rossi G. Palliative embolization for metastases of the spine. Eur J Orthop Surg Traumatol. 2016;26(3):247–52.

64. Mavrogenis AF, Rossi G, Rimondi E, Papagelopoulos PJ, Ruggieri P. Embolization of bone tumors. Orthopedics. 2011;34(4):303–10.

65. Rossi G, Mavrogenis AF, Rimondi E, Braccaioli L, Calabrò T, Ruggieri P. Selective embolization with N-butyl cyanoacrylate for metastatic bone disease. J Vasc Interv Radiol. 2011;22(4):462–70.

66. Harty JA, Brennan D, Eustace S, O'Byrne J. Percutaneous cementoplasty of acetabular bony metastasis. Surgeon. 2003;1(1):48–50.

67. Scaramuzzo L, Maccauro G, Rossi B, Messuti L, Maffulli N, Logroscino CA. Quality of life in patients following percutaneous PMMA acetabuloplasty for acetabular metastasis due to carcinoma. Acta Orthop Belg. 2009;75:484–9.

68. Delloye C, Banse X, Brichard B, et al. Pelvic reconstruction with a structural pelvic allograft after resection of a malignant bone tumor. J Bone Joint Surg Am. 2007;89:579–87.

69. Wunder JS, Ferguson PC, Griffin AM, Pressman A, Bell RS. Acetabular metastases: planning for reconstruction and review of results. Clin Orthop Relat Res. 2003;415S:187–97.

70. Harrington KD. Orthopaedic management of extremity and pelvic lesions. Clin Orthop. 1995;312:136–47.

71. Hoell S, Dedy N, Gosheger G, Dieckmann R, Daniilidis K, Hardes J. The Burch-Schneider cage for reconstruction after metastatic destruction of the acetabulum: outcome and complications. Arch Orthop Trauma Surg. 2012;132(3):405–10.

72. Levine AM, Aboulafia AJ. Pathologic fractures. In: Browner BD, Levine AM, Jupiter JB, Trafton PG, Krettek C, editors. Skeletal trauma: basic science, management, and reconstruction. Philadelphia: Saunders Elsevier; 2008. p. 453–512.

73. Pant R, Moreau P, Ilyas I, Paramasivan ON, Younge D. Pelvic limb-salvage surgery for malignant tumors. Int Orthop. 2001;24:311–5.

74. Cascella M, Muzio MR, Viscardi D, Cuomo A. Features and role of minimally invasive palliative procedures for pain management in malignant pelvic diseases: a review. Am J Hosp Palliat Care. 2017;34:524–31.

75. Carrafiello G, Laganà D, Mangini M, Fontana F, Dionigi G, Boni L, Rovera F, Cuffari S, Fugazzola C. Microwave tumors ablation: principles, clinical applications and review of preliminary experiences. Int J Surg. 2008;6(Suppl 1):S65–9.

76. Castaneda Rodriguez WR, Callstrom MR. Effective pain palliation and prevention of fracture for axial-loading skeletal metastases using combined cryoablation and cementoplasty. Tech Vasc Interv Radiol. 2011;14(3):160–9.

77. Goetz MP, Callstrom MR, Charboneau JW, Farrell MA, Maus TP, Welch TJ, Wong GY, Sloan JA, Novotny PJ, Petersen IA, Beres RA, Regge D, Capanna R, Saker MB, Grönemeyer DH, Gevargez A, Ahrar K, Choti MA, de Baere TJ, Rubin J. Percutaneous image-guided radiofrequency ablation of painful metastases involving bone: a multicenter study. J Clin Oncol. 2004;22(2):300–6.

78. Hillen TJ, Anchala P, Friedman MV, Jennings JW. Treatment of metastatic posterior vertebral body osseous tumors by using a targeted bipolar radiofrequency ablation device: technical note. Radiology. 2014;273(1):261–7.

79. Lane MD, Le HB, Lee S, Young C, Heran MK, Badii M, Clarkson PW, Munk PL. Combination radiofrequency ablation and cementoplasty for palliative treatment of painful neoplastic bone metastasis: experience with 53 treated lesions in 36 patients. Skelet Radiol. 2011;40(1):25–32.

80. Pusceddu C, Sotgia B, Fele RM, Ballicu N, Melis L. Combined microwave ablation and cemento-plasty in patients with painful bone metastases at high risk of fracture. Cardiovasc Intervent Radiol. 2016;39(1):74–80.

81. Rosenthal D, Callstrom MR. Critical review and state of the art in interventional oncology: benign and metastatic disease involving bone. Radiology. 2012;262(3):765–80.

82. Toyota N, Naito A, Kakizawa H, Hieda M, Hirai N, Tachikake T, Kimura T, Fukuda H, Ito K. Radiofrequency ablation therapy combined with cementoplasty for painful bone metastases: initial experience. Cardiovasc Intervent Radiol. 2005;28(5):578–83.

83. Joo B, Park MS, Lee SH, Choi HJ, Lim ST, Rha SY, Rachmilevitch I, Lee YH, Suh JS. Pain palliation in patients with bone metastases using magnetic resonance-guided focused ultrasound with conformal bone system: a preliminary report. Yonsei Med J. 2015;56(2):503–9.

84. Liberman B, Gianfelice D, Inbar Y, Beck A, Rabin T, Shabshin N, Chander G, Hengst S, Pfeffer R, Chechick A, Hanannel A, Dogadkin O, Catane R. Pain palliation in patients with bone metastases using MR-guided focused ultrasound surgery: a multicenter study. Ann Surg Oncol. 2009;16(1):140–6. https://doi.org/10.1245/s10434-008-0011-2. Epub 2008 Nov 11.

85. Tempany CM, McDannold NJ, Hynynen K, Jolesz FA. Focused ultrasound surgery in oncology: overview and principles. Radiology. 2011;259(1):39–56.

Pathologic Versus Impending Fracture

11

Maria Silvia Spinelli and Andrea Piccioli

Abstract

The constant improvement of medical therapies has led to the longer survival of patients affected by carcinoma and a consequent increase in the number of patients with bone metastasis. In the natural history of bone metastatic patients they Skeletal Related Events (SREs) are likely to occur. SREs are: pathologic fracture of the long bones, the need of surgical procedures on the bone, spinal compression, and radiotherapy on the bone. SREs have a well-documented negative impact on clinical outcomes and on pain, reduce the quality of life and survival, and increase morbidity. The most frequent complication among SREs is the pathological fracture, which is defined as a fracture that occurs spontaneously or with a low-energy trauma in the site of a preexisting bone lesion. For the patient with bone metastasis, a pathological fracture is always a dramatic event and should be considered a matter of urgency in the orthopedic treatment of these patients. The aim of a high quality of care is to prevent a pathologic fracture; given that the bone lesions are known, these should be treated before the bone fractures with a preventive osteosynthesis. This imminent risk of fracture that may occur in daily activities is a specific diagnosis and is given the name impending fracture.

The aim of this chapter is to focus on different aspects of pathologic and impending fracture, including diagnostic and clinical aspects, the impact on survival and on health resource utilization.

Keywords

Pathologic fracture · Impending fracture · Bone metastasis · Survival estimation · Economic burden

Pathologic fracture is a dramatic event that occurs in the history of patients affected by metastatic carcinoma and is a part of the complex of events known as skeletal-related events (SREs). Healey and Brown [1] in their review published in 2000 demonstrate how SREs represent a critical moment and clearly clarify the negative impact of the fracture on the patient's quality of life. SREs are the pathologic fracture of the long bones, surgical procedures on the bone, spinal compression, and radiotherapy on the bone [2]. SREs have a well-documented negative impact on clinical outcomes and on pain, reduce the

M. S. Spinelli (✉)
Traumatology and Orthopaedic Unit,
"Fatebenefratelli - Isola Tiberina" Hospital,
Rome, Italy

A. Piccioli
General Direction of Health Program, Italian Ministry of Health, Rome, Italy

© Springer International Publishing AG, part of Springer Nature 2019
V. Denaro et al. (eds.), *Management of Bone Metastases*, https://doi.org/10.1007/978-3-319-73485-9_11

quality of life and survival, and increase morbidity [3, 4]. The constant improvement of medical therapies has led to the longer survival of patients affected by carcinoma and a consequent increase in the number of patients with bone metastasis [5–7]. The epidemiological data for the US population [8] shows an incidence of 279,679 bone metastases per year. Projecting this data on to the Italian population figure for 2010 gives an incidence of bone metastasis of 64,293 cases per year. Currently there are no certain figures for the number of metastatic patients treated surgically in Italy. The only document on the epidemiology of bone metastasis was published under the patronage of the Italian Society of Orthopaedics and Traumatology (SIOT) by the Bone Metastasis Study Group on the basis of the data of the "Muscolo-Skeletal Sarcoma Group" of Piemonte, who, extrapolating data from the clinical records of patients with a diagnosis of bone metastasis, identify 4157 patients for 2010 [9]. The total number of such patients includes both those treated

surgically, with any type of surgical procedure and any type of clinical need (13% of the total), and patients not treated surgically (87% of the total) (Figs. 11.1, 11.2, and 11.3).

These data must be considered an underestimation since they include only inpatients and not those who are treated as outpatients with radiotherapy or with any other outpatient treatment for bone metastases. However, such a low percentage of patients treated with surgery shows how the orthopedic surgeon is still only marginally involved in the treatment of patients with bone metastases and how such patients are sent to other therapies rather than being given the possibility to evaluate surgical treatments that may impact positively on their quality of life.

The pathological fracture is defined as a fracture that occurs spontaneously or with a low-energy trauma in the site of a preexisting bone lesion [9]. For the patient with bone metastasis, a pathological fracture is always a dramatic event and should be considered a matter

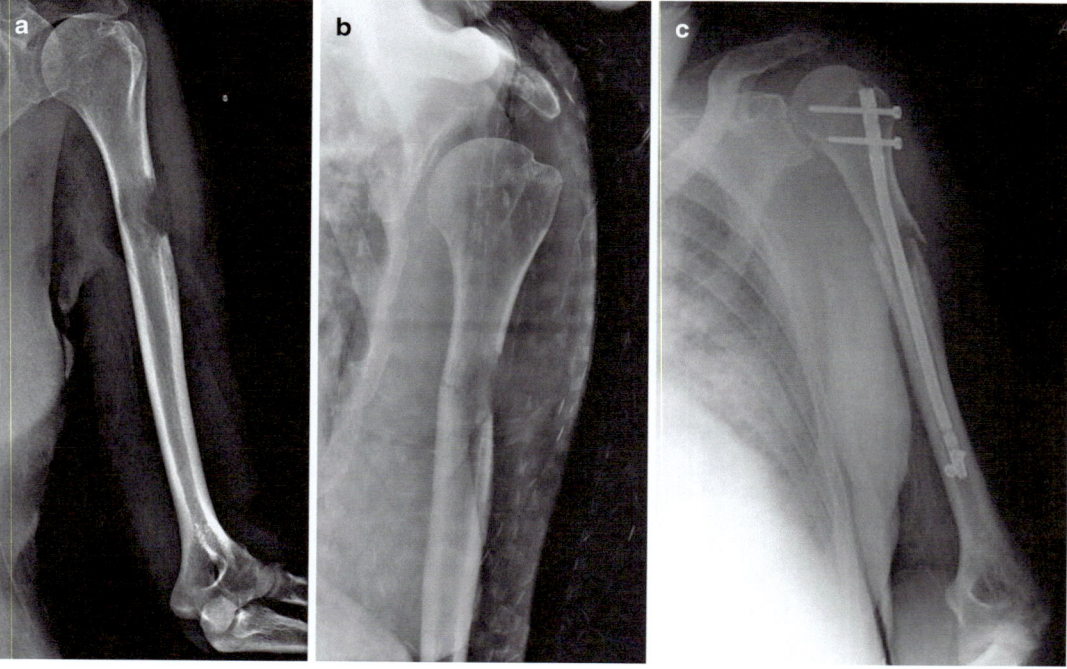

Fig. 11.1 (**a**) Impending fracture in a 57-year-old patient with clear cell carcinoma affected by multiple visceral and bone metastasis. (**b**) Pathologic fracture of the humerus due to an untreated impending fracture. (**c**) Osteosynthesis of the humerus with a nail

Fig. 11.2 (**a, b**) A
68-year-old patient with
multiple metastases
from prostate cancer,
complaining functional
pain on his left femur
after a rotational
movement. X-rays show
an osteoblastic lesion of
the proximal femur, but
no fracture are clearly
visible on the distal part
of the femur

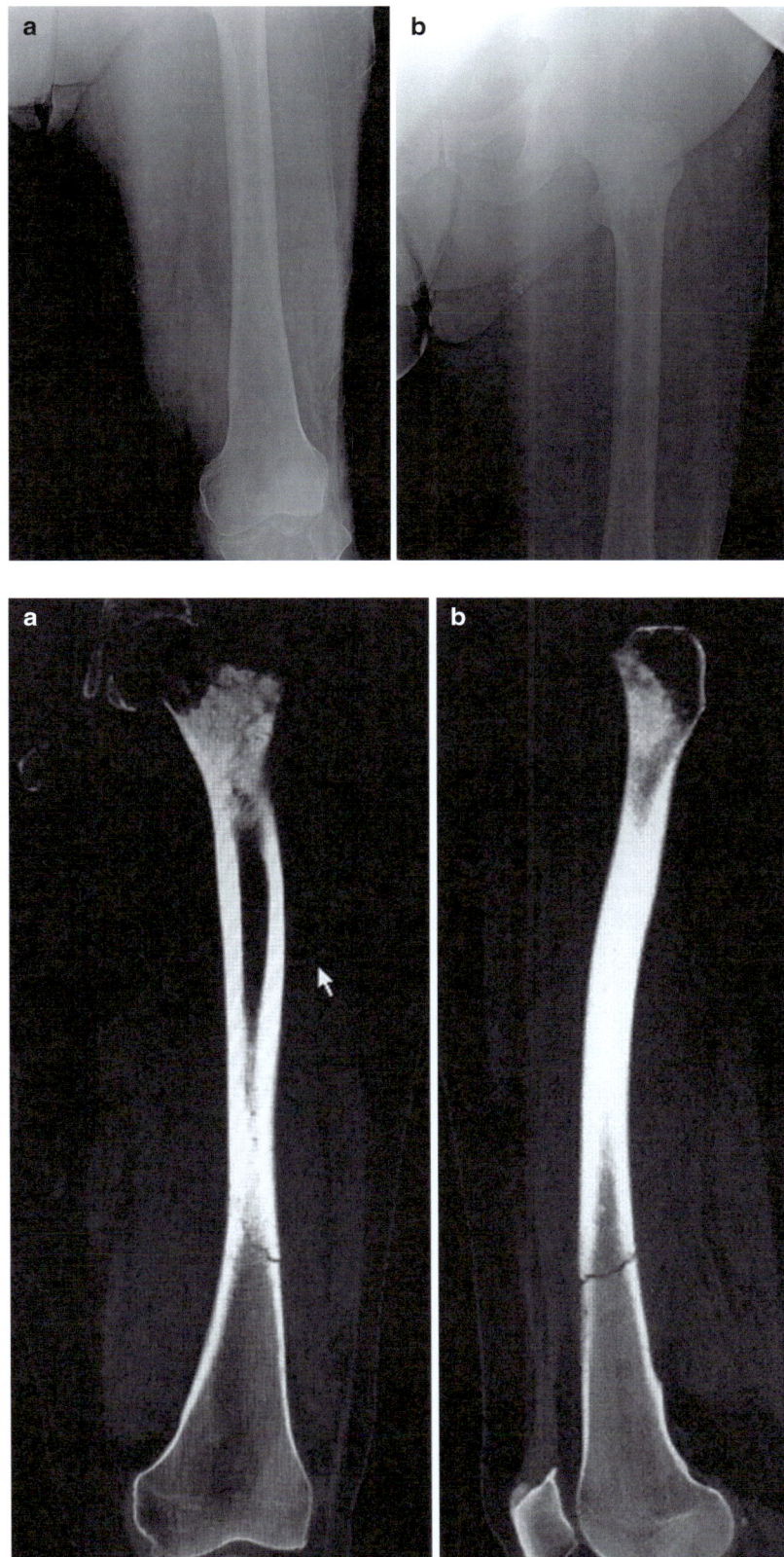

Fig. 11.3 (**a, b**)
CT-scans show an
undisplaced incomplete
pathologic fracture of
the mid-distal third of
the femur

of urgency in the orthopedic treatment of these patients [10]. Its principles of treatment are not the same as those for traumatic fractures, since the presence of tumor cells impairs bone healing, which is therefore independent of the surgical treatment adopted but depends on the primary diagnosis, and thus on the histologic type of tumor and on the adjuvant therapies. The rate of healing for pathologic fracture is very low, reported at around 35%, and in some histologic types, such as lung carcinoma, is very rare [11, 12].

The goal of surgical treatment, therefore, is not to allow the fracture to heal but to convert the bone segment from an open system to a closed one, to restore the bone resistance to bending and torsional forces, and to allow weight-bearing and restore function as quickly as possible. As we develop knowledge in this field, we understand how the primary task of the orthopedic surgeon is to preserve autonomy and the quality of life. The aim of a high quality of care is to prevent a pathologic fracture; given that the bone lesions are known, these should be treated before the bone fractures with a preventive osteosynthesis.

The fracture risk of a bone with a secondary lesion is clear to all the doctors who deal with these patients in the multidisciplinary team. First among these is the oncologist, who will work closely with the expert in orthopedic oncology regarding fracture risk. This imminent risk of fracture that may occur in daily activities is a specific diagnosis and is given the name impending fracture.

11.1 Impending Fracture

The impending fracture "is a state of the bone where a pathologic fracture appears almost certain if no preventive action is taken" [13]. Many studies on bone biomechanics have shown that the mineral component gives high resistance to axial compressive forces, while the mineral and protein component gives resistance to bending forces (compression + tension). The major weakness of the bone is during torsional forces [1]. A hole in the bone of 6 mm, similar to the one per-

formed to carry out a bone biopsy, has been demonstrated to reduce the bone strength in terms of torsion by 50%. This is the reason why in a secondary osteolytic bone lesion a pathologic fracture could be caused by a simple everyday activity that does not require high energy, such as putting on a coat in the case of the humerus or rotating the leg to get up from the bed in that of the femur. The diagnosis of impending fracture was defined in the previously cited paper of Healey as "controversial" [1], and even today there are no objective guidelines for predicting fracture in a metastatic bone. Even if there is no doubt as to the efficacy and benefit of a preventive osteosynthesis, this seems to be dependent largely on the surgeon's experience and linked to subjective parameters.

The history of classification systems for impending fracture begins in the 1980s with Fidler, who presented a case series of 66 patients [14]. When cortical involvement for secondary lesions was <50%, 2,3% of the subjects experienced a pathologic fracture, whereas when cortical involvement was >75%, 80% of patients experienced a fracture. In 1987 Menck [15] published a paper in which pathologic fracture occurred in 62 of 67 patients with a ratio equal or greater of 0,60 between metastasis width and bone diameter, or when the size of the lesion was >13 mm in the femoral neck and >30 mm in other parts of the same segment, or when bone involvement was equal or greater than 50%. These metric parameters were measured using standard X-rays. These elements were all confirmed in the more widely known criteria of Harrington [16], bone cortical disruption >50%, length of the lesion >2.5 mm, pathologic fracture of the lesser trochanter, and persistent pain on weight bearing after radiation therapy. Though we have here a confirmation of the metric parameters seen previously, Harrington introduced a new parameter as an indicator for fracture risk: pain. The integration of this element into the clinical evaluation is very important because the shape of a metastatic lesion on X-ray evaluation alone can be very unclear, with blurred edges that do not permit a precise evaluation for a surgical indication as preventive osteosynthesis.

A score for the symptomatologic factor was subsequently included in the most famous scoring system for impending fracture, drawn up by Mirels in 1989 [17]. It is a scoring system of 12 points divided into 4 factors (site, radiographic aspect, bone involvement, pain). Each factor has a grade of three points. If the total score is greater than 8, preventive osteosynthesis is strongly recommended; if the overall score is 7, it is up to the surgeon to decide on the basis of the evaluation of additional factors. In his report on 78 patients, those with a score greater than 9 presented a fracture in 33% of the cases, while with a score of 8 the figure was 15%. The advantage of Mirels' scoring system, which has been for years and still is the one most commonly used, is that is easy to remember and apply and shows a good interdisciplinary reliability. The limit of the Mirels scale, however, was shown in its only external validation, conducted by Damron et al. [18], in which it demonstrated a sensibility of 91% and a specificity of 35%, which in clinical practice means a tendency to an overestimation of pathological fracture and thus to the carrying out of unnecessary surgical procedures. The pain is the main factor that guides surgeon's evaluation for surgical decision, either when under load or persistent, but a weakness of this approach is that it may be easily hidden by the kind of good medical therapy that is very often prescribed for these types of patients. In recent studies, high and accurate prediction of the fracture risk is achieved with CT scan with finite element software [19–22], but their use is limited in day-to-day practice when we have to decide whether there is a need for surgery or not.

11.2 The Economic Impact of Pathologic Fracture

The prevalence and increasing incidence of metastatic bone patients will be a huge economic burden on the health system and will impact on health resources in a way that requires consideration in relation to surgical treatment.

The first multicentric retrospective observational study conducted in Europe was published in 2015 [23], with the aim of evaluating the costs and the impact on health resources in economic terms of the management of SREs in patients affected by bone metastasis. The countries involved were Germany, Spain, Italy, and the United Kingdom. The total number of patients involved in the study was 478. The costs included in the analysis covered those linked to the length of inpatient stay, outpatient attendances, and the procedures themselves. Sixty-six percent of the patients underwent radiotherapy. Only 7% of the patients were treated for spinal compression and 10% with other surgical procedures to the bone. Although these last two represent the minority of the procedures carried out, the study shows that they contribute most of the economic burden because they involve prolonged inpatient stay, which was the factor with the major economic impact on health resources. A second European multicentric retrospective study involved eight countries (Austria, the Czech Republic, Finland, Greece, Portugal, Sweden, and Switzerland) [24]. This study analyzed health resource utilization (HRU), focusing on the following parameters: the number and length of inpatient stays and the number of procedures, outpatient visits, and day-hospital admissions. The data were analyzed both before the SRE event (about 3.5 months) and after the SRE (3 months). The results show that the skeletal event is always associated with an increase in HRU in the number and length of inpatient stays. However, the increase differed according to the type of SRE. Surgical procedures to the long bone and spinal cord compression impacted for three times more than radiotherapy. These two factors, however, demonstrated the same impact, with the procedure to the long bone having a greater impact compared to those on other bones, probably owing to the longer immobilization period and to the greater need for more surgical procedures. The data from Portugal and Finland showed that pathologic fractures were the most relevant factor impacting on HRU because of the longer impatient stay involved. This result reflects the fact that the decision to proceed with surgical treatment is not dictated by international guidelines but is still open to subjective evaluation which in the end impacts on both economic health resources and the quality of care.

Both studies concluded by suggesting that to reduce the economic impact of SREs on health resources, it would be desirable to prevent every situation that leads to a major cost and prolonged hospitalization, i.e., pathologic fracture and spinal cord compression.

The diagnosis that should be formulated is thus that of impending fracture, and this should be treated accordingly [25].

A more focused analysis regarding the need for preventive osteosynthesis to save health costs was conducted on the US population [26] in a study whose goals were expressed in two questions: 1) Is there a difference in costs between patients treated for a pathologic fracture and patients treated with a preventive osteosynthesis? 2) Do these patients… differ in terms of HRU? The variables of the study were total amount of direct costs for each episode, days of hospitalization, condition at discharge, and postoperative mortality at 1 year. The results of the study show that total costs were greater for pathologic fracture, with an increase of 41% in direct costs compared to preventive procedure. One other statistically significant difference between the two groups was the length of hospitalization, which was longer for patients with pathologic fracture. All these results strongly indicate the advantage of preventive surgery, that is, the treatment of the impending fracture. However, we have seen that the scores used today overestimate the case for surgery and the risk of fracture, thus making them an imprecise tool. Comparative data on the complications and costs of the management of patients with overtreatment for impending fracture are lacking.

11.3 Pathologic Fracture and Survival

One final issue that is gaining an increasingly important place in the discussion about the treatment of bone metastasis is the impact of pathologic fracture on survival.

It is obvious how the event of pathological fracture impacts negatively on the metastatic patient's quality of life and also on his or her psychological state [27]; less clear, however, is the impact on survival. Does the occurrence of pathological fracture reduce life expectancy? The study by Nathan et al. [28] is the first to assess the impact of the most used prognostic factors and to place among them the surgeon's estimation of survival. Among these factors, however, pathological fracture is not included. The results of the study show that using the Cox regression analysis the following were found to be independent predictors for survival: the diagnosis, ECOG performance status, the number of metastases, the presence of visceral metastases, hemoglobin, the estimated survival time.

Oefelein et al. [29] found in their study on 195 patients with non-metastatic prostate cancer that bone fracture correlates negatively with overall survival. A study conducted on a much bigger number of patients is that of Saad et al. [30], which analyzes the data from three double-blind randomized control trials in phase 3 of zoledronic acid, from an international multicentric database, in adult patients with bone metastasis. The aim of these trials was not to evaluate the link between pathologic fracture and patient survival but the efficacy of zoledronic acid in these patients. The analysis conducted on a sample of 3059 patients with multiple myeloma, breast cancer, non-small cell lung carcinoma (NSCLC), prostate, and other solid tumors shows that the pathological fracture is related to an increased risk of death. In patients with breast cancer, this increased risk reached the highest value (32%), while the risk of death in patients with multiple myeloma and prostate cancer was lower, at around 20%. The correlation between pathologic fracture and increased risk of death was not seen in patients with non-small cell lung carcinoma (NSCLC) and other solid tumors, but this result is probably due to the short survival of these patients. These data underline how preventive treatment is an important therapeutic target. The same paper evaluates the different impact of vertebral and non-vertebral fractures on the risk of death in patients with breast cancer: in models unadjusted with regard to the variables, a statistically significant difference was seen between fractured subjects and non-fractured for both vertebral and non-vertebral. In models where the data were adjusted for previous SRE and ECOG performance status, non-vertebral fractures maintained a statistically significant correlation with the risk of death, while vertebral fractures showed an increased risk trend.

An interesting fact is provided by the study of Forsberg et al. [31, 32], in which the authors present the variables that have an impact on survival in patients with bone metastases, this time including pathological fracture and using the Bayesian statistical method of ordering the variables in degrees of influence over the primary outcome, that is, survival at 3 and 12 months, in a graphical representation, the so-called Bayesian network. The influence of the variables does not seem to have the same impact if the patient's survival is 12 or 3 months, meaning that different factors impact more greatly as survival decreases. Pathologic fracture appears at the second degree of relationship with survival in the 12-month model; at the first degree, the following variables are linked to survival: the preoperative hemoglobin, the diagnosis of the primary tumor, the number of metastases, and the surgeon's estimate of survival. In the 3-month survival model, pathological fracture is linked to survival at the first degree, signifying a greater impact, together with hemoglobin, the performance status, preop lymphocytes costs, and the surgeon's estimate. These data suggest that if the fracture occurs when survival is already low, it can have a negative impact on survival, while with longer survival estimates, it is other factors that influence survival more, such as the diagnosis and the number of metastases, factors that are irrelevant in the survival at 3 months (the number of metastases appears at the fourth degree and the diagnosis at the third).

Conclusions

The skeletal complications that occur in patients with bone metastases from carcinoma have a serious impact on the prognosis of survival and on the patient's quality of life. The pathologic fracture, in particular, is a dramatic event since it limits patients' autonomy and mobility, creates severe bone pain, and requires surgery and hospitalization with long periods of rehabilitation. The ways to prevent this are either through pharmacological therapy with bisphosphonates or denosumab or through surgery [33]. Surgical treatment should be considered for both impending and pathologic fracture. The prevention of pathologic fracture with the surgical treatment of an impending fracture is crucial in the decision-making process in bone metastatic patients and also has economic benefits in the management of the health resource and decreases the burden of the costs associated with the treatment of this patients' population.

References

1. Healey JH, Brown HK. Complications of bone metastases: surgical management. Cancer. 2000;88(12 Suppl):2940–51.
2. Matza LS, Van Brunt K, Chung K, Brazier J, Braun AH, Currie B, et al. Health state utilities for skeletal-related events associated with bone metastases. J Clin Oncol Off J Am Soc Clin Oncol. 2011; 29(15_suppl):e16620.
3. Yong M, Jensen AØ, Jacobsen JB, Nørgaard M, Fryzek JP, Sørensen HT. Survival associated with bone metastases and skeletal-related events in breast cancer patients: a population-based cohort study in Denmark (1999 - 2007). J Clin Oncol Off J Am Soc Clin Oncol. 2009;27(15_suppl):e22210.
4. Fryzek JP, Cetin K, Nørgaard M, Jensen AØ, Jacobsen J, Sørensen HT. The prognostic significance of bone metastases and skeletal-related events (SREs) in prostate cancer survival: a population-based historical cohort study in Denmark (1999-2007). J Clin Oncol Off J Am Soc Clin Oncol. 2009;27(15_suppl):5160.
5. Zustovich F, Pastorelli D. Therapeutic management of bone metastasis in prostate cancer: an update. Expert Rev Anticancer Ther. 2016;16(11):1199–211.
6. Zhiyu W, Rui Z, Shuai W, Hui Z. Surgical treatment of patients with lung cancer and bone metastases: a prospective, observational study. Lancet (Lond Engl). 2016;388(Suppl 1):S42.
7. Mokdad AH, Dwyer-Lindgren L, Fitzmaurice C, Stubbs RW, Bertozzi-Villa A, Morozoff C, et al. Trends and patterns of disparities in cancer mortality among US counties, 1980-2014. JAMA. 2017; 317(4):388–406.
8. Li S, Peng Y, Weinhandl ED, Blaes AH, Cetin K, Chia VM, et al. Estimated number of prevalent cases of

metastatic bone disease in the US adult population. Clin Epidemiol. 2012;4:87–93.

9. Piccioli e coll. Documento siot sul trattamento delle metastasi ossee. GIOT; 2012.

10. Manglani HH, Marco RA, Picciolo A, Healey JH. Orthopedic emergencies in cancer patients. Semin Oncol. 2000;27(3):299–310.

11. Piccioli A, Rossi B, Scaramuzzo L, Spinelli MS, Yang Z, Maccauro G. Intramedullary nailing for treatment of pathologic femoral fractures due to metastases. Injury. 2014;45(2):412–7.

12. Piccioli A, Maccauro G, Scaramuzzo L, Graci C, Spinelli MS. Surgical treatment of impending and pathological fractures of tibia. Injury. 2013;44(8): 1092–6.

13. Piccioli A, Spinelli MS, Maccauro G. Impending fracture: A difficult diagnosis. Injury. 2014;45(Suppl 6):S138–41.

14. Fidler M. Incidence of fracture through metastases in long bones. Acta Orthop Scand. 1981;52(6):623–7.

15. Menck H, Schulze S, Larsen E. Metastasis size in pathologic femoral fractures. Acta Orthop Scand. 1988; 59(2):151–4.

16. Harrington KD. Impending pathologic fractures from metastatic malignancy: evaluation and management. Instr Course Lect. 1986;35:357–81.

17. Mirels H. Metastatic disease in long bones. A proposed scoring system for diagnosing impending pathologic fractures. Clin Orthop. 1989;249:256–64.

18. Damron TA, Morgan H, Prakash D, Grant W, Aronowitz J, Heiner J. Critical evaluation of Mirels' rating system for impending pathologic fractures. Clin Orthop. 2003;415(Suppl):S201–7.

19. Liebl H, Garcia EG, Holzner F, Noel PB, Burgkart R, Rummeny EJ, et al. In-vivo assessment of femoral bone strength using Finite Element Analysis (FEA) based on routine MDCT imaging: a preliminary study on patients with vertebral fractures. PLoS One. 2015; 10(2):e0116907.

20. Koivumäki JEM, Thevenot J, Pulkkinen P, Kuhn V, Link TM, Eckstein F, et al. Ct-based finite element models can be used to estimate experimentally measured failure loads in the proximal femur. Bone. 2012;50(4):824–9.

21. Bessho M, Ohnishi I, Matsumoto T, Ohashi S, Matsuyama J, Tobita K, et al. Prediction of proximal femur strength using a CT-based nonlinear finite element method: differences in predicted fracture load and site with changing load and boundary conditions. Bone. 2009;45(2):226–31.

22. Crawford RP, Cann CE, Keaveny TM. Finite element models predict in vitro vertebral body compressive strength better than quantitative computed tomography. Bone. 2003;33(4):744–50.

23. Hechmati G, Cure S, Gouépo A, Hoefeler H, Lorusso V, Lüftner D, et al. Cost of skeletal-related events in European patients with solid tumours and bone metastases: data from a prospective multinational observational study. J Med Econ. 2013;16(5):691–700.

24. Body J-J, Pereira J, Sleeboom H, Maniadakis N, Terpos E, Acklin YP, et al. Health resource utilization associated with skeletal-related events: results from a retrospective European study. Eur J Health Econ HEPAC Health Econ Prev Care. 2016;17(6): 711–21.

25. Spinelli MS, Campi S, Sacchetti FM, Rossi B, Di Martino A, Giannini S, et al. Pathologic and impending fractures: biological and clinical aspects. J Biol Regul Homeost Agents. 2015;29(4 Suppl):73–8.

26. Blank AT, Lerman DM, Patel NM, Rapp TB. Is prophylactic intervention more cost-effective than the treatment of pathologic fractures in metastatic bone disease? Clin Orthop Relat Res. 2016;474(7): 1563–70.

27. Piccioli A. CORR Insights®: what factors are associated with quality of life, pain interference, anxiety, and depression in patients with metastatic bone disease? Clin Orthop. 2017;475:508–10.

28. Nathan SS, Healey JH, Mellano D, Hoang B, Lewis I, Morris CD, et al. Survival in patients operated on for pathologic fracture: implications for end-of-life orthopedic care. J Clin Oncol Off J Am Soc Clin Oncol. 2005;23(25):6072–82.

29. Oefelein MG, Ricchiuti V, Conrad W, Resnick MI. Skeletal fractures negatively correlate with overall survival in men with prostate cancer. J Urol. 2002;168(3):1005–7.

30. Saad F, Lipton A, Cook R, Chen Y-M, Smith M, Coleman R. Pathologic fractures correlate with reduced survival in patients with malignant bone disease. Cancer. 2007;110(8):1860–7.

31. Forsberg JA, Wedin R, Bauer HCF, Hansen BH, Laitinen M, Trovik CS, et al. External validation of the Bayesian Estimated Tools for Survival (BETS) models in patients with surgically treated skeletal metastases. BMC Cancer. 2012;12:493.

32. Forsberg JA, Sjoberg D, Chen Q-R, Vickers A, Healey JH. Treating metastatic disease: which survival model is best suited for the clinic? Clin Orthop. 2013;471(3):843–50.

33. Ibrahim T, Ricci M, Scarpi E, Bongiovanni A, Ricci R, Riva N, et al. RANKL: a promising circulating marker for bone metastasis response. Oncol Lett. 2016; 12(4):2970–5.

Osteosynthesis in Metastatic Disease of Long Bones

12

Primo Daolio, Vincenzo Ippolito, Barbara Rossi, Eleonora Marini, and Stefano Bastoni

Abstract

Prompt evaluation and effective treatment of long bone metastasis are a priority in the management of cancer patients. The main goals are to achieve local tumor control, pain relief, prevention and treatment of fractures, and maintenance of patient independence and quality of life.

Prognosis estimate, cross-sectional extent of bone destruction, and anatomic site of the bone lesion are clinical and radiographic features used by orthopedic surgeons in the decision-making process.

Treatment principles are the same regardless of the skeletal location. A construct should ideally provide enough stability to allow immediate full weight-bearing with enough durability to last the patients expected lifetime. Adequate mechanical stabilization by intramedullary interlocking nailing or plating and screws may address the vast majority of lesions of long bone diaphyseal and meta-diaphyseal portion in the presence of an adequate proximal and distal bone stock for fixation.

However, there are many additional aspects to consider in this setting as the need for biopsy, the evaluation of the extent of bone destruction and stability of the implant, dedicated and specific instruments for tumor surgery, the risk of perioperative bleeding and consideration to preoperative selective arterial embolization, cancer sensitivity and timing of postoperative radiation, possible tumor curettage, and use of local adjuvant and cement to improve tumor control and mechanical strength of the construct.

Keywords

Long bones metastasis · Impending fracture · Pathological fracture · Intramedullary nailing · Plating

12.1 Introduction

Goals of the surgical treatment of long bone metastasis are pain control and relief, function restoration, and prevention of tumor progression and complications for the patient lifespan [1–3]. For most cancer patients, a pathological fracture heralds the end-stage of their disease; on the other hand, the improvement of early diagnosis and the implementation of multidisciplinary therapies for primary tumors have resulted in prolonged life

P. Daolio (✉) · E. Marini · S. Bastoni
Centro di Chirurgia Oncologica Ortopedica Istituto Ortopedico "Gaetano Pini", Milan, Italy
e-mail: primoandrea.daolio@gpini.it

V. Ippolito
Clinica Ortopedica Policlinico Universitario, Padua, Italy

B. Rossi
UOC Ortopedia, Ospedale Gubbio-Gualdo Tadino, Gubbio, Italy

expectancy, thus increasing the incidence of bone metastases and skeletal-related events of patients with metastatic disease.

Surgery for bone metastatic cancer is generally indicated for patients with an expected survival at least of 3–6 months, although clinical judgment remains a key factor and may lead to more individualized management outside this timeframe [4].

When life expectancy related to histotype, staging, and general health condition is poor, the treatment aims to be palliative for pain control and prevention or treatment of mechanical complications. Conversely, if the patients' prognosis is favorable, the treatment of the metastases should be more aggressive and long-lasting and therefore can follow the principles of excisional surgery [5]. Regarding to the use of osteosynthesis in the treatment of long bone metastases, it is well known that the curative purpose is effectively achieved when the fixation is combined to wide or marginal resection or curettage and cement reconstruction. Therefore, the surgical strategy will depend on both the prognostic factors and the biological and mechanical features of metastatic disease and is conditioned by five key points [3–5]: (1) prognosis, good or poor; (2) histotype and its chemo-radio sensitivity, sensitive or resistant; (3) number of lesions, solitary or multiple; (4) location in the bone segment, diaphysis or metaepiphysis; and (5) pathological fracture, actual or impending.

12.2   Clinical and Prognostic Evaluation

The most common site for pathological fractures is the femur, followed by the humerus, and the tibia [1, 6–8]. Clinical course of long bone metastatic disease is variable, but pain is the most common symptom and complaint at onset. It is usually described as a night pain, typically deep and gnawing. Sharp pain increasing with weight-bearing is a concern for impending pathological fractures. Painless lesions are usually diagnosed during routinely follow-up at bone scan or CT-PET in patients with a known history of car-

cinoma. However, in 5–10% of cancer patients, a bone metastasis can be discovered as an incidental finding, thereby representing the first onset of a primary carcinoma. In a consecutive retrospective series of 139 pathological fractures, of which 36 from metastases, Hu et al. [9] focus on the statistically significant presence of prodromes before actual fracture in metastatic patients such as lump, soreness, and swelling. The evaluation of past medical history is mandatory along with a physical examination of the involved limb and palpation of the principal lymph node chains (axillary, supraclavicular, and inguinal).

Life expectancy evaluation is a key factor to conceive the feasibility of prophylactic fixation in case of impending fracture. Several prognostic factors can help the prediction of life expectancy as shown by the study of Forsberg et al. [10]: Eastern Cooperative Oncology Group (ECOG) "performance status" [11], presence of visceral metastasis, surgeon's estimate patient survival, number of bone metastasis, hemoglobin concentration, absolute lymphocyte count, and completed pathological fracture. A multicenter Italian and American scientific collaboration has recently resulted in the validation of Bayesian method to assess that the presence of a pathological fracture affects more significantly the survival of patient with worst prognosis (<12 months) than patients with better life expectancy (>12 months); in other words, patient selection and meticulous considerations of expected survival, benefits, and potential risk from surgical choice are a paramount concern [10, 12].

12.3   Evaluation of Mechanical Stability

Along with the prognosis, the assessment of the risk of fracture is important for the choice of the most appropriate surgical procedure. As well as preventing complete fractures, surgery at the stage of impending fracture is of significantly shorter duration and often technically simpler [2]. Evaluation of the mechanical stability is challenging even for an experienced surgeon. Plain radiographs provide the insight into the

Table 12.1 Studies defining the fracture risk in the setting of impending fracture evaluation

Authors	Recommendations for prophylactic fixation
Fidler [14]	>50% cortical destruction
Harrington [15]	– Lesion >25 mm – >50% cortical destruction – Persistent pain after radiation therapy
Mirels [16]	Variable points: (1), (2), (3) *Site*: Upper limb (1), lower limb (2), peritrochanteric (3) *Pain*: Mild (1), moderate (2), functional (3) *Lesion type*: Blastic (1), mixed (2), lytic (3) *Size as a proportion of shaft diameter*: <1/3 (1) 1/3–2/3 (2) >2/3 (3) >9 points = high risk of fracture

structural integrity of cortex and the presence of an alteration in the intracortical and medullary bone. Computed tomography (CT) scan defines in a detailed way the cortical structure and the extent of cortical compromise. Magnetic resonance imaging (MRI) shows the intramedullary extent of the tumor and any soft tissue extension. MRI is valuable to find spot lesions at the femoral neck or in the trochanter region, not well detected at a standard X-ray study [13]. Metastasis located at the long bones requires plain radiographs, CT, and/or MRI of the entire extent of the bone to exclude the possibility of additional lesions and aimed to the surgical planning. Missed metastasis, proximal or distal to the level of fixation, could determine pathological fractures at weight-bearing at the surgical treated extremity.

Although neither objective criteria nor guidelines exist, several studies have provided clinical and radiographic parameters to provide an algorithm for prophylactic fixation (Table 12.1).

12.4   Preoperative Planning

It is important to confirm the diagnosis of bone metastasis with a biopsy. A lesion in a patient with a known primary tumor should not be assumed to be from the patient's known primary tumor. Most of all, a biopsy is recommended if a bone lesion is solitary and if the primary tumor is unknown. Biopsy may be performed with a fine needle, a CT-guided or open procedure. In case of uncertain diagnosis when a surgical fixation has been planned for an impending or displaced pathological fracture, an open biopsy with frozen section should be performed immediately before the fixation, and the surgeon should not proceed until the pathology report has confirmed the metastatic disease. If the frozen specimen is inconclusive, the operative time should be stopped until the definitive pathology report is returned [17].

Angiography can be used preoperatively to embolize hypervascular lesions such as clear cell kidney carcinoma, thyroid, and liver carcinomas or myeloma reducing intraoperative bleeding at the time of fixation, thereby minimizing the postoperative anemia [18]; embolization can be expected to be effective in approximately 90% of cases [19, 20].

Bone pain could be treated by narcotic analgesics and radiation therapy, usually external beam irradiation. Also bisphosphonates have been shown to impact on pain and to contribute to the reconstitution of the bone stock [3, 21]. As Cheung [17] shortly assessed, the surgical indication and the kind of fixation should suit the following conditions: acceptable perioperative life risk and a shorter recovery time than the expected patient life; the construct must ensure immediate functionality, mechanical resistance to potential metastatic progression in the bone segment, and postoperative radiotherapy.

12.5   Treatment

12.5.1   General Considerations and Principles

The indications for operative treatment of long bone metastasis include impending and pathological fractures and intractable pain [3, 7, 8]. Patient's survival, the location of the lesion, skeletal complications, and response to nonsurgical therapies guide the choice of the surgical procedure (Fig. 12.1).

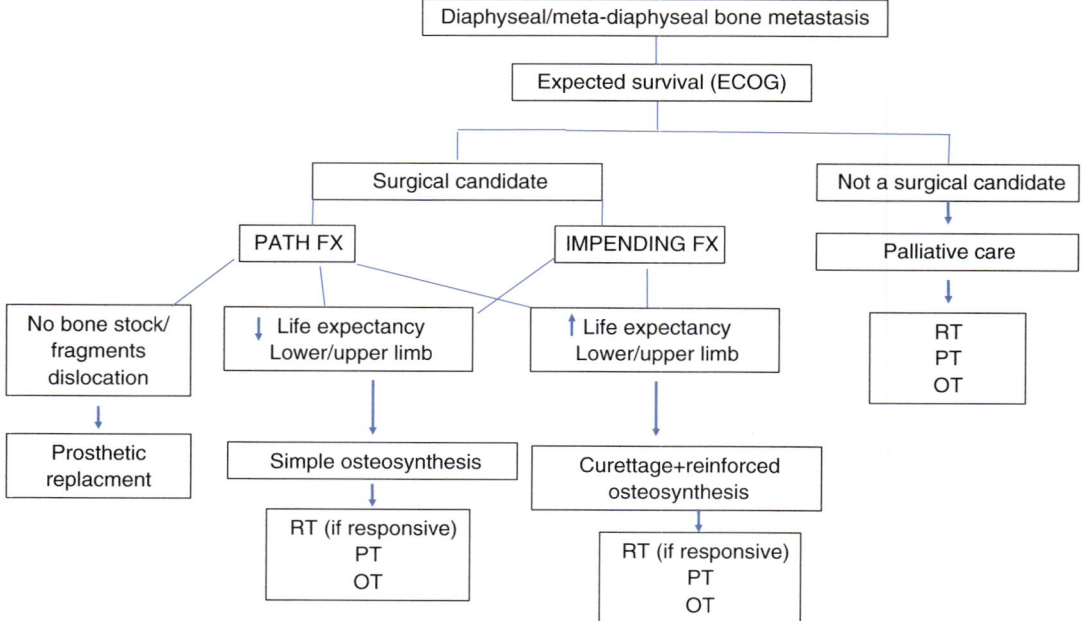

Fig. 12.1 Treatment strategy for long bone metastasis. *RT* radiation therapy, *PT* pain therapy, *OT* osteoprotective therapy

A construct should ideally provide enough stability to allow immediate restoring of the function, with enough durability to overcome the patients expected survival, which may be prolonged for patients with breast, prostate, or renal cancer [3, 6]. The procedures used for osteosynthesis are conceived to ensure early full weight-bearing of the lower extremities and to stabilize the upper extremities to allow common activities.

Plating, as a load-bearing device, is suggested in metaphyseal and epiphyseal lesions in the case of intact articular surface and sufficient adjacent bone stock [22]. Indeed, plate fixation requires adequate cortical bone proximal and distal to the fracture. Fixation with side plates is appropriate for lesions located at the upper extremity, for example, the humeral diaphysis, which is not subjected to considerable weight-bearing, or in places where it is difficult to use an intramedullary device such as the proximal tibial metaphysis. Conversely, reamed intramedullary nails have a neutral axis almost identical to that of the bone in which they are placed [23]. Considering that a normal bone healing cannot

be expected, this load-sharing device, with a small moment arm and low transmission of torque, can withstand the mechanical loads and support the entire length of the affected bone [3, 22]. Intramedullary nailing is the most accepted method of fixation in diaphyseal metastasis, because of its ease of insertion, less invasiveness and limited bleeding, load-sharing properties, and low costs [24, 25]. Cemented or not, reamed or not, intramedullary fixation should be long enough to reinforce the entire length of the bone and to prevent the breakdown from potential contiguous lesions. The nail should be of the greater possible diameter, proximally and distally locked with static holes and interlocking screws to control distraction and torsion stresses, and to early gain function [13, 22, 26].

Simple closed osteosynthesis, without open curettage, may be considered for patients in a poor general health condition, and for lesions with favorable predicted response to radiotherapy. Closed nailing is done in patients affected by impending or actual pathological fractures with minimal bone destruction and fragment displacement.

Fractures involving the proximal femur are the most common surgical issues in the management of long bone metastasis. Of all long bone pathologic fractures, 60% involve the femur. Of these, 80% involve the proximal portion: the femoral neck (50%), the subtrochanteric region (30%), and the intertrochanteric region (15%) [27]. Anterograde reconstruction nail is recommended to prophylactically and simultaneously stabilize the neck, intertrochanteric region, and shaft. Reconstruction nailing provides resistance to torsional stresses as well as to angular displacement through the full length of the femur, and fixation with static screws gives the adequate stability to allow for immediate postoperative function [13, 24]. Tanaka et al. [25], among 186 surgically treated femoral metastasis cases, retrospectively reviewed 80 consecutive nailing procedures in 75 patients, including 14 pathological and 66 impending fractures. In this cohort, only three intramedullary nails broke through their proximal parts, where the fracture site was in the subtrochanteric region; the 2- and 3-year postoperative survivals were 14.2% and 8.4%, respectively, whereas the implant survival rate was 94.0% at both 2 and 3 years; however, it dropped to 62.8% at 50 months. They proposed a much broader indication for the use of intramedullary devices including the trochanteric part of the femur as a sufficient fixation system for a few years, demonstrating several advantages and wider indications compared to prosthetic reconstruction implants, and sufficient durability and revision options.

A more aggressive approach, as reinforced osteosynthesis with cement augmentation, is indicated in patients with a good prognosis and in case of scarce response to adjuvant therapy. Open exposure may be required in cases of pathological fractures with considerable bone destruction. Bone cement increases the structural stability, enables the patient to withstand the stress of immediate motion and function, and enhances the local control after debulking of the tumor; the disadvantages include longer surgical times, risk of wound healing compromise, and local bleeding [4, 5]. Pairing intralesional curettage with the use of local adjuvant treatment, such as liquid nitrogen, alcohol and phenol, and argon probes,

improves the debulking of the tumor deposit and helps to prevent the local progression of disease. Cementing requires the use of low-viscosity PMMA, minimal pressurization, clean canals, and adequate patient hydration to reduce the risk of fat emboli [17, 18].

Immediate functionality of the construct is important in this setting because the patient's lifespan may be limited.

Therefore, construct that rely on allograft healing, bone healing, and ingrowth into stems and cups are discouraged in favor of cemented constructs. Large destructive lesions, intra- or periarticular, may require prosthetic replacement [28].

Indications for different implants and features to obtain adequate stabilization of long bone metastases are summarized in Table 12.2.

Table 12.2 Options and features of osteosynthesis for long bone metastases

Construct	Indication	Features
Plating	Proximal humerus, distal femur, distal tibia and distal humerus <50% diameter, radio and ulna	Adequate length Periarticular
	Open surgery, curettage or tumor resection, use of cement	
	Preexisting implants or prosthesis	
Nailing	All diaphyseal lesion, femoral neck, and trochanteric impending lesion	Anterograde, long, interlocking, recon, reamed, greater diameter, flexible in radio and ulna
	Patients with poor prognosis	
Cemented osteosynthesis (nail or plate)	Patients with good prognosis	Low-viscosity PMMA, low pressurization, repeated clean canals
	Clear cell kidney carcinoma and thyroid histotype (CHT-RT resistance)	
	Trend in pathological fracture more than impending	

12.6 Impending and Complete Pathologic Fracture

From the Scandinavian Skeletal Metastasis Registry for patients with skeletal metastasis of the extremities surgically treated between 1999 and 2009, the complete fracture was the major reason for surgery in 74.2% of the cases while an impending fracture in 18.3% of cases [8].

The pathologic fracture is one of the adverse prognostic factors in the lifespan of a metastatic patient [29]. General indications for surgery are a life expectancy of 1–3 months for a fracture of a weight-bearing bone and 3 months or more for fracture of a non-weight-bearing segment; adequate bone stock to support the construct; a benefit from surgery in terms of pain, patient mobilization, and general care [1].

Although potentially simpler than stabilization of an actual fracture, prophylactic fixation of an impending fracture requires peculiar considerations and planning.

Plating with cement augmentation is the surgical choice for metaphyseal and epiphyseal lesions, but it requires an intact articular surface and sufficient bone stock to stabilize the interested bone portion. At least one intact cortex is required to achieve rigid fixation and allow full weight-bearing in a short time postoperatively in this setting [30]. Intramedullary nailing is the most common treatment for diaphyseal lesions at risk of fracture of the upper and lower limbs.

It is contraindicated when there is a substantial periarticular involvement, when the bone stock is inadequate (a load-bearing device such as endoprosthetic replacement is preferable in these cases), and when the life expectancy is less than 6 weeks (Fig. 12.2).

Usually it is recommended to completely excise the metastatic cancer deposit, followed by using local adjuvants (alcohol, liquid nitrogen, phenol, peroxide) to sterilize the lesion cavity. The defect, after performing the curettage should be filled with cement [31].

It is important to preserve the soft tissue attachments to the bone and articular surfaces to improve its function and to lower the infection risk in immune-depressed patients.

Fractures involving different portions of long bones are treated with different forms of fixation (Table 12.3). In general, intramedullary devices are the choice in pathological fracture allowing to stabilize all the anatomical segments reducing the risk of failure due to progression of the disease and permitting an easier return to normal life [26].

If epiphyseal and diaphyseal lesions benefit from well-established fixation systems (prosthetic replacement for epiphyseal fractures and intramedullary nail for diaphyseal fractures), metaphyseal fractures provide a more significant surgical challenge [32].

There are instances in which nailing is contraindicated, such as sclerotic lesions or when there are metaphyseal fragments that cannot be reduced

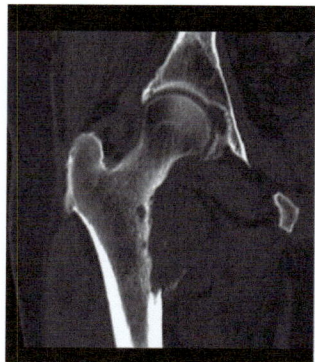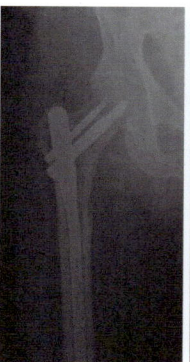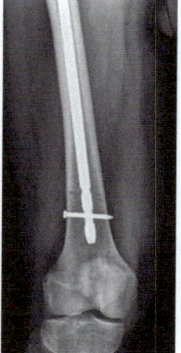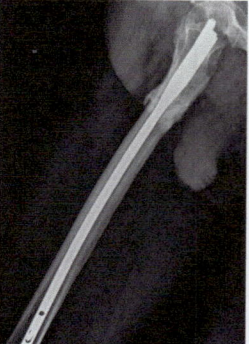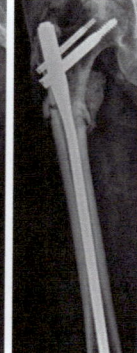

Fig. 12.2 Proximal femur metastatic impending fracture lesion in lung tumor. Last pictures show 6 months' follow-up

Table 12.3 Osteosynthesis options by segmental location

Bones	Site	Fracture	Osteosynthesis
Femur	Proximal (trochanteric)	Impending	Long cephalomedullary nail
		Complete	Cemented long cephalomedullary nail
	Diaphysis	Impending	Long cephalomedullary nail (with or without cement)
		Complete	
	Distal	Impending	Distal femoral plate
		Complete	Cemented distal femoral plate
Humerus	Proximal	Impending	Plate or long proximal humeral nail
		Complete	Cemented long proximal humeral nail
	Diaphysis	Impending	Long humeral nail (with or without cement)
		Complete	
	Distal	Impending	Distal humeral plate
		Complete	Cemented distal humeral plate
Tibia	Proximal	Impending	Proximal tibial plate or cemented K-wires
		Complete	Cemented proximal tibial plate
	Diaphysis	Impending	Long cephalomedullary nail (with or without cement)
		Complete	
	Distal	Impending	Cemented distal tibial plate
		Complete	
Radio	Proximal	Impending	Small fragment T plate
		Complete	
	Diaphysis	Impending	Small fragment plate or flexible nail (with or without cement)
		Complete	
	Distal	Impending	Distal radius plate (with or without cement) or wrist fusion to ulna
		Complete	
Ulna	Proximal	Impending	Olecranon plate
		Complete	
	Diaphysis	Impending	Small fragment plate or flexible nail (with or without cement)
		Complete	
	Distal	Impending	Small fragment plate (with or without cement) or resection
		Complete	
Fibula	Proximal	Impending	Not surgical
		Complete	
	Diaphysis	Impending	
		Complete	
	Distal	Impending	Distal fibular plate or retrograde screw
		Complete	Distal fibular plate or ankle fusion
Phalanx	Any	Any	Small fragment plate vs K-wire fixation

without opening the site of fracture that are not permitting a good stabilization of the fracture site. In these setting plating is more indicated (Fig. 12.3). When the bone stock at the fracture site of a metaphyseal unique lesion is inadequate, it is important to consider the prosthetic replacement. This could guarantee a better stability and debulking of local disease. Diaphyseal fractures are best treated with intramedullary nailing. To stabilize the fracture, it is recommended to use a long, interlocking nail and to cement the defect.

When the fracture involves both the diaphyseal and metaepiphyseal portion, a cemented prosthetic replacement is the best device to stabilize the fracture sites.

There is not a universal nail or plate in orthopedic oncology. Titanium is traditionally the material of choice for fixation constructs, and it reduces the infective risk in patient candidates to postoperative radiotherapy and chemotherapy. Carbon-fiber-reinforced (CFR) implants have been recently proposed as very valuable

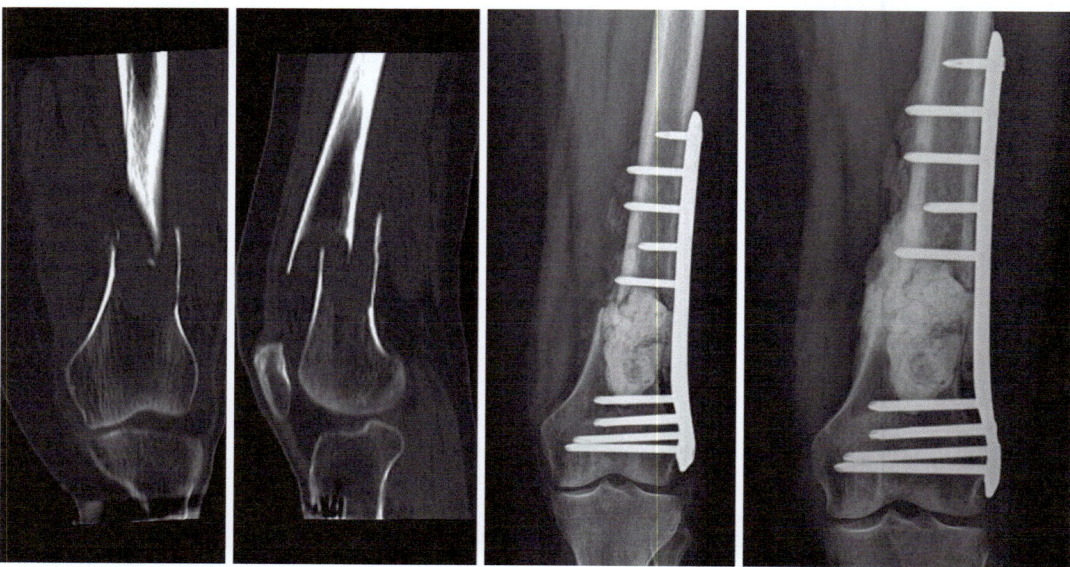

Fig. 12.3 Pathological fracture in patient affected by multiple myeloma. After surgery X-ray. Last picture shows 2 years' follow-up

devices for osteosynthesis in musculoskeletal tumors, due to their peculiar biomechanical strength and for their advantages in combination with adjuvant radiotherapy and fracture monitoring during follow-up [33, 34]. It is not surprising that the first clinical application of a CFR-PEEK nail has been described for the treatment of long bone metastases. Collis et al. [33] reported the first case and technique of CFR nailing for treatment of a humeral metastasis from melanoma; the authors remarked the definition of "the invisible nail," focusing on its radiolucent properties. Zimel et al. [34] qualitatively and semiquantitatively assessed the differences between CFR-PEEK and titanium implant artifact seen on the MRI and CT imaging follow-up for recurrent oncologic disease in a phantom simulation. Moreover, the authors described the clinical application of CFR nails in eight cancer patients, reporting no immediate or short-term postoperative complications nor implant failure; the lower MRI distortion immediately adjacent to the implant allowed a better visualization of the surrounding marrow space, cortex, and bone–muscle interface.

IlluminOss® Photodynamic Bone Stabilization System (IlluminOss® Medical GmbH, Germany) is an innovative percutaneous stabilization device for diaphyseal fragility fractures of not weight-bearing long bones. This mini-invasive procedure incorporates the use of an inflatable polyethylene terephthalate (Dacron®) walled balloon catheter that is inserted into the previously reamed canal and then infused with a liquid monomer, so the balloon expansion fills the intramedullary canal with patient-specific anatomical conformation. The monomer-filled balloon is cured in situ and on demand using a fiber optic light source resulting in a stable and radiotransparent implant [35]. Overall complication rate, surgical time, and costs make IlluminOss® System a reliable system to stabilize pathological fractures and lytic lesions in the upper limb (Fig. 12.4). No intramedullary devices are to date available for the radial and ulnar shaft. Similarly to CFR devices, IlluminOss® System is radiotransparent, and moreover, it allows placement of locking screws anywhere along the length of the implant. Even if it is a good solution for diaphyseal bone, metaepiphyseal lesions are at high fracture risk with this technique and often require ancillary stabilization with plate and screws.

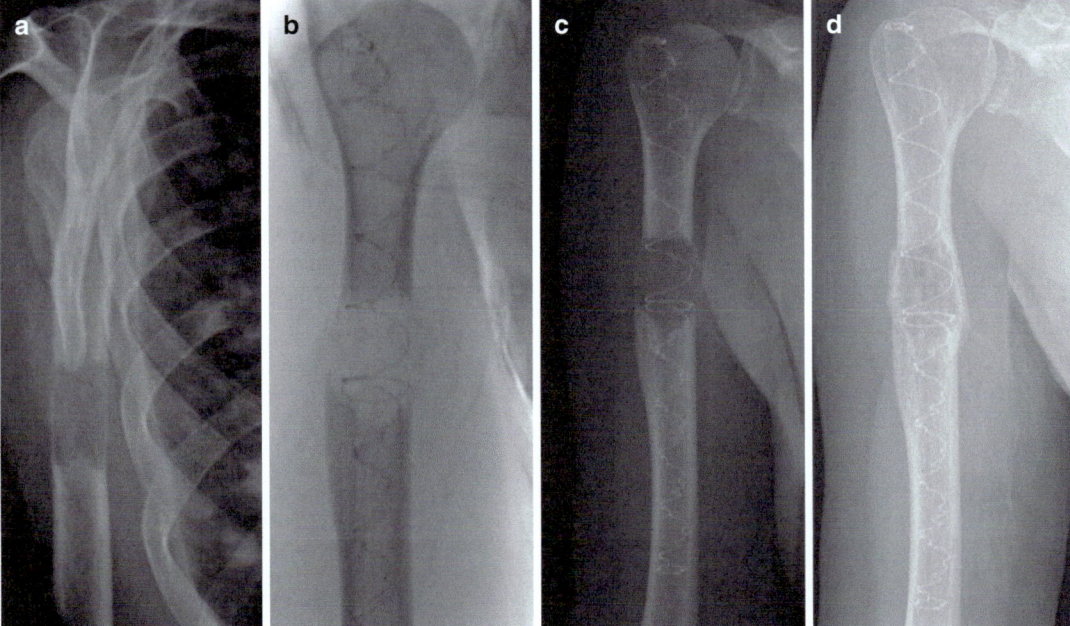

Fig. 12.4 Clinical case of a patient with a pathologic fracture of the humerus due to a metastasis from a solid tumor (**a**), fluoroscopic intraoperative picture of the Illuminoss® implant (**b**); 1-week postoperative X-ray (**c**); 90-day postoperative X-ray (**d**), after the performance of radiotherapy, showing partial healing of the fracture (Courtesy of IlluminOss Medical, Inc. East Providence, Rhode Island, USA)

12.7 Postoperative Treatment and Care

Following intramedullary fixation, early weight-bearing is encouraged as tolerated by the patient. The use of antibiotics therapies and deep vein thrombosis prophylaxis is dictated by postoperative course and by the level of mobility and comorbidities. Passive and active range of motion exercises of the adjacent joints should be performed as soon as possible as determined on the basis of the wound healing and the patient's ability. Early discharge from the hospital will generally enhance the patient's motivation and minimize the interruption of an ongoing oncological protocol.

Postoperative clinical and radiographic follow-up is then undertaken. Radiation therapy usually follows at 3–4 weeks from surgery, provided wound healing is complete. Townsend et al. [36] found that 15% of patients treated with surgery alone required a second surgery because of increasing pain or loss of fixation due to tumor progression, but only 3% of patients who received postoperative radiation therapy needed additional surgical procedures. The radiation field should cover the site of disease, the operative field, and also the entire fixation device.

The most frequent complications are wound dehiscence, deep infection, and fracture due to tumor progression otherwise post-actinic.

In case of plating and screws, the patient can be mobilized except for full weight-bearing that is prohibited indicatively for 30 days or more, depending on the progression of fracture healing.

12.8 Complications and Risk of Failure

Complications are reported in 11% (61/554) of plate and nailing procedures in the Scandinavian Sarcoma Group cohort: systemic complications, wound infections, deep infections, nail brakes, fractures next to implant, and nerve injuries, non-unions, and technical errors/immediate fails [8].

The long survival after surgery is the most important risk factor for failure of osteosynthesis secondary to disease progression, implant failure, or loss of fixation [22]. Failed surgery depends on implant breakage, tumor progression, stress fracture, and poor surgery.

By comparing different surgical procedures from a series of 57 patients with bone metastases secondary to breast cancer, Wegener et al. [7] assess that the procedure (nail, standard, or tumor endoprosthesis) had no impact on survival and the complication rate was 11%.

From the Scandinavian series, in plating and nailing procedure group, there were 6.1% reoperations because of either local tumor progression or failure of fixation [8].

Conclusions

Patients with metastatic disease at long bones pose a management challenge. A multimodality approach is mandatory in caring for these patients: oncologists, radiation therapists, radiologists, and pathologists' cooperation is needed to estimate the therapeutic program and their life expectancy. Because surgery has most frequently a palliative role for patients with limited life expectancy, unnecessary reoperations due to complications resulting from hardware failure are unwarranted. This should be kept in mind in surgical osteosynthesis, like intramedullary nailing and plating: a patient's survival should not exceed the durability of the construct.

References

1. Healey JH, Brown HK. Complications of bone metastases: surgical management. Cancer. 2000;88(12 Suppl): 2940–51.
2. Katzer A, Meenen NM, Grabbe F, Rueger JM. Surgery of skeletal metastases. Arch Orthop Trauma Surg. 2002;122(5):251–8. Epub 2001 Dec 4
3. Bickels J, Dadia S, Lidar Z. Surgical management of metastatic bone disease. J Bone Joint Surg Am. 2009;91:1503–16. Review
4. Capanna R, Campanacci DA. The treatment of metastases in the appendicular skeleton. J Bone Joint Surg Br. 2001;83(4):471–81.
5. Capanna R, Piccioli A, Di Martino A, Daolio PA, Ippolito V, Maccauro G, et al. Management of long bone metastases: recommendations from the Italian Orthopaedic Society bone metastasis study group. Expert Rev Anticancer Ther. 2014;14(10): 1127–34.
6. Swanson KC, Pritchard DJ, Sim FH. Surgical treatment of metastatic disease of the femur. J Am Acad Orthop Surg. 2000;8(1):56–65.
7. Wegener B, Schlemmer M, Stemmler J, Jansson V, Dürr HR, Pietschmann MF. Analysis of orthopedic surgery of bone metastases in breast cancer patients. BMC Musculoskelet Disord. 2012;13:232.
8. Ratasvuori M, Wedin R, Keller J, Nottrott M, Zaikova O, Bergh P, Kalen A, Nilsson J, Jonsson H, Laitinen M. Insight opinion to surgically treated metastatic bone disease: Scandinavian Sarcoma Group Skeletal Metastasis Registry report of 1195 operated skeletal metastasis. Surg Oncol. 2013;22(2):132–8.
9. Hu YC, Lun DX, Wang H. Clinical features of neoplastic pathological fracture in long bones. Chin Med J. 2012;125(17):3127–32.
10. Forsberg JA, Wedin R, Bauer HCF, Hansen BH, Laitinen M, Trovik CS, et al. External validation of the Bayesian Estimated Tools for Survival (BETS) models in patients with surgically treated skeletal metastases. BMC Cancer. 2012;12:493.
11. Conill C, Verger E, Salamero M. Performance status assessment in cancer patients. Cancer. 1990;65(8): 1864–6.
12. Piccioli A, Spinelli MS, Forsberg JA, Wedin R, Healey JH, Ippolito V, et al. How do we estimate survival? External validation of a tool for survival estimation in patients with metastatic bone disease-decision analysis and comparison of three international patient populations. BMC Cancer. 2015;15:424.
13. Maccauro G, Muratori F, Liuzza F, Rossi B, Logroscino CA. Anterograde femoral nail for the treatment of femoral metastases. Eur J Orthop Surg Traumatol. 2008; 18:509–13.
14. Fidler M. Prophylactic internal fixation of secondary neoplastic deposits in long bones. Br Med J. 1973;1(5849):341–3.
15. Harrington KD. New trends in the management of lower extremity metastases. Clin Orthop. 1982;169: 53–61.
16. Mirels H. Metastatic disease in long bones: a proposed scoring system for diagnosing impending pathologic fractures. Clin Orthop. 2003;415(Suppl):S4–13.
17. Cheung FH. The practicing orthopedic surgeon's guide to managing long bone metastases. Orthop Clin North Am. 2014;45(1):109–19.
18. Randall RL, Aoki SK, Olson PR, Bott SI. Complications of cemented long-stem hip arthroplasties in metastatic bone disease. Clin Orthop. 2006;443:287–95.

19. Sun S, Lang EV. Bone metastases from renal cell carcinoma: preoperative embolization. J Vasc Interv Radiol. 1998;9(2):263–9.
20. Layalle I, Flandroy P, Trotteur G, Dondelinger RF. Arterial embolization of bone metastases: is it worthwhile? J Belg Radiol. 1998;81(5):223–5.
21. Jehn CF, Diel IJ, Overkamp F, Kurth A, Schaefer R, Miller K, et al. Management of metastatic bone disease algorithms for diagnostics and treatment. Anticancer Res. 2016;36(6):2631–7.
22. Dijstra S, Wiggers T, van Geel BN, Boxma H. Impending and actual pathological fractures in patients with bone metastases of the long bones. A retrospective study of 233 surgically treated fractures. Eur J Surg. 1994;160(10):535–42.
23. Jacofsky DJ, Frassica D, Frassica F. Metastatic disease to bone. Hosp Physician. 2004;39:21–8.
24. Sharma H, Bhagat S, McCaul J, Macdonald D, Rana B, Naik M. Intramedullary nailing for pathological femoral fractures. J Orthop Surg (Hong Kong). 2007;15(3):291–4.
25. Tanaka T, Imanishi J, Charoenlap C, Choong PF. Intramedullary nailing has sufficient durability for metastatic femoral fractures. World J Surg Oncol. 2016; 14:80.
26. Ward WG, Holsenbeck S, Dorey FJ, Spang J, Howe D. Metastatic disease of the femur: surgical treatment. Clin Orthop. 2003;415(Suppl):S230–44.
27. Sim FH. Metastatic bone disease of the pelvis and femur. Instr Course Lect. 1992;41:317–27.
28. Chan D, Carter SR, Grimer RJ, Sneath RS. Endoprosthetic replacement for bony metastases. Ann R Coll Surg Engl. 1992;74(1):13–8.
29. Nathan SS, Healey JH, Mellano D, Hoang B, Lewis I, Morris CD, et al. Survival in patients operated on for pathologic fracture: implications for end-of-life orthopedic care. J Clin Oncol Off J Am Soc Clin Oncol. 2005;23(25):6072–82.
30. Harrington KD. Impending pathologic fractures from metastatic malignancy: evaluation and management. Instr Course Lect. 1986;35:357–81.
31. Harrington KD, Sim FH, Enis JE, Johnston JO, Diok HM, Gristina AG. Methylmethacrylate as an adjunct in internal fixation of pathological fractures. Experience with three hundred and seventy-five cases. J Bone Joint Surg Am. 1976;58(8): 1047–55.
32. Forsberg JA, Wedin R, Bauer H. Which implant is best after failed treatment for pathologic femur fractures? Clin Orthop. 2013;471(3):735–40.
33. Collis PN, Clegg TE, Seligson D. The invisible nail: a technique report of treatment of a pathological humerus fracture with a radiolucent intramedullary nail. Injury. 2011;42(4):424–6.
34. Zimel MN, Hwang S, Riedel ER, Healey JH. Carbon fiber intramedullary nails reduce artifact in postoperative advanced imaging. Skeletal Radiol. 2015;44(9):1317–25.
35. Gausepohl T, Pennig D, Heck S, Gick S, Vegt PA, Block JE. Effective management of bone fractures with the Illuminoss® photodynamic bone stabilization system: initial clinical experience from the European Union Registry. Orthop Rev (Pavia). 2017;9(1): 6988.
36. Townsend PW, Rosenthal HG, Smalley SR, Cozad SC, Hassanein RE. Impact of postoperative radiation therapy and other perioperative factors on outcome after orthopedic stabilization of impending or pathologic fractures due to metastatic disease. J Clin Oncol Off J Am Soc Clin Oncol. 1994;12(11):2345–50.

Spinal Metastases: Diagnosis and Management

13

Vincenzo Denaro and Alberto Di Martino

Abstract

The management of the patient affected by spinal metastases requires an integrated multidisciplinary approach. Surgery and radiotherapy being the mainstay of the treatment of these fragile patients, clinical and surgical trials are required to determine which patients will benefit most from these treatments when affected by metastatic epidural spinal cord compression. In recent years, a newer and more important role for radiotherapy is emerging for these patients; in particular, stereotactic radiosurgery is used as an adjuvant to the decompressive surgery for management of these patients.

Keywords

Spinal metastases · Surgery · Radiation therapy · Separation surgery · IONM

13.1 Introduction

The spine is the most common bony site for solid tumor metastases [1, 2], and nearly 5–10% of patients with systemic cancer will eventually develop spinal metastases during life [3]. Moreover, between 30 and 70% of patients affected by cancer will show spinal metastases at autopsy studies [4].

The incidence of symptomatic spinal metastases has recently increased in association with the improvement in the general condition and the overall prognosis of cancer patients [5]. Determining the histology of the primary tumor is crucial to determine the prognosis and the management of these patients. Breast cancer, prostate cancer, non-small cell lung carcinomas, renal cell carcinomas, and thyroid cancer account for nearly 80% of spinal metastases [1]. The histotype also affects the nature of the metastases, which can be osteolytic, sclerotic, or mixed.

Spinal metastases mostly affect the dorsal spine followed by the lumbar and cervical spine and the lumbosacral junction [6]. The neoplastic tissue usually affects the posterior half of the vertebral body, while the anterior portion and the posterior structures are involved in a later stage during the progress of the disease or can be spared [4]. The growth of the neoplastic tissue leads to a progressive structural disruption of the vertebral body, determining a loss of stability and

V. Denaro · A. Di Martino (✉)
Department of Orthopaedics and Trauma Surgery,
University Campus Bio-Medico of Rome,
Rome, Italy
e-mail: a.dimartino@unicampus.it

an eventual compression of the neural structures in the spinal canal [7].

In one out of four cases, spinal metastases are asymptomatic, and the diagnosis of the spinal involvement is incidental [8]. In the remaining cases, the first and often most relevant symptom is severe mechanical pain. Pain in patients with spinal metastases is a frequent complaint, but it is also non-specific and frequently underestimated. Clinically, the fixed local pain depends on the local growth of the tumor with consequent stretching of the periosteum; mechanical pain is related to the structural failure, and it is secondary to a progressive invasion of the vertebral body with an eventual pathologic fracture. The neurological symptoms are a direct consequence of either the pathologic fracture of the vertebral bodies or of the direct extension of the tumor mass within the spinal canal [9]. These are associated to the violation of the epidural space and to the compression of the neurological structures in the spinal canal (spinal cord, cauda equina, nerve roots) [7, 10, 11]; nearly 10% of patients with spinal metastases will develop neurological deficits with weakness, sensory loss, intense pain, and compromise of the sphincteric function; these are often associated to a segmental loss of stability at the affected level [12–15].

Identifying the most appropriate treatment in patients with vertebral metastases can be a demanding task [16, 17] and requires consideration of patients' general health conditions and of several characteristics of the metastatic disease [18]. Corticosteroid therapy is the first-line therapy in most of these patients, before the definitive surgical management is performed. Both high- and low-dose corticosteroid regimens have been studied, but, to date, the best dosage has not been determined [19, 20]. Together with the advances of chemotherapy, radiotherapy, and immunotherapy, new techniques and combined surgical approaches have been developed for the patients with spinal involvement by metastases.

Newer instrumentation systems can improve the chance to stabilize and reconstruct different tracts of the spine, contributing to improve the outcome of surgery in this patient population [21–26]. Surgery aims to improve the patient's quality of life and to indirectly improve the life

expectancy by reducing the complications related to pain and neurological compromise which directly or indirectly may result in the death of the patient. These are achieved by the control of pain after spinal stabilization and by the improvement of the neurological functions through the decompression of the spinal canal.

The complete removal of the mass is required for selected patients with very good prognosis in presence of a solitary metastasis, even though this requires a more aggressive surgery [27–29]. Indeed, the complete excision of the tumor mass may require a more complex surgery and staged or combined surgical approaches, which can determine complications on the neighboring vascular, myeloradicular, and visceral structures [30–32]. In other patients, debulking of the tumor mass and indirect decompression of the neural structures allow to improve the patients' neurological status.

After tumor removal or decompression, the surgeon must stabilize the operated segments by the use of spinal instrumentation to restore the segmental stability. The surgeon will need to adapt the surgical approach and the type of fixation to the individual requirements.

In all cases, surgery represents the best option when possible to maximize the chances of recovery [33–37]: in selected patients with neurological deficits (young patients with localized disease and good general health status) decompressive surgery followed by stabilization through instrumentation and followed by radiation therapy is associated to an increased chance of ambulation [38].

13.2   Medical Evaluation and Imaging

Early diagnosis and appropriate definition of the clinical status of the patient affected by metastatic spinal disease are important because the functional outcome after treatment depends on the neurologic condition at the time of presentation.

Patient evaluation begins with a detailed medical history, clinical examination, and directed laboratory tests [39]. Determination of the general health and nutritional status is part of the pre-operative assessment of the patient with cancer, since all of these factors may affect healing and infection risk. The assessment and documentation of any bowel/bladder function, motor weakness, and sensory deficits are routinely included in the preoperative evaluation of the patients candidate to surgery. Complete laboratory studies should be performed, and any electrolyte imbalance, coagulopathy, and neutropenia should be corrected if required. Nutritional optimization should be pursued in patients with recognized malnutrition [39].

The most common symptom in patients with metastatic spine tumors is back pain, which can anticipate the development of any neurologic symptom by weeks or months. The pain can be tumor-related or mechanical [40]. Tumor-related pain typically occurs at night or early morning and improves during the day. It is caused by inflammatory mediators or by the stretching of the periosteum of the vertebral body by the tumor [40]. Mechanical pain results from a structural abnormality of the spine, such as a pathologic compression fracture resulting in instability. It is related to movement and loads and may be exacerbated by sitting or standing positions. The consequence of a thoracolumbar compression fracture is often kyphosis, and patients typically show severe pain in recumbence; they can give a history of sleeping upright to avoid extension of the unstable kyphosis and to decrease pain [40].

Advances in imaging techniques have improved the sensitivity in detecting spinal metastases. The goal of imaging is early diagnosis and tumor characterization in terms of anatomical relationships and content; as a parallel matter, diagnostic imaging techniques should give identity to any distant metastases and show recurrent tumor following instrumentation. Understanding the advantages and disadvantages of different imaging modalities can assist the clinician in patient screening and plan the most appropriate treatment [40]. Often, multiple modalities are used in conjunction to tailor the treatment on the patient's pathology [41, 42].

Standard radiographs are considered insensitive to screen for asymptomatic spinal metasta-

ses [43], and in Western countries, most patients are referred to the spine specialist after a routine total body CT scan or an MRI. In fact, the visualization of a radiolucent defect on plain radiographs requires a 50–70% destruction of the vertebral body; moreover, the metastatic tumor often infiltrates the bone marrow of the vertebral body without destroying the cortical bone. X-rays are currently more often used to assess the presence of deformity in case of any alignment modification, on either the sagittal (kyphosis) or coronal (scoliosis) plane. They give the unique chance to perform weight-bearing imaging, usually not possible by MRI or CT scans. Dynamic flexion and extension films can detect instability, although these are rarely performed in spinal metastases patients [40, 44].

CT scan provides an excellent resolution of cortical and trabecular bone and has a higher sensitivity compared to plain radiographs in detecting both osteolytic and osteosclerotic metastases. Moreover, CT is the screening tool for skeletal metastasis since it is used to evaluate the treatment response at the time of staging or restaging other organs: this reduces the burden of imaging to the patient. Despite the limited soft tissue resolution of CT compared to MRI, CT can show bone marrow metastases before the bone destruction occurs, which results in an earlier diagnosis. CT is also the diagnostic imaging of choice to guide a percutaneous biopsy when required. Clinical trials have also demonstrated a role for CT in evaluating sclerotic changes within a metastatic deposit which can occur in response to chemo/radiotherapy treatment [43].

MRI helps in assessing the metastatic spread to the bone marrow; moreover, it allows an estimation of the extension of tumor out of the bone marrow and its involvement of the surrounding structures. Moreover, it is the technique of choice in suspected cases of spinal cord compression from pathologic vertebral body fractures, since it clearly demonstrates any compression of the spinal cord and the eventual related myelopathy [43]. Another advantage of MRI is that it can be used to distinguish between osteoporotic and pathologic vertebral compression fractures [43].

CT and MRI and conventional radiographs study the structure of a lesion within the bone. Conversely, nuclear medicine techniques are aimed at the evaluation of the function of the bone or tumor cells [43]. These can use osteotropic and oncotropic radioisotopes. Osteotropic radioisotopes include technetium 99-labeled diphosphonates (usually methylene diphosphonate 99mTc-MDP) and 18F labeled sodium fluoride (NaF), that are used in positron emission tomography (PET) imaging. Oncotropic radioisotopes have direct uptake into malignant cells; these are classified as either specific or non-specific. Those specific oncotropic agents investigate bone metastases from neuroendocrine tumors [43]. Skeletal scintigraphy, single-photon emission CT, PET, and hybrid imaging techniques are now common parts of clinical practice in patients with symptomatic spinal metastases, and the recent improvements in reconstruction techniques are enabling low-dose image acquisitions while maintaining excellent contrast resolution [43].

13.3 Integrated Treatment of the Patient with Spinal Metastases

The treatment of the patient with spinal metastases is typically multidisciplinary: it requires a team made by an orthopedic, a radiologist, a radiotherapist, a physiatrist, an oncologist, and a pain management consultant. The principal aims of the treatment are prevention and cure of the spinal cord compression, pain control, improvement of the quality of life, preservation or restoration of the segmental stability, and achievement of a local control of a metastatic lesion. The treatment can include surgery, radiotherapy alone, radiotherapy plus systemic chemotherapy, surgery plus radiotherapy, hormone therapy, and medical therapy.

This latter, not including pain therapy, includes corticosteroids and bisphosphonates or denosumab. Corticosteroid therapy is often added in patients with spinal metastases and neurological compromise. Dexamethasone decreases the vasogenic edema typical of acute spinal cord compression to stabilize or improve neurologic status in some patients. It also relieves the tumor-related pain. The most appropriate dosage of the drug in patients with acute spinal cord compression is still a matter of debate. Common sense suggests the application of high-dosage corticosteroid therapy in nonambulating patients, while low dose of corticosteroid therapy is suggested in patients with incomplete neurological lesion to balance drug-related complications [45, 46]. It has been suggested that the high dosage of dexamethasone (100 mg as loading dose and then 96 mg per day) may be administered to patients that cannot walk or to those with rapidly progressive neurological symptoms. An intermediate dosage (10 mg as loading dose and then 16 mg per day) is administered in ambulatory patients with little or nondevelopmental symptoms [40]. In patients with an undiagnosed spinal mass, the administration of steroids prior to a biopsy should be avoided because of the oncolytic effect for certain tumors such as lymphomas. Bisphosphonates and denosumab are drugs that inhibit osteoclastic activity and suppress bone resorption. In combination with systemic antitumor therapy, these can reduce or delay skeletal events, such as pathologic fractures [38, 40].

Spinal orthoses are important in the treatment of patients with spinal metastasis, in the perioperative period, in the support of patients undergoing radiotherapy and chemotherapy, and in those patients not suitable for surgery because of the overall general health status [47–49].

The type of orthoses changes depending on the affected site and to the grade of instability. The choice is based on three parameters: the type of lesion, the level of the lesion, and the function of the orthoses (kinetic immobilization, immobilization, and static support) [50].

Surgery and radiotherapy are the mainstays of the management of patient with symptomatic spinal metastases (Table 13.1). Radiotherapy is advised as the first-line treatment when the tumor is sensitive, when the segmental instability is not clear, when the neurological picture is stable, in case of reduced life expectancy, and in case of spinal cord compressions lasting more than

Table 13.1 Indications for surgery or radiotherapy in the spinal metastasis patient

Radiotherapy	Surgery
Sensitive tumor	Spinal deformity that causes pain and/or neurological compression
Local pain	Spinal instability
Intradural spinal cord compression	Progressive neurological deficit
Life expectancy <3–6 months	No response to radiotherapy: relapse/new deficit during RT
Non-operable patient	Bone fragment dislocated causing neural compression
Long-lasting complete neurological deficit	Unknown primary tumor

48–72 h [15]. If the patient is not operable and the tumor histotype is not sensitive to radiotherapy and oncology therapies, the management of pain should be considered.

Surgery is advised for spinal metastasis in the oligometastatic patient, in those patients whose primary tumor has a good prognosis with long life expectancy (e.g., in case of renal cancer or hormone-sensitive tumor such as breast cancer and prostate cancer), for those with intractable pain, and in the case of onset of neurological deficits, as in the case of compression of the myeloradicular structures by the tumor. The surgical indications are conditioned by type and staging of the primary tumor, general health status of the patient, chance for fixation and reconstruction, and by the surgeons' experience [51].

In general, the surgical treatment of metastatic spine tumors may involve two contrasting surgical strategies: palliative surgery with neural decompression and spine stabilization or attempt of locally curative (and more aggressive) surgery, consisting of complete tumor resection and stabilization.

The improvements in surgical techniques and spinal instrumentation systems has positively affected the management of patients with spinal metastases or metastatic spinal cord compression [52]. Modern bar and screw instrumentation systems are derived by the original plate and screw fixation systems conceived by Roy-Camille (Fig. 13.1) [53]. These address the issue of the postsurgical instability after the decompressive

procedures have been performed, being either laminectomy alone, surgical tumor debulking, or en bloc resection [15].

Palliative surgery is aimed to the decrease of local pain, to the stabilization of the affected spinal segment, and to the prevention of further damage to the neurological structures. It is the treatment of choice in most patients with disseminated neoplastic disease and compromised conditions with initial neurological deficits, especially for those with tumors with worse prognosis (e.g., lung cancer, visceral, or brain metastasis) and a pathologic fracture.

Decompression and stabilization is the less aggressive "open" surgical technique. It does not necessarily include an approach aimed at the tumor. It is performed in order to decompress the circumference of the spinal cord and stabilize the spine. It is the procedure of choice in cases of neurological compromise consequently to a pathological fracture in progress but also in conditions in which the metastasis appears sensitive to radiotherapy or responsive to chemotherapy or hormonal therapy.

It has been demonstrated that in patients with short life expectancy and good general health status, it is possible to perform a stabilization at the thoracolumbar level by realizing an "internal bracing," represented by a posterior spinal construct of rods and laminar hooks (Fig. 13.2) and, in selected cases, screws (Fig. 13.3) [15, 24]. This stabilization, associated to the segmental decompression by laminectomy, is associated to clinical and neurological improvement of patients affected by multiple metastatic lesions of the thoracolumbar spine, not eligible for complete tumor removal [54, 55]; moreover, in selected patients it can represent the first stage of a circumferential approach after postsurgical adjuvant treatment. This less aggressive surgical approach can be indicated to improve patient care and quality of life and has proven its effectiveness in the management of patients with neurological symptoms and poor-to-intermediate prognosis [21, 56].

The role of fixation in the setting of epidural spinal cord compression is also confirmed by the work of Patchell et al. [34] that compared radiation therapy alone versus surgical decompression and

Fig. 13.1 Lateral (**a**) and anterior posterior (**b**) radiographs of the first Roy-Camille plate and pedicle screws implant ever used in Italy; it was implanted by the senior author (VD) in 1979 for stabilization after dorsal laminectomy for a spinal metastasis

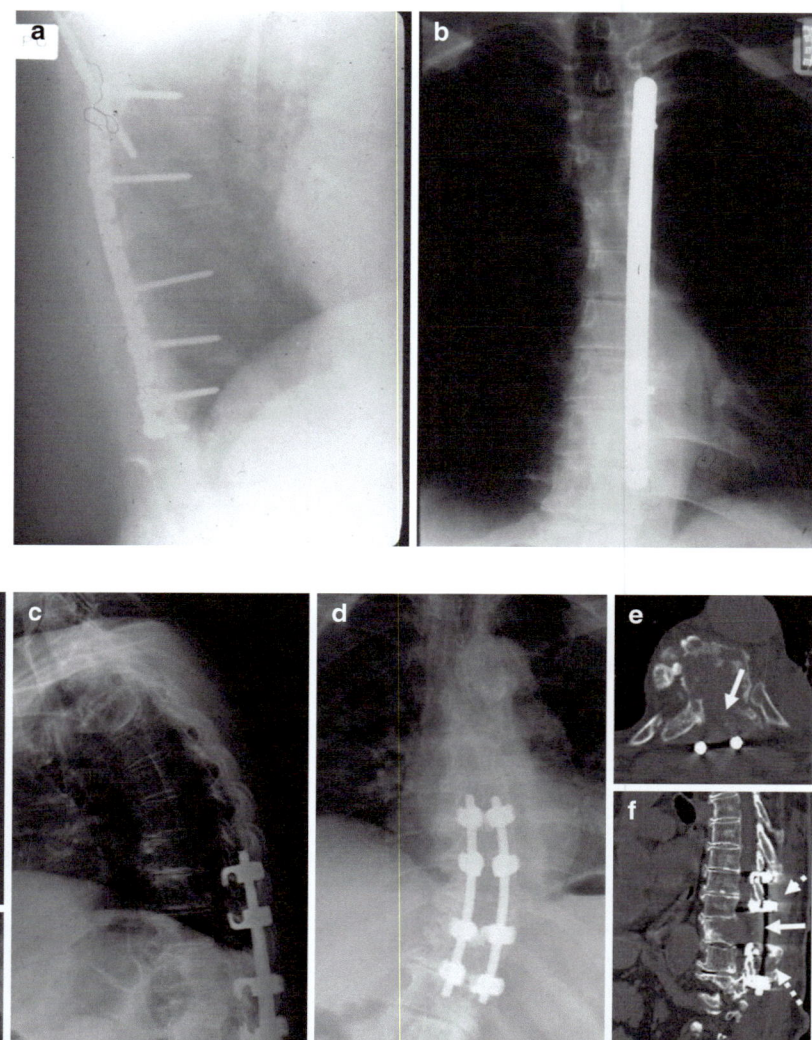

Fig. 13.2 Sagittal (**a**) and axial (**b**) T2-weighted MRI of an 80-year old patient with unknown primary malignancy, showing anterior and posterior spinal cord compression by a tumor mass. Surgery consisted of posterior laminectomy, biopsy, and segmental stabilization with laminar hooks and longitudinal bars (**c, d**) without correction of the patients' scoliosis. The biopsy showed a lung adenocarcinoma, and adjuvant chemotherapy and radiotherapy were started. Three months axial (**e**) and sagittal (**f**) CT scans show the widening of the spinal canal (arrow) after segmental laminectomy at the affected level and positioning of the laminar hooks (dash arrows)

stabilization combined with postoperative radiation therapy; in the study, surgical treatment proved the superiority in recovering or keeping ambulation. After this study, others were performed, with controversial results. It has recently been compared the therapeutic efficacy of surgery (with or without adjuvant radiotherapy) to radiotherapy alone in the treatment of metastatic spinal cord

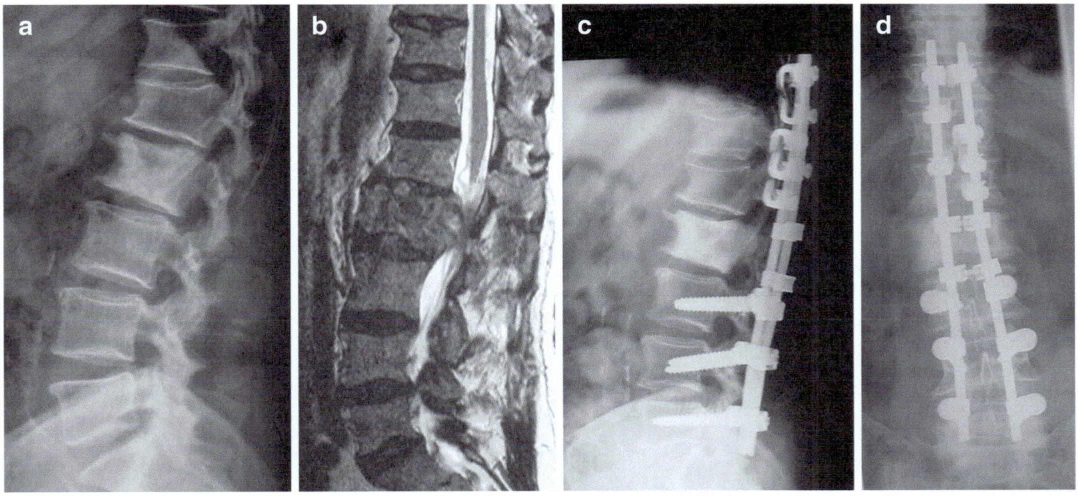

Fig. 13.3 (**a**) L2 osteosclerotic lesion in a 72-year old patient affected by prostate cancer. (**b**) Sagittal T2-weighted MRI shows the pathologic fracture with metastatic epidural spinal cord compression. Surgery consisted of posterior laminectomy and segmental stabilization with a hybrid construct with pedicle screw, laminar hooks, and longitudinal bars (**c, d**)

compression. It was found that compared to radiotherapy alone, surgery (with or without adjuvant radiotherapy) was associated to an improvement of the ability to ambulate, to a higher relief in pain and in higher 1-year survival [51].

The complete resection of the tumor is the procedure of choice in the treatment of primary tumors and sometimes can be performed in the case of isolated vertebral metastases of tumors resistant to chemotherapy and radiation treatments, with little or no visceral involvement of the disease, and in those patients with good medium to long-term life expectancy. It can be performed through a surgical posterior approach only or through a combination of different approaches (Fig. 13.4). The complete tumor removal allows for an optimal local control since the risk of local recurrence is minimal, but it can be demanding for both the patient and the surgeon and should be reserved only for selected cases due to its high morbidity.

Most often, spinal metastatic lesions are managed by intralesional excision/removal ("debulking") of the tumor, which allows the surgeon to remove the greatest possible amount of tumor, to decompress the spinal cord, and to reduce the size of the tumor mass and is followed by fixation and reconstruction of the bone loss. This procedure is anticipated by an adequate surgical planning that often includes preoperative arterial embolization and is included in the multidisciplinary treatment approach of the metastatic disease, being usually followed by radiation therapy course and adjuvant chemotherapy. In fact, the aim of this procedure is the removal of the tumor mass to ease or improve the local effect of other therapies [14] (Fig. 13.5).

Percutaneous procedures, like vertebroplasty (VP) or kyphoplasty (KP), are indicated for the treatment of refractory pain to medical therapies and vertebral body fractures without neurological involvement, whether they due to trauma, osteoporosis or tumors [57]. The advantages of VP and KP are immediate pain relief, improved functional capacity, and the chance to perform biopsy. However, these have mechanical and not oncological purposes. In addition to that, there are complications related to the leakage of cement in the spinal canal.

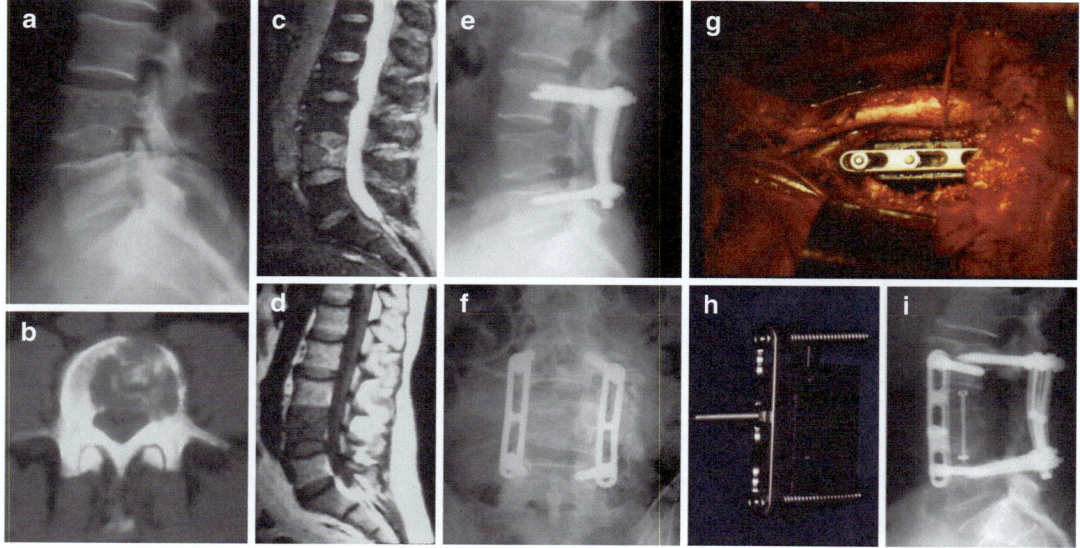

Fig. 13.4 Lateral X-ray (**a**), axial CT scan (**b**), and sagittal T2 and T1 MRI (**c**, **d**) showing pathologic fracture of the L4 vertebra of a patient whose biopsy showed an undifferentiated adenocarcinoma. Surgery consisted of a posterior L4 laminectomy and instrumentation with Steffee plates (**e**, **f**), followed by corpectomy via an anterior approach (**g**), followed by reconstruction by a first-generation carbon fiber MESH and plate (**h**), allowing for circumferential stabilization (**i**)

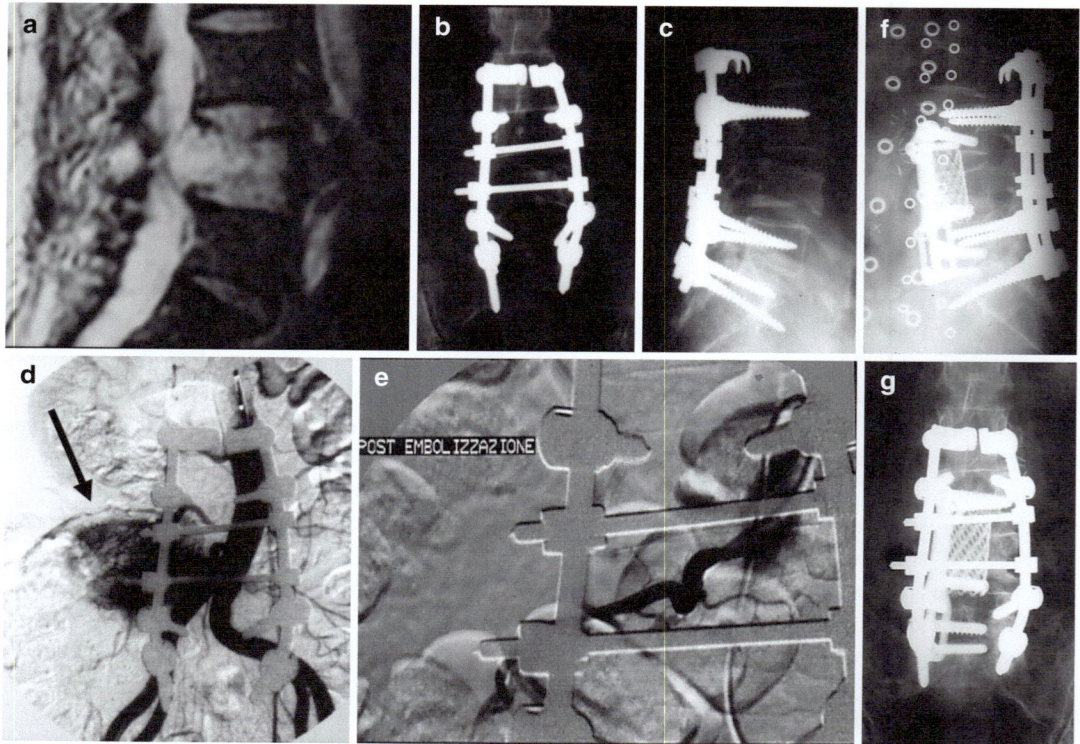

Fig. 13.5 Sagittal T2 MRI (**a**) showing pathologic fracture of the L4 vertebra of a patient whose biopsy was nondiagnostic. Surgery consisted of a posterior L4 laminectomy and instrumentation with pedicle screws, hooks, and bars (**b**, **c**). The biopsy showed a thyroid cancer. After arterial embolization (**d**, **e**), a corpectomy via an anterior approach followed by reconstruction by a titanium MESH and plate was performed (**f**, **g**)

13.4 Complications of Spine Surgery in the Metastatic Patient

The perioperative complication rate in the surgery of spinal metastases is relatively high and ranges from 5 to 76% in the different studies [58]. Intra- or postoperative complications, including the ones related to prolonged chemotherapy, radiotherapy, and chronic use of steroids, remain high despite the improvement in medical and surgical techniques. Ibrahim et al. in a multicentric study of 223 patients operated for spinal metastasis found an overall surgical perioperative mortality rate of 5.8%, and both minor and major morbidity occurred in 21% of patients [26].

Complications in the patient operated for spinal metastases are usually classified into surgical-related and medical complications. Medical complications are related to the general health status of the patient; as an example, delirium and pneumonia are between the most common medical complications. Surgical-related complications include dural tears, wound dehiscence, infections, and neurological deficits. Risk factors for the development of surgical-related complications include age, multilevel spinal metastases, preoperative irradiation, surgery performed by low-volume surgeons, and presence of preoperative myelopathy. Neurological deterioration is between the most feared complications related to this surgery, since spinal tumor surgery carries the risk of new neurological deficits in the postoperative period. It has been demonstrated that in patients with neurological deficits and neoplastic pachymeningitis, there is a reduced chance to improve the neurological picture after surgery, despite an appropriate decompression [14].

Only a paucity of studies have explored the utility of intraoperative neurophysiological monitoring and mapping (IONM) to assess the functional integrity of the spinal cord nerve roots during spinal tumor surgery. A recent systematic review has shown a positive role of IONM as a tool in the workup for spinal tumor surgery. However, it has been observed that individual monitoring and mapping techniques have insufficient sensitivity and specificity. Conversely, multimodal IONM has been found to be more sensitive and specific for anticipating neurological injury during spinal tumor surgery [59] and should be used in this setting if available.

Reoperations in the setting of surgery for spinal metastases can reach up to 20% of cases, but some patients may not sustain repeat surgery because of the general health status. Surgical site infection, failure of instrumentation, local recurrence, hematoma evacuation, and refracture are between the most common causes for revision surgery [58].

Conclusions

The management of the patient affected by spinal metastases requires an integrated multidisciplinary approach. Surgery and radiotherapy being the mainstay of the treatment of these fragile patients, clinical and surgical trials are required to determine which patients will benefit most from these treatments when affected by metastatic epidural spinal cord compression. In recent years, a newer and more important role for radiotherapy is emerging for these patients; in particular, stereotactic radiosurgery is used as an adjuvant to the decompressive surgery in those patients that can be candidate to the so-called separation surgery [51].

Laufer et al. [60] reported the results of separation surgery in MESSC patients, followed by stereotactic radiosurgery. It consists of a laminectomy followed by epidural tumor resection circumferentially starting from normal dural planes. The posterior longitudinal ligament is resected to obtain a margin on the anterior dura and to achieve spinal cord decompression, by partial vertebral body resection. If more than 50% of the vertebral body is resected, vertebral body replacement is performed with polymethylmethacrylate or titanium or PEEK cages [51]. High-dose postoperative stereotactic radiosurgery, indipendently from tumor hystology and radiosensitivity, allows for local control of the diesease. Prospective studies are needed to confirm the bounty of this technique.

References

1. Tubiana-Hulin M. Incidence, prevalence and distribution of bone metastases. Bone. 1991;12(Suppl 1):S9–10.
2. Durr HR, Maier M, Pfahler M, Baur A, Refior HJ. Surgical treatment of osseous metastases in patients with renal cell carcinoma. Clin Orthop Relat Res. 1999;367:283–90.
3. Sundaresan N, Digiacinto GV, Hughes JE. Surgical treatment of spinal metastases. Clin Neurosurg. 1986;33:503–22.
4. Fornasier VL, Horne JG. Metastases to the vertebral column. Cancer. 1975;36:590–4.
5. Schuster JM, Grady MS. Medical management and adjuvant therapies in spinal metastatic disease. Neurosurg Focus. 2001;11(6):e3.
6. Raque GH Jr, Vitaz TW, Shields CB. Treatment of neoplastic diseases of the sacrum. J Surg Oncol. 2001;76:301–7.
7. Gasbarrini A, Boriani S, Capanna R, Casadei R, Di Martino A, Spinelli MS, Papapietro N, Piccioli A, The Italian Orthopaedic Society Bone Metastasis Study Group. Management of patients with metastasis to the vertebrae: recommendations from the Italian Orthopaedic Society (SIOT) Bone Metastasis Study Group. Expert Rev Anticancer Ther. 2014;14:143–50.
8. Coleman RE. Clinical features of metastatic bone disease and risk of skeletal morbidity. Clin Cancer Res. 2006;12(20 Pt 2):6243s–9s.
9. Coleman RE. Skeletal complications of malignancy. Cancer. 1997;80(8 Suppl):1588–94.
10. Vrionis FD, Miguel R. Management of spinal metastases. Semin Pain Med. 2003;11:25–33.
11. Dewald RL, Bridwell KH, Prodromas C, Rodts MF. Reconstructive spinal surgery as palliation for metastatic malignancies of the spine. Spine. 1985;10:21–6.
12. Galasko CSB. Spinal instability secondary to metastatic cancer. J Bone Joint Surg. 1991;73B:104–8.
13. Brihaye J, Ectors P, Lemort M, Van Houtte P. The management of spinal epidural metastases. Adv Tech Stand Neurosurg. 1988;16:121–76.
14. Denaro V, Di Martino A, Papalia R, Denaro L. Patients with cervical metastasis and neoplastic pachymeningitis are less likely to improve neurologically after surgery. Clin Orthop Relat Res. 2011;469:708–14.
15. Di Martino A, Vincenzi B, Denaro L, Barnaba SA, Papalia R, Santini D, Tonini G, Denaro V. 'Internal bracing' surgery in the management of solid tumor metastases of the thoracic and lumbar spine. Oncol Rep. 2009;21:431–5.
16. Tomita K, Kawahara N, Kobayashi T, Yoshida A, Murakami H, Akamuru T. Surgical strategy for spinal metastases. Spine. 2001;26(3):298–306.
17. Sundaresan N, Steinberger AA, Moore F, et al. Indications and results of combined anterior-posterior approaches for spine tumor surgery. J Neurosurg. 1996;85(3):438–46.
18. Damron TA, Sim FH. Surgical treatment for metastatic disease of the pelvis and the proximal end of the femur. Instr Course Lect. 2000;49:461–70.
19. Vecht CJ, Haaxma-Reiche H, van Putten WLJ, et al. Initial bouls of conventional versus high-dose dexamethasone in metastatic spinal cord compression. Neurology. 1989;39:1255–7.
20. Helweg-Larsen S, Mouridsen H, et al. Effect of high-dose dexamethasone in carcinomatous metastatic spinal cord compression treated with radiotherapy: a randomized trial. Eur J Cancer. 1994;30A:22–7.
21. Bauer H. Posterior decompression and stabilization for spinal metastases: analysis of sixty-seven consecutive patients. J Bone Joint Surg Am. 1997;79A:514–22.
22. Bilsky MH, Boakye M, Collignon F, Kraus D, Boland P. Operative management of metastatic and malignant primary subaxial cervical tumors. J Neurosurg Spine. 2005;2:256–64.
23. Denaro V, Denaro L, Papalia R, Marinozzi A, Di Martino A. Surgical management of cervical spine osteoblastomas. Clin Orthop Relat Res. 2007;455:190–5.
24. Denaro V, Gulino G, Papapietro N, Denaro L. Treatment of metastasis of the cervical spine. Chir Organi Mov. 1998;83:127–37.
25. Ghogawalw Z, Mansfield FL, Borges LF. Spinal radiation before surgical decompression adversely affects outcomes of surgery for symptomatic metastatic spinal cord compression. Spine. 2001;26:818–24.
26. Ibrahim A, Crockard A, Antonietti P, et al. Does spinal surgery improve the quality of life for those with extradural (spinal) osseous metastases? An international multicenter prospective observational study of 223 patients. J Neurosurg Spine. 2008;8:271–8.
27. Sundaresan N, Digiacinto GV, Hughes JE, Cafferty M, Vallejo A. Treatment of neoplastic spinal cord compression: results of a prospective study. Neurosurgery. 1991;29(5):645–50.
28. Sundaresan N, Rosen G, Boriani S. Primary malignant tumors of the spine. Orthop Clin N Am. 2009;40:21–36.
29. Vieweg U, Meyer B, Schramm J. Tumour surgery of the upper cervical spine – a retrospective study of 13 cases. Acta Neurochir. 2001;143:217–25.
30. Bauer HCF, Wedin R. Survival after surgery for spinal and extradural metastases. Prognostication in 241 patients. Acta Orthop Scand. 1995;66:143–6.
31. Landreneau RJ, Weigelt JA, Meier DE, et al. The anterior operative approach to the cervical vertebral artery. J Am Coll Surg. 1995;180:475–80.
32. McPhee IB, Williams RP, Swanson CE. Factors influencing wound healing after surgery for metastatic disease of the spine. Spine. 1998;23:726–32.
33. Kitchel SH, Eismont FJ, Green BA. Closet subarachnoid drainage for management of cerebrospinal fluid leakage after an operation to the spine. J Bone Joint Surg Am. 1989;71:984–7.

34. Patchell RA, Tibbs PA, Regine WF, et al. Direct decompressive surgical resection in the treatment of spinal cord compression caused by metastatic cancer: a randomized trial. Lancet. 2005;366:643–8.

35. Riew DK, Khanna N. Treatment of cerebrospinal fluid leaks. In: Vaccaro AR, Betz RR, Zeidman SM, editors. Principles and practice of spine surgery. St. Louis: C.V. Mosby; 2002. p. 727–43.

36. Sorenson PS, Helweg-Larsen S, Mouridsen H, et al. Effect of high-dose dexamethasone in carcinomatous metastatic spinal cord compression treated with radiotherapy: a randomized trial. Eur J Cancer. 1994;30A:22–7.

37. Weigel B, Maghsudi M, Neumann C, et al. Surgical management of symptomatic spinal metastases. Postoperative outcome and quality of life. Spine. 1999; 24:2240–6.

38. Zheng GZ, Chang B, Lin FX, Xie D, Hu QX, Yu GY, Du SX, Li XD. Meta-analysis comparing denosumab and zoledronic acid for treatment of bone metastases in patients with advanced solid tumours. Eur J Cancer Care (Engl). 2016. https://doi.org/10.1111/ecc.12541. [Epub ahead of print].

39. Ecker RD, Endo T, Wetjen NM, Krauss WE. Diagnosis and treatment of vertebral column metastasis. Mayo Clin Proc. 2005;80(9):1177–86.

40. Bilsky MH, Lis E, Raizer J, Lee H, Boland P. The diagnosis and treatment of metastatic spinal tumor. Oncologist. 1999;4:459–69.

41. Liu T, Xu JY, Xu W, Bai YR, Yan WL, Yang HL. Fluorine-18 deoxyglucose positron emission tomography, magnetic resonance imaging and bone scintigraphy for the diagnosis of bone metastases in patients with lung cancer: which one is the best? A meta-analysis. Clin Oncol (R Coll Radiol). 2011;23: 350–8.

42. Maralani PJ, Lo SS, Redmond K, Soliman H, Myrehaug S, Husain ZA, Heyn C, Kapadia A, Chan A, Sahgal A. Spinal metastases: multimodality imaging in diagnosis and stereotactic body radiation therapy planning. Future Oncol. 2017;13:77–91. https://doi.org/10.2217/fon-2016-0238.

43. O'Sullivan GJ, Carty FL, Cronin CG. Imaging of bone metastasis: an update. World J Radiol. 2015; 7(8):202–11.

44. Bastawrous S, Bhargava P, Behnia F, Djang DSW, Haseley DR. Newer PET application with an old tracer: role of 18F-NaF skeletal PET/CT in oncologic practice. Radiographics. 2014;34:1295–316. https://doi.org/10.1148/rg.345130061.

45. Denaro L, Di Martino A, et al. Cervical spine bone tumor surgery. Berlin Heidelberg: Springer; 2010. p. 165–74.

46. Gasbarrini A, Casadei R, Papapietro N. Il trattamento delle metastasi vertebrali. GIOT. 2012;38:188–93.

47. Denaro V. Stenosis of the cervical spine. Berlin: Springer; 1994.

48. Denaro V, Denaro L, Albo E, Papapietro N, Piccioli A, Di Martino A. Surgical management of spinal fractures and neurological involvement in patients with myeloma. Injury. 2016;47(Suppl 4):S49–53. https://doi.org/10.1016/j.injury.2016.07.047. Epub 2016 Aug 6.

49. Chen B, Xiao S, et al. Comparison of the therapeutic efficacy of surgery with or without adjuvant radiotherapy versus radiotherapy alone for metastatic spinal cord compression: a meta-analysis. World Neurosurg. 2015;6:1066–73.

50. Agabegi SS, Asghar FA, Herkowitz HN. Spinal orthoses. J Am Acad Orthop Surg. 2010;18(11):657–67.

51. Di Martino A, Caldaria A, De Vivo V, Denaro V. Metastatic epidural spinal cord compression. Expert Rev Anticancer Ther. 2016;12:1–10.

52. Zairi F, Marinho P, Bouras A, Allaoui M, Assaker R. Recent concepts in the management of thoracolumbar spine metastasis. J Neurosurg Sci. 2013;57(1):45–54.

53. Denaro V, Di Martino A. Cervical spine surgery: an historical perspective. Clin Orthop Relat Res. 2011;469(3):639–48. https://doi.org/10.1007/s11999-010-1752-3.

54. Roy-Camille R, Judet TH, Saillant G, Mamoudy P, Denaro V. Tumeurs du rachis. Encicl med-Chir Techniquee Chirurgicales. Orthopedie. 1982;11: 44–165.

55. Denaro V. Treatment of metastases and systemic tumors of the cervical spine. Neuroorthopedics. 1988;6: 101–10.

56. Shimizu K, Shikata J, Iida H, Iwasaki R, Yoshikawa J, Yamamuro T. Posterior decompression and stabilization for multiple metastatic tumors of the spine. Spine. 1992;17:1400–4.

57. Cappuccio M, Gasbarrini A, et al. Vertebroplasty in the treatment of vertebral metastases: clinical cases and review of the literature. Eur Rev Med Pharmacol Sci. 2007;11(2):91–100.

58. Luksanapruksa P, Buchowski JM, Zebala LP, Kepler CK, Singhatanadgige W, Bumpass DB. Perioperative complications of spinal metastases surgery. Clin Spine Surg. 2017;30(1):4–13.

59. Scibilia A, Terranova C, Rizzo V, Raffa G, Morelli A, Esposito F, Mallamace R, Buda G, Conti A, Quartarone A, Germanò A. Intraoperative neurophysiological mapping and monitoring in spinal tumor surgery: sirens or indispensable tools? Neurosurg Focus. 2016;41(2):E18. https://doi.org/10.3171/2016.5.FOCUS16141.

60. Laufer I, Iorgulescu JB, Chapman T, Lis E, Shi W, Zhang Z, et al. Local disease control for spinal metastases following "separation surgery" and adjuvant hypofractionated or highdose single-fraction stereotactic radiosurgery: outcome analysis in 186 patients. J Neurosurg Spine. 2013;18:207–14.

Megaprosthesis for Metastasis of the Lower Limb

14

Carmine Zoccali, Dario Attala, Alessandra Scotto, and Roberto Biagini

Abstract

In the past, the surgical approach to bone metastasis had the sole purpose to solve a biomechanical problem because the patient would die for systemic disease progression. Intramedullary nailing was the mainstay of the treatment, and its aim was allowing the patient to stand, with local tumor control achieved by radiotherapy [1, 2]. The improvement of medical therapy, radiotherapy and new diagnostic techniques have led to an increment of global life expectancy in bone metastatic patients, so complications related to the first surgery, often requiring further surgeries, are more common (Fig.1) [3, 5].

Today, the surgeon has to take the possibility of a long survival into account, moreover if the patient has just one bone metastatic disease; this means performing more resections with wide margins and prosthetic reconstruction than before [6].

Resection has to be considered after taking account of several factors which have to be evaluated from a multidisciplinary point of view and

considering life expectancy: the oncologist, the orthopedic surgeon, the pathologist, the radiotherapist and the anesthesiologist are the main protagonists. The final decision has to be taken by the patient, once correctly informed about advantages and disadvantages of the possible procedures [7].

14.1 Introduction

In the past, the surgical approach to bone metastasis had the sole purpose to solve a biomechanical problem because the patient would die for systemic disease progression. Intramedullary nailing was the mainstay of the treatment, and its aim was allowing the patient to stand, with local tumor control achieved by radiotherapy [1, 2].

The improvement of medical therapy, radiotherapy, and new diagnostic techniques has led to an increment of global life expectancy in bone metastatic patients, so complications related to the first surgery, often requiring further surgeries, are more common (Fig. 14.1) [3, 4].

Today, the surgeon has to take the possibility of a long survival into account, above all if the patient has just a single localization of bone metastatic disease; this means performing more resections with wide margins and prosthetic reconstruction than before [5].

C. Zoccali · D. Attala · R. Biagini (✉)
Oncological Ortopedics,
Regina Elena National Cancer Institute, Rome, Italy
e-mail: biagini@ifo.it

A. Scotto
School of Medicine,
Tor Vergata University, Rome, Italy

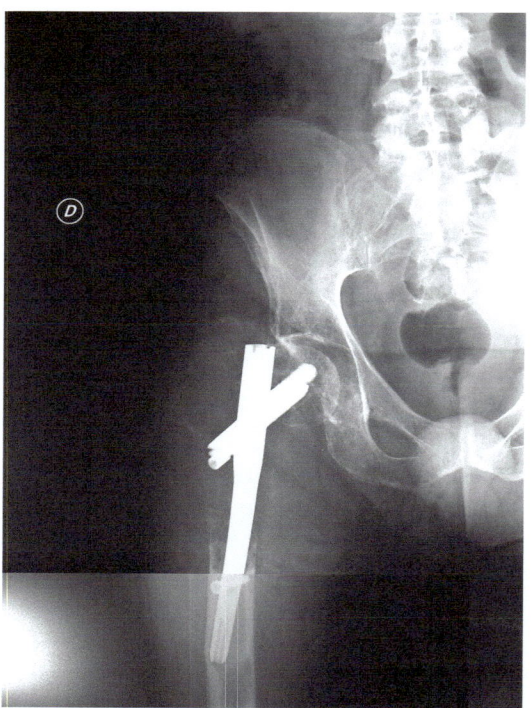

Fig. 14.1 An intramedullary nail failure because of a local lung metastasis progression in a long survivor

Indeed, it is hypothesized that an intralesional violation of the metastasis can increase its biological activity because of the growth factors associated to bleeding and hematoma.

14.2   Indications for Resection

Resection has to be considered after taking account of several factors which have to be evaluated from a multidisciplinary point of view and considering life expectancy: the oncologist, the orthopedic surgeon, the pathologist, the radiotherapist, and the anesthesiologist are the main protagonists. The final decision has to be taken by the patient, once correctly informed about advantages and disadvantages of the possible procedures [6].

The main factors that have to be considered are:

– The histology: renal, breast, and prostate tumors are considered favorable histologies, while lung and gastric cancers are considered unfavorable [6].

– The time since the extirpation of the primary tumor: in case of metastasis and primary tumor synchrony, the power of indication is low; otherwise, the longer is the time since the extirpation of the primary tumor, the stronger is the indication for wide resection.
– The number of metastasis: when the secondary lesion is solitary, the indication is strong; the power rapidly decreases with the number of lesions [6–9].
– Presence of visceral metastases: visceral metastases are a relative contraindication for wide surgery [6].
– The availability of other systemic adjuvant therapies: indeed, the existence of other therapies such as chemotherapy, immunotherapy, and bisphosphonates increases the possibilities that the patient may be a long survivor.
– The availability of local adjuvant therapy: if the metastasis is radiosensitive, an intralesional surgery, like an intramedullary nail stabilization for long bones, could be more indicated because the adjuvant local therapy can decrease the risk of local progression; otherwise, in case of radioresistant histologies (for instance, kidney), resection can be considered in order to decrease the risk of local progression after intralesional surgery.
– Comorbidities: global health status is always to be considered; sometimes resections are very stressful surgeries that can expose the patient to a high complication rate [10–12].
– The site of the metastasis: the more accessible it is, the stronger the indication. A patient with a solitary lesion of the proximal femur presents a stronger indication for resection than a patient with a solitary lesion of a vertebra. The approaches to the spine and the acetabular areas in the pelvis are considered high demanding procedures [6]. Nevertheless, some studies sustain that global survival is independent from the site of metastasis [13].

14.3   Estimation of Fracture Risk

In bone metastasis, indication for surgery is often directly related to the risk of fracture.

Table 14.1 Mirels' scoring system

	1	2	3
Location	Upper extremity	Lower extremity	Intertrochanteric
Radiographic appearance	Blastic	Mixed	Lytic
Size	<1/3	1/3–2/3	>2/3
Pain	Mild	Moderate	Severe and functional

It depends on several factors as the site of metastasis, its size, if it is osteoblastic or osteolytic.

The most used system is the Mirels' classification [14]; it consists of four items: location of the metastasis, its nature and radiographic appearance, its size related to the diameter of the entire segment, and the presence of pain. Each item is scaled from 1 to 3.

For total score of 7 or less, observation and radiation therapy is advisable; for total score of 9 or more, prophylactic fixation is suggested; if the score is 8, the indication is uncertain, and it should be valued based on clinical conditions as well.

In multimetastatic patients, even if the treatment of these lesions usually does not directly modify their survival, if the patient is constricted to bed because of the risk of fractures, he or she is exposed to complications that could interfere with medical therapies, thus decreasing survival [15, 16].

14.4 General Surgical Consideration

- In metastatic patients, the reconstruction is often sacrificed to reduce the risk of infection; indeed, in case of complications, it could be difficult to start chemotherapy with a negative influence on the patient's survival [17, 18].
- In metastatic patients, the prosthetic intramedullary stem should be as long as possible to stabilize the entire segment in case of future, more distant metastases [19].
- In metastatic patients, the prosthetic intramedullary stem should always be cemented to decrease the risk of mobilization in case of further metastases or in case of radiotherapy [19].

In this chapter, we analyze resection and prosthesis reconstruction in the different segments at the lower limb.

14.5 Proximal Femur Resection and Prosthetic Reconstruction

The proximal femur is the most common site of metastasis, after the spine [20]. The proximal third, and particularly the neck, is the preferential site, exposing the patient to a high risk of pathological fractures. Indeed, that risk has to be valued especially in the inferior limbs to give the indication for surgery.

Indications: in addition to general considerations for resection, in the proximal femur, the precise site of the metastasis has to be considered to evaluate the prosthetic reconstruction. If the lesion is in the femoral head or in the neck, the indication for resection and reconstruction is stronger because the risk of cut out is important.

Surgery is usually performed via a lateral approach, removing the biopsy track en bloc with the tumor. Unfortunately, pelvic-trochanteric tendon insertions are frequently sacrificed, with a consequent instability and loss of function. Some authors advocate the use of trevira tubes to increase joint stability and function by reattaching soft tissue [21].

Reconstruction is usually performed with a modular endoprosthesis which is assembled to reach the size of the resection (Fig. 14.2) [22–24].

The replacement of the acetabular surface is only suggested in young patients with a long life expectancy, to decrease the risk of pain or in case of its metastatic involvement, otherwise endoprosthetic reconstruction should be preferred to decrease the risk of postoperative complications that could interfere with systemic therapies [25].

In multimetastatic patients the intramedullary stem should be as long as possible to reinforce the entire femur, stabilizing the segment also in case of the onset of further distal metastasis. If

Fig. 14.2 An intra-operative picture showing a modular endoprosthesis replacing the proximal 12 cm of the femur

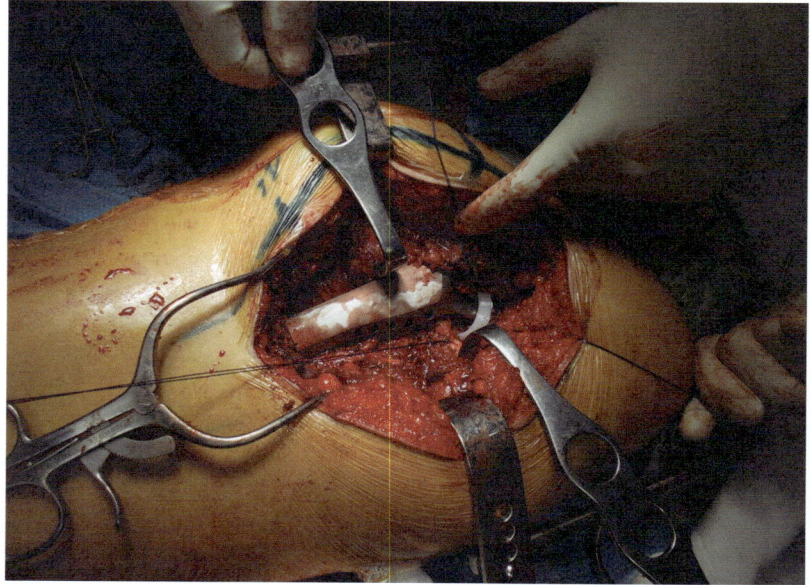

Fig.14.3 A modular prosthesis useful to reconstruct the proximal femur when the tumor is located in the femoral head or neck, sparing the lesser and greater trochanters; on the right the postoperative X-Ray

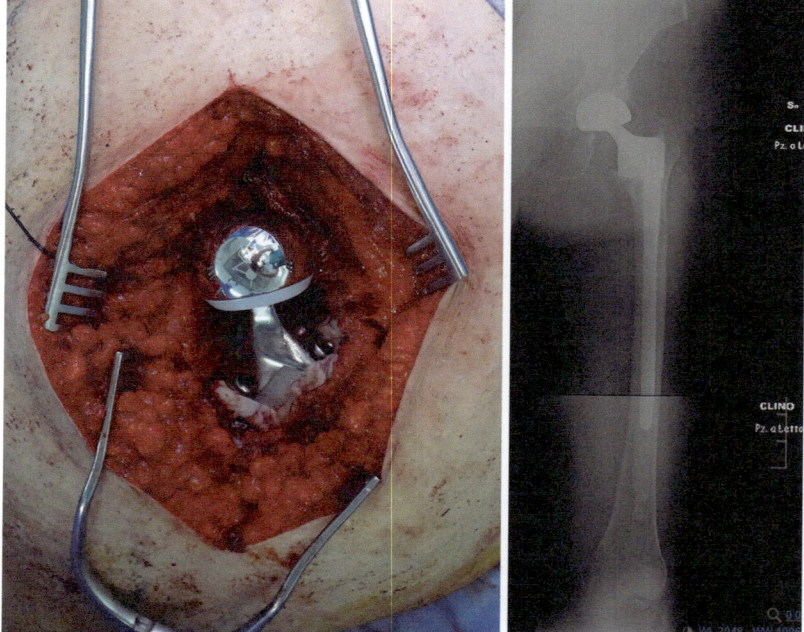

the lesion is located in the femoral neck or in the femoral head, the greater and the lesser trochanters can be spared, maintaining the muscular insertions (Fig. 14.3) [26].

An ideal modular prosthesis should allow a minimal resection, arming the entire femur when necessary; it should be cemented to assure grip even in case of further metastases.

Resection also has to be preferred in case of multimetastatic patients when the disease extends to the femoral head and neck; intramedullary nailing can complicate with proximal screw cut out.

Results: the patients who undergo proximal femur resection usually present a lower function than those who go through intramedullary stabilization; it is reasonable to wear a pelvic brace to reduce the risk of dislocation [27];

Nevertheless, the percentage of satisfaction is quite consistent, in particular with lesions located at the femoral head and neck, where it is possible to spare muscles' insertions. Bischel and Böhm, in 2010, published a series of 31 resections and prosthetic reconstruction of the proximal femur and reported a mean postoperative Musculoskeletal Tumor Society score of 62.4% and an increase of the mean Karnofsky index from 44.2% preoperatively to 59.7% postoperatively [19].

The main complications are infections (6–20% of cases) and dislocations (4–10%) [28]; some authors advocate the use of trevira tubes to reduce the risk of dislocation, and sustaining it does not increase the infection ratio, but more studies are necessary to confirm this aspect [19, 21, 29].

14.6   Femoral Diaphysis Resection and Reconstruction

Indications: indication for resection of the diaphyseal femur is rare. Reconstruction can be performed with a diaphyseal prosthesis (Fig. 14.4) or by a homograft filled with cement and stabi-

lized with plate and screws [30]. In this case, as in the humerus, a potential limitation is the need to have a sufficient length of healthy canal, proximally and distally to the resected segment, to allow the insertion of the intramedullary stem. A possible solution is to use a diaphyseal homograph filled with cement to reach the sufficient length to stabilize the prosthesis stem.

Surgery: The surgical approach is lateral; pay attention to recognizing and isolating neurovascular bundles in case of very distal resections.

Results: no specific data is available in literature; however, it is reasonable to sustain that the functional outcome is directly related to the muscles spared.

14.7   Distal Femur Resection and Prosthesis Reconstruction

Indications: indication for resection and prosthetic reconstruction of the distal femur is rare. When a metastasis is located at the distal part of the femur, resection can be necessary even in multimetastatic patients because it may be impossible to stabilize the segment with an intramedullary nail (Fig. 14.5).

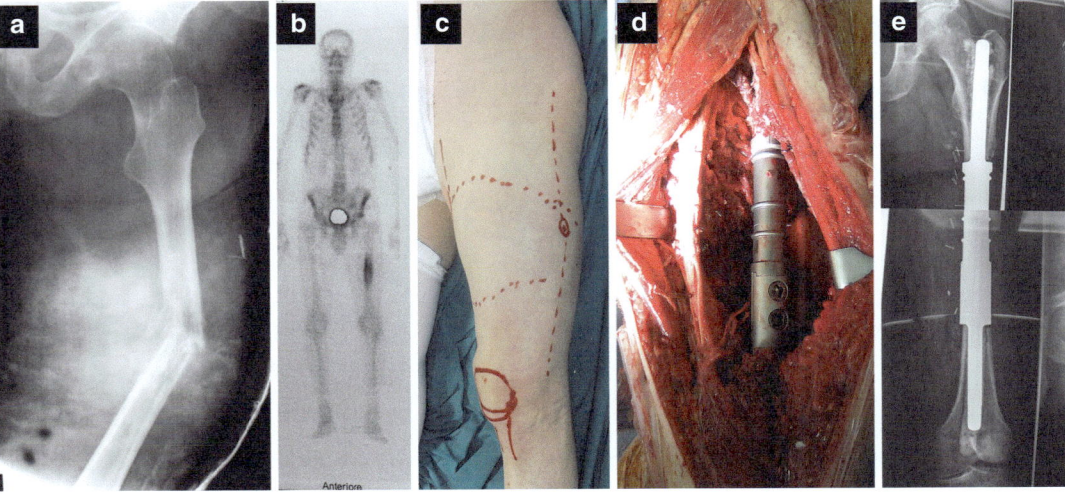

Fig.14.4 A patient affected by a diaphyseal pathological fracture of the left femur from kidney metastasis (**a**); the bone scan, previously performed, evidenced a solitary bone lesion (**b**); (**c**) the patient in supine position; the longitudinal dashed line corresponds to the surgical incision; (**d**) the prosthesis after reconstruction; (**e**) postoperative X-Ray

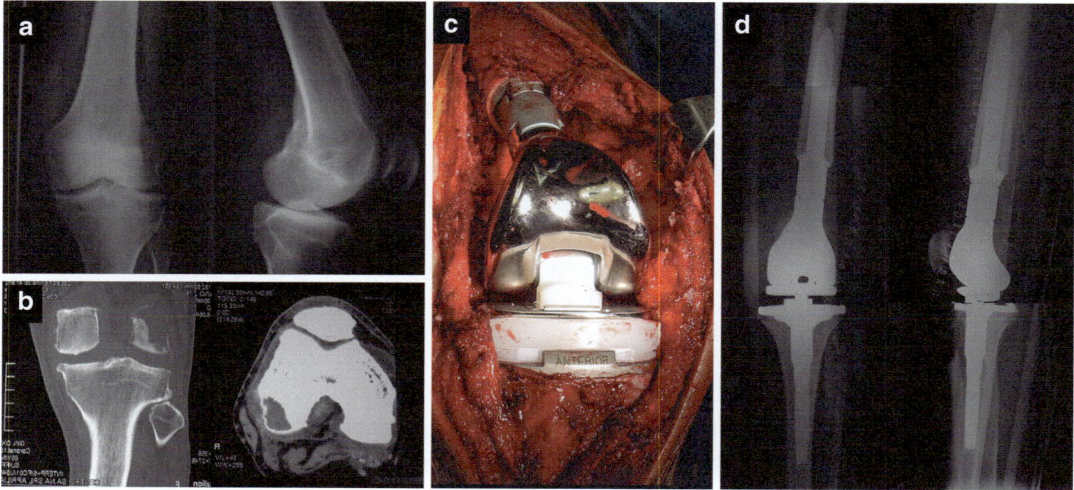

Fig.14.5 (**a**, **b**) Preoperative X-Ray and CT scan showing a renal metastasis of the lateral femoral condyle; (**c**) the prosthesis inserted in situ; (**d**) postoperative X-ray

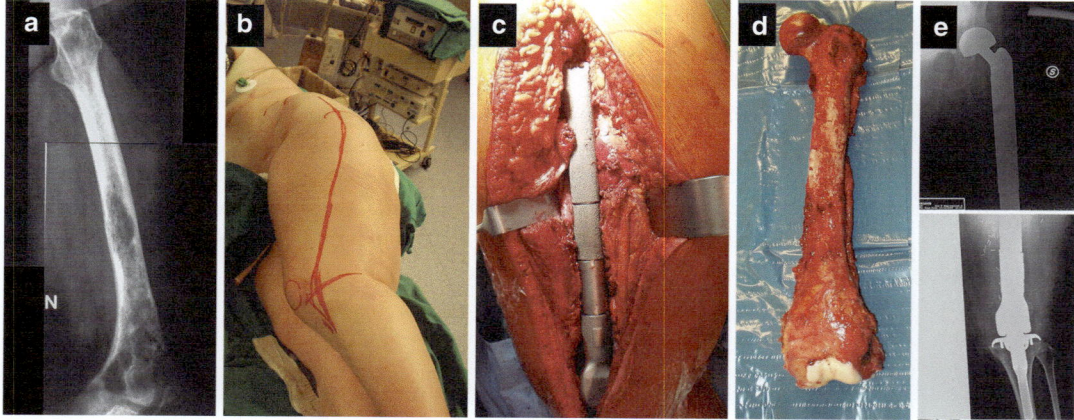

Fig. 14.6 (**a**) A solitary extensive metastasis of the left femur from breast cancer; (**b**) the surgical access; (**c**) the prosthesis in situ after resection; (**d**) The resected femur; (**e**) postoperative X-Ray

Surgery: The access is lateral and prolonged distally, laterally to the patella and the patellar tendon, till the tibial tuberosity. The insertion of the femoral bicep should be cut to allow a better view and isolation of the popliteal vessels, paying attention to spare the external popliteal nerve.

Results: Pala et al. recently reported satisfactory results for knee megaprosthesis, considering resections for distal femur and for proximal tibia tumors together; they presented a mean MSTS score of 84%, with no difference between sites of localization [31]. Also, for distal femur as for proximal femur, the most frequent cause of failure is infection; aseptic

loosening is the second most commune complication [32].

14.8 Total Femur Resection and Prosthetic Reconstruction

It is a very unusual indication which has to be accurately evaluated considering the high risk of complications such as infections. The surgery is performed with a lateral approach, extended for the whole length of the thigh and prolonged down to the tibial tuberosity (Fig. 14.6). The residual function is directly related to the muscular sparing. Because of the extension of the surgical approach, the infection rate is consistent and should be considered the main limit to the indication.

14.9 Proximal Tibial Resection and Prosthesis Reconstruction

Indications: rarely, in case of lesions located at the proximal part of the tibia, resection and prosthetic reconstruction can be indicated, especially in case of a single metastasis. Sometimes resection can even be necessary in multimetastatic patient where the osteolysis is too proximal or when minimally invasive techniques are not possible to be performed.

Surgery: the surgical approach is medial, with the incision starting from the medial aspect of the distal femur and prolonged distally along the medial tibial edge. Unfortunately, sacrificing the pes anserinus tendons to have access to the popliteal neurovascular bundles is often necessary. It is recommended to completely identify and isolate the popliteal vessels, the bifurcation, and the subsequent anterior and posterior tibial rami. Sometimes the anterior tibial vessels can be involved by the tumor; these can be ligated in young patients with a good chance to keep a valid distal vascular supply by the posterior tibial artery; however, in older patients ligation of the anterior tibial artery could determine a distal necrosis since the posterior tibial artery may not be sufficient to sustain the distal perfusion in the case of a preexistent vascular disease. In that case, an artery bypass could be considered, but the results are low, and the risk of secondary amputation should be taken into account.

14.10 Tibial Diaphysis Resection and Reconstruction

Indications: lesions located in the tibial diaphysis are usually treated by the implant of an intramedullary locked nail. However, in long survivors, surgical resection could be suitable. Resection can also be indicated in case of radioresistant metastasis to decrease the risk of further local progression and secondary amputation. Prosthesis reconstruction is demanding, and results are quite poor because often soft tissues are not sufficient to ensure an adequate prosthesis coverage, and a surgical flap could be necessary; a sufficient segment of healthy medullary canal is obviously necessary for proximal and distal stem insertion.

Surgery: the surgical approach is anterior and the incision has to be valued considering both the tumor and the skin closure. Particular attention has to be paid to spare the anterior vascular bundle during the section of the interosseous membrane.

Results: no specific data for reconstruction after bone metastasis resection at this site is available in literature; nevertheless, Sewell et al. published a series of 18 patients who underwent tibial diaphyseal prosthetic replacement after primitive bone tumor. They reported aseptic loosening and periprosthetic fractures in four and two patients, respectively, with a mean Musculoskeletal Tumor Society score of 76.7% [33].

14.11 Distal Tibia Resection and Prosthesis Reconstruction

Indications: lesions located in the distal tibia are rare; in most cases these are treated conservatively; furthermore, resection and prosthesis reconstruction is technically difficult, and only specialized centers have a sufficient experience.

Surgery: the incision is anterior and tailored on the specific patient; the anterior neurovascular bundle is isolated and retracted to decrease the risk of distal necrosis. After resection, the reconstruction is performed with a tibial component with an intramedullary stem, and a distal talar component whereof the stem is inserted in the talus and the calcaneus (Fig. 14.7).

Results: no specific data after metastasis resection in this region is available in literature; also in this case, the main problem is the anterior prosthesis coverage, so a surgical flap could be advocated to reduce the suture tension. In our opinion, the risk of infection and mobilization of the distal stem, introduced in the talar and calcaneus bone, are the main dangers.

Fig. 14.7 Postoperative
X-ray showing distal
tibia prosthesis

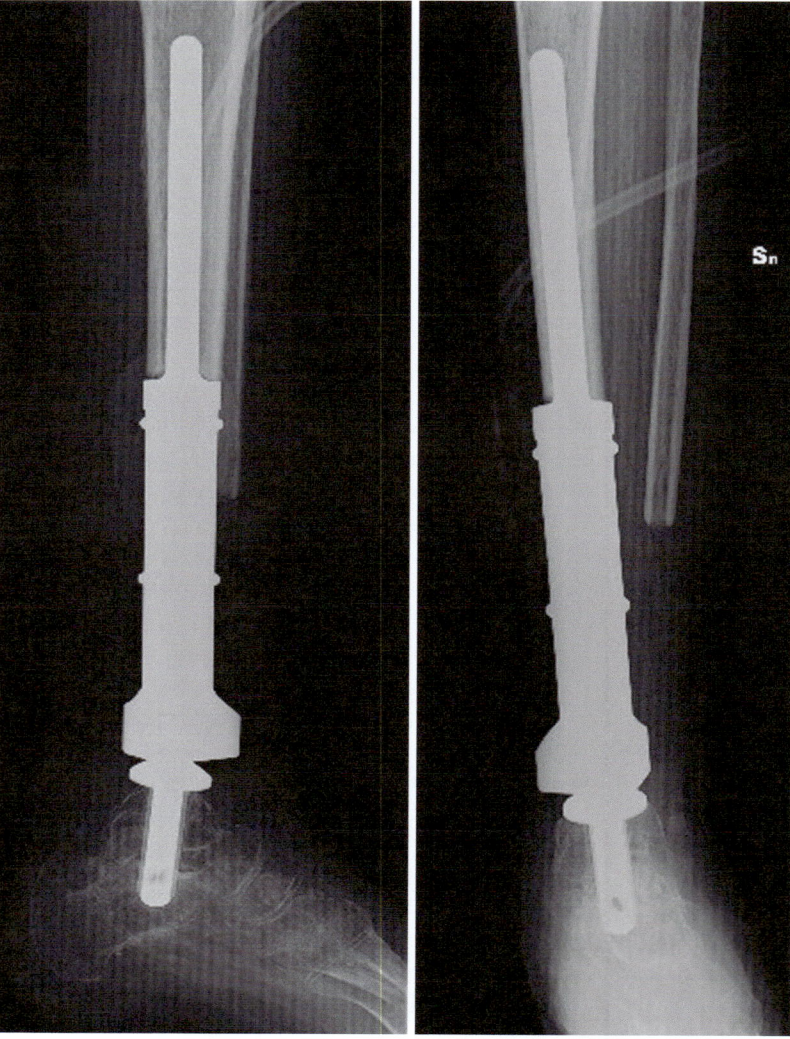

Shekkeris et al. published the result of a cohort of six patients who underwent prosthesis reconstruction after resection of primitive distal tibia bone tumor. They reported two below-knee amputations for persistent infection. For the other four cases, the mean Musculoskeletal Tumor Society score was 70% [34].

References

1. Durandeau A, Geneste R. Surgical treatment of metastatic fractures and metastases of the long bones. Apropos of 73 cases. Rev Chir Orthop Reparatrice Appar Mot. 1977;63(5):501–17.
2. Futani H, Kamae S, Atsui K, Yoh K, Tateishi H, Maruo S. Successful limb salvage of pathological fracture of the distal tibia caused by cancer metastasis. J Orthop Sci. 2002;7(2):262–6.
3. Coleman RE. Clinical features of metastatic bone disease and risk of skeletal morbidity. Clin Cancer Res. 2006;12(20 Pt 2):6243s–9s.
4. Forsberg JA, Eberhardt J, Boland PJ, Wedin R, Healey JH. Estimating survival in patients with operable skeletal metastases: an application of a Bayesian belief network. PLoS One. 2011;6:e19956.
5. Gao H, Liu Z, Wang B, Guo A. Clinical and functional comparison of endoprosthetic replacement with intramedullary nailing for treating proximal femur metastasis. Chin J Cancer Res. 2016;28(2):209–14.
6. Nathan SS, Healey JH, Mellano D, Hoang B, Lewis I, Morris CD, et al. Survival in patients operated on

for pathologic fracture: implications for end-of-life orthopedic care. J Clin Oncol. 2005;23(25):6072–82.

7. Chan D, Carter SR, Grimer RJ, Sneath RS. Endoprosthetic replacement for bony metastases. Ann R Coll Surg Engl. 1992;74:13–8.

8. Bauer HC, Wedin R. Survival after surgery for spinal and extremity metastases: prognostication in 241 patients. Acta Orthop Scand. 1995;66:143–6.

9. Coleman RE, Rubens RD. The clinical course of bone metastases from breast cancer. Br J Cancer. 1987; 55:61–6.

10. Oken MM, Creech RH, Tormey DC, Horton J, Davis TE, McFadden ET, et al. Toxicity and response criteria of the Eastern Cooperative Oncology Group. Am J Clin Oncol. 1982;5(6):649–55.

11. Masutani M, Tsujino I, Fujie T, Yamaguchi M, Miyagi K, Yano T, et al. Moderate dose-intensive chemotherapy for patients with non-small cell lung cancer: randomized trial, can it improve survival of patients with good performance status? Oncol Rep. 1999;6(5):1045–50.

12. Mani S, Todd MB, Katz K, Poo WJ. Prognostic factors for survival in patients with metastatic renal cancer treated with biological response modifiers. J Urol. 1995;154(1):35–40.

13. Bohm P, Huber J. The surgical treatment of bony metastases of the spine and limbs. J Bone Joint Surg Br. 2002;84:521–9.

14. Mirels H. Metastatic disease in long bones: a proposed scoring system for diagnosing impending pathologic fractures. Clin Orthop Relat Res. 2003; 415(Suppl):S4–13.

15. Zacherl M, Gruber G, Glehr M, Ofner-Kopeinig P, Radl R, Greitbauer M, et al. Surgery for pathological proximal femoral fractures, excluding femoral head and neck fractures: resection vs. stabilisation. Int Orthop. 2011;35(10):1537–43.

16. Camnasio F, Scotti C, Peretti GM, Fontana F, Fraschini G. Prosthetic joint replacement for long bone metastases: analysis of 154 cases. Arch Orthop Trauma Surg. 2008;128(8):787–93.

17. Kapoor SK, Thiyam R. Management of infection following reconstruction in bone tumors. J Clin Orthop Trauma. 2015;6(4):244–51.

18. Rossi B, Zoccali C, Toma L, Ferraresi V, Biagini R. Surgical site infections in treatment of musculoskeletal tumors: experience from a single oncologic orthopedic institution. J Orthop Oncol. 2016;2:108.

19. Bischel OE, Böhm PM. The use of a femoral revision stem in the treatment of primary or secondary bone tumours of the proximal femur: a prospective study of 31 cases. J Bone Joint Surg Br. 2010;92(10):1435–41.

20. Campanacci M. Bone and soft tissue tumors. New York: Springer; 1999.

21. Gosheger G, Hillmann A, Lindner N, Rödl R, Hoffmann C, Bürger H, et al. Soft tissue reconstruction of megaprostheses using a trevira tube. Clin Orthop Relat Res. 2001;393:264–71.

22. Guzik G. Results of the treatment of bone metastases with modular prosthetic replacement-analysis of 67 patients. J Orthop Surg Res. 2016;11(1):20.

23. Henrichs MP, Krebs J, Gosheger G, Streitbuerger A, Nottrott M, Sauer T, et al. Modular tumor endoprostheses in surgical palliation of long-bone metastases: a reduction in tumor burden and a durable reconstruction. World J Surg Oncol. 2014; 12:330.

24. Chandrasekar CR, Grimer RJ, Carter SR, Tillman RM, Abudu A, Buckley L. Modular endoprosthetic replacement for tumours of the proximal femur. J Bone Joint Surg Br. 2009;91(1):108–12.

25. Haentjens P, de Neve W, Casteleyn PP, Opdecam P. Massive resection and prosthetic replacement for the treatment of metastases of the trochanteric and subtrochanteric femoral region bipolar arthroplasty versus total hip arthroplasty. Acta Orthop Belg. 1993; 59(Suppl 1):367–71.

26. Cho HS, Lee YK, Ha YC, Koo KH. Trochanter/calcar preserving reconstruction in tumors involving the femoral head and neck. World J Orthop. 2016;7(7): 442–7.

27. Manoso MW, Frassica DA, Lietman ES, Frassica FJ. Proximal femoral replacement for metastatic bone disease. Orthopedics. 2007;30(5):384–8.

28. Calabró T, Van Rooyen R, Piraino I, Pala E, Trovarelli G, Panagopoulos GN, et al. Reconstruction of the proximal femur with a modular resection prosthesis. Eur J Orthop Surg Traumatol. 2016;26(4):415–21.

29. Winkelmann W. Reconstruction of the proximal femur with the MUTARS® system. Orthopade. 2010; 39(10):942–8.

30. Benevenia J, Kirchner R, Patterson F, Beebe K, Wirtz DC, Rivero S, et al. Outcomes of a modular intercalary endoprosthesis as treatment for segmental defects of the femur, tibia, and humerus. Clin Orthop Relat Res. 2016;474:549–50.

31. Pala E, Trovarelli G, Calabrò T, Angelini A, Abati CN, Ruggieri P. Survival of modern knee tumor megaprostheses: failures, functional results, and a comparative statistical analysis. Clin Orthop Relat Res. 2015;473(3):891–9.

32. Pala E, Trovarelli G, Angelini A, Ruggieri P. Distal femur reconstruction with modular tumour prostheses: a single institution analysis of implant survival comparing fixed versus rotating hinge knee prostheses. Int Orthop. 2016;40(10):2171–80.

33. Sewell MD, Hanna SA, McGrath A, Aston WJ, Blunn GW, Pollock RC, et al. Intercalary diaphyseal endoprosthetic reconstruction for malignant tibial bone tumours. J Bone Joint Surg Br. 2011;93(8): 1111–7.

34. Shekkeris AS, Hanna SA, Sewell MD, Spiegelberg BG, Aston WJ, Blunn GW, et al. Endoprosthetic reconstruction of the distal tibia and ankle joint after resection of primary bone tumours. J Bone Joint Surg Br. 2009;91(10):1378–82.

Metastases to the Pelvis

15

Eduardo J. Ortiz-Cruz, Manuel Peleteiro-Pensado,
Irene Barrientos-Ruiz, and
Rafael Carbonell-Escobar

Abstract

The optimal surgical treatment of bone metastases may be complex and require multimodality
treatment strategies to achieve optimal outcomes. We describe the surgical indications of
these patients, mainly in the periacetabular zone.

15.1 Introduction

Metastatic bone disease (MBD) to the pelvis is a
challenging problem that affects the patient's quality of life (QOL) and is more frequently encountered by orthopedic surgeons. Pelvic metastases
cause pain, pathologic fractures, and limit the ability to ambulate independently. Due to the relatively large dimension of the pelvic cavity, tumors
at that location usually reach a significant size
before symptoms appear.

Some locations of metastases within the pelvis have no important impact on pelvic stability
and function (e.g., ilium and pubis), but tumors
located at the posterior ilium may carry a risk for
lumbosacral integrity, and tumors of the acetabulum may impair the hip function and the weight-
bearing of extremity. Engagement of the
acetabular region entails a major risk for pathological fracture due to the high mechanical loads.

The optimal treatment of bone metastases
may be complex and require multimodality treatment strategies to achieve optimal outcomes, and
these patients need multidisciplinary approach.

15.2 Treatment Planning

The selected procedure should offer an adequate
treatment to the patient in order to achieve the
best possible quality of life (QOL) while eluding
an under- or overtreatment. Factors associated
with poor QOL include loss of limb function,
being bedridden, *and* the occurrence of pathologic fractures. There are three types of treatment: nonoperative treatment, minimally invasive
palliative procedures, and surgical treatment.

The treatment depends on the patient's symptoms, prognosis, patient class [1], histological
type, and the site of the metastasis, bone loss,
performance status, patients, and family goals.

15.2.1 Minimally Invasive Palliative Procedures

Radiation therapy is effective in providing relief
from painful bone metastasis with a global pain
response rate as 60%, and therefore the external

E. J. Ortiz-Cruz (✉) · M. Peleteiro-Pensado ·
I. Barrientos-Ruiz ·
R. Carbonell-Escobar
Orthopaedic Oncology Unit,
Orthopaedic Surgery Department,
Hospital Universitario La Paz, Madrid, Spain
e-mail: rcarbonell@alumni.unav.es

© Springer International Publishing AG, part of Springer Nature 2019
V. Denaro et al. (eds.), *Management of Bone Metastases*, https://doi.org/10.1007/978-3-319-73485-9_15

irradiation is the standard care for patients with localized bone pain and palliation of the majority of these patients [2, 3].

However, patients who have recurrent pain at a site previously irradiated may not be eligible for further radiation therapy, and if they are not candidates for surgery, the advances in interventional radiology add to our armamentarium a palliative treatment of their symptoms [4].

The most frequent techniques are radiofrequency ablation, microwave ablation, cryoablation, and cementoplasty, which could be used in combination with the previous techniques [5–10].

15.2.2 Surgical Treatment

Surgical management of MBD is typically reserved for lesions with the highest risk of fracture and some solitary metastases. Curative resection is rare for bone metastasis, except for selected patients with isolated involvement; MBD requires mainly a palliative approach.

Although these procedures have a high rate of complications, the improvement of the quality of life could justify the surgical risks [11].

15.2.2.1 We Need to Know

The management of pelvic tumors is a challenge for orthopedics oncologists due to the complex anatomy of the pelvis and the need to have extensive exposures. The decision to proceed with surgery can be difficult for the clinician and the patient, as the risks of surgery may outweigh the expected benefits of improvement in pain and function.

The surgeon needs to understand the next issues and allow to answer some questions that are formulated in the next paragraphs:

– Comprehend the anatomic classification by Enneking. This classification is based on the resected region of the pelvis: type I, ilium; type II, periacetabular; type III, pubis; and resection of sacrum type IV resection [12] (Fig. 15.1).
– Comprehend the patients "classes," which are essential to distinguish which patients require a surgical treatment. Capanna and Campanacci [1] introduced a protocol in long bone metastases, which provide an aim to look for a suitable treatment and working for pelvic metastases too. The patients were divided into four classes: (1) solitary lesion with good prognosis, (2)

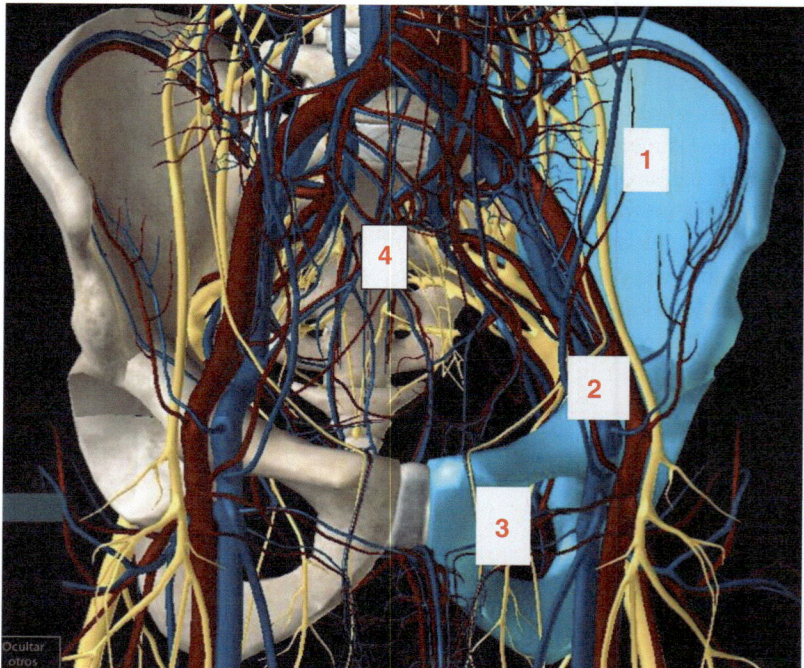

Fig. 15.1 Anatomic classification by Enneking. Type I, ilium; type II, periacetabular; type III, pubis; and type IV, sacrum resection

pathologic fracture, (3) impending fracture, and (4) osteoblastic lesions at all sites; osteolytic or mixed lesions in non-weight-bearing bones such as the fibula, ribs, sternum, or clavicle; osteolytic lesions in major bones with no impending fracture; and lesions in the iliac wing, anterior pelvis, or scapula.

Patients included in classes 1, 2, and 3 should have been referred to oncology orthopedic surgeon for possible surgical treatment. Class 4 patients are treated mainly conservatively by chemotherapy, hormonotherapy, and/or radiation therapy. Diphosphonates, narcotic analgesia, radiation therapy, and protected weight-bearing are the first steps in this nonsurgical management. The radiotherapy should not be indicated before surgery because of problems with wound healing that can occur.

- Recognize the zones of the pelvis those are at risk for mechanical failure and require surgery.
  - According to Muller and Cappanna, zones 1 and 3 are comparable to non-weight-bearing and expendable bones of the extremity (clavicle, sternum, and fibula). Zone 2 equals to the articular part of long bones (humerus, femur, and tibia), and those are the lesions with a high risk for mechanical failure.
  - Metastatic lesions in zones 1 and 3 (pubic rami, ischia, iliac wings) do not compromise the mechanical stability of the pelvic ring, and most of them don't require surgery and are not amenable to reconstruction. Patients with lesions in these locations often are managed with nonoperative treatment, in the form of medical and radiation therapy or with resection only. In contrast, the condition of patients with metastatic lesions about the acetabulum that result in progressive functional pain, hip protrusion, pathologic fracture, and inability to ambulate often is improved by operative reconstruction [13].
- Patient prognosis and an estimation of survival will help dictate the best treatment indication [14, 15].
- It is important to understand the metastatic acetabular classifications described by Harrington [16] and Issack et al. [17] in order to select the best type of surgical management.
- Nonetheless, there is significant risk of morbidity and mortality that had to take in mind. Wood and coworkers [18] accomplished a systematic review of the literature in patients with MBD to the long bones and/or pelvis/acetabulum treated surgically, and they found a surgical advantage if the surgery is done and well indicated.
- If the indication for surgery is made, which type of surgery is the best for the patient? What type of margin and what type of reconstruction? Regard which resection has to be indicated, after analysis of the literature; there are few data available to compare the outcome of wide resection and intralesional resection for pelvic metastases.
- Ruggieri et al. [19] evaluate the role of intralesional/marginal resection compared to wide resection, and they didn't found difference in survival between wide resection and intralesional/marginal resection even in patients with solitary metastases. However, if the wide margin and reconstruction is suitable for the patient with solitary metastases, this indication is probably the best option in order to attempt to increase the survival mainly if the metastases are coming from thyroid and renal carcinomas. Preoperative embolization of these tumors is strongly recommended to reduce intraoperative blood loss.

15.2.3 Surgical Planning

Surgeries are rarely required for complete or impending pathologic fractures of the pelvis other than for those involving the acetabulum.

Surgical resection of the metastatic disease of the acetabulum should fulfill three aims:

1. Tumor resection
2. Bone defect reconstruction
3. Stabilization of the skeletal segment

15.2.4 Periacetabular Defects

Periacetabular tumors may cause severe debilitating pain with hip dysfunction and pathologic fractures often lead to protrusion acetabuli (Fig. 15.2). Small metastatic lesions to the acetabulum may be managed by radiation alone and intralesional resection to strengthen the acetabular roof and cement packing augmentation reinforcement with Steinman pins, or the use of a hip or pelvic prosthesis [20], and also with percutaneous bone packing. Bone cement raises the resistance of the acetabulum and allows loading of the limb (Fig. 15.3a, b).

When larger lesions have an intact medial wall but have significant acetabular defect, they can be reconstructed with a total hip arthroplasty augmented by cement and screws fixation.

Surgery is required for those lesions that compromise the load transfer from the lower limb to spine. These lesions affect the superior and medial acetabular walls, as well as the medial column of the pelvis and the posterior ilium in the region of the sacroiliac joint.

– Posterior ilium lesions not involving the acetabulum can be treated by intralesional resection and cement reconstruction (Fig. 15.3b).

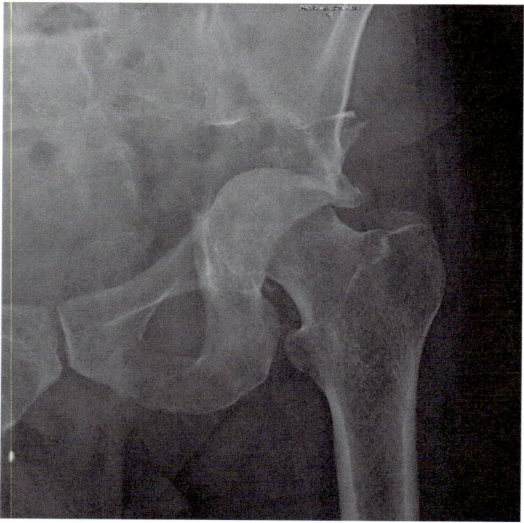

Fig. 15.2 AP radiograph of a 72-year-old male that shows protrusion acetabuli, secondary by thyroid cancer, with hip pain since 3 months ago. Probably he needed a previous surgery, before protrusion acetabuli were identified

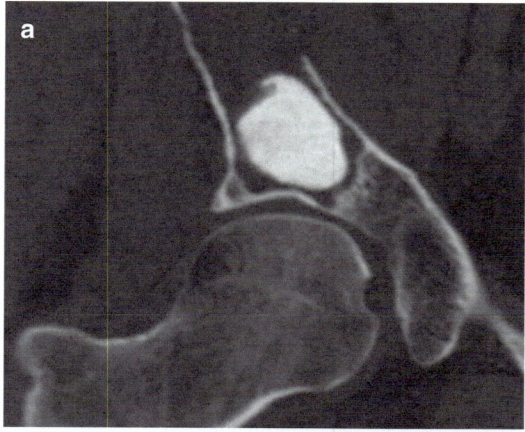

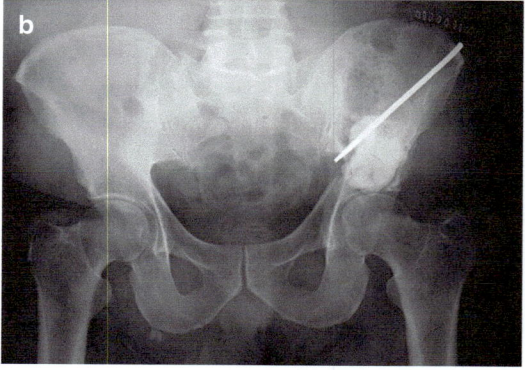

Fig. 15.3 AP radiographs that show percutaneous bone packing (**a**) and open intralesional resection and bone packing reinforced with a Steinman pin (**b**)

– Acetabular lesions that are contained (with an intact medial wall) can be reconstructed by a cemented arthroplasty. Protrusio acetabular cups compensate for deficiencies of the medial wall (MEC: Type 2), while cement and pin fixation (modified Harrington method) can be used effectively to reconstruct large defects in the acetabular column and dome (MEC Type 1 and 2) [21].
– In addition to classified metastatic disease of the acetabulum, Harrington described the surgical technique of reconstructing the pelvic ring with multiple pins, cement, cage, and a cemented total hip replacement. Since then, the method has been validated, and modifications of the technique have been proposed [22].
– A long-stem femoral component is often used, not just to complete the total hip reconstruction but also to prevent against pathologic fracture of the femur in the case of disease

progression. However, long cemented femoral stems may lead to adverse events such as hypotension or desaturation that are thought to be secondary to embolic phenomena.

- Cemented components are commonly favored in the setting of metastatic bone disease, as the associated use of radiation therapy will limit the degree of bony ingrowth with noncemented prostheses.

Type 3 and 4 may require resection or reconstruction with an acetabular prosthesis. Stemmed acetabular implants (ice cream cone prosthesis or pedestal cup) allow anchorage of the acetab-

ular cup into the posterior ilium with the stem (Fig. 15.4a, b). Modular tumor prostheses are being increasingly used.

Alternatively, a custom made pelvic prosthesis may be used and joint reconstruction using bone allografts; however, they are burdened with a high rate of complications.

If the acetabulum is not possible to reconstruct, but a significant amount of iliac crest is available, a saddle prosthesis implant can be used, which acts as a yoke type device using the iliac crest as a fulcrum. These devices can fail by dislocation or by fracture of the remaining iliac crest.

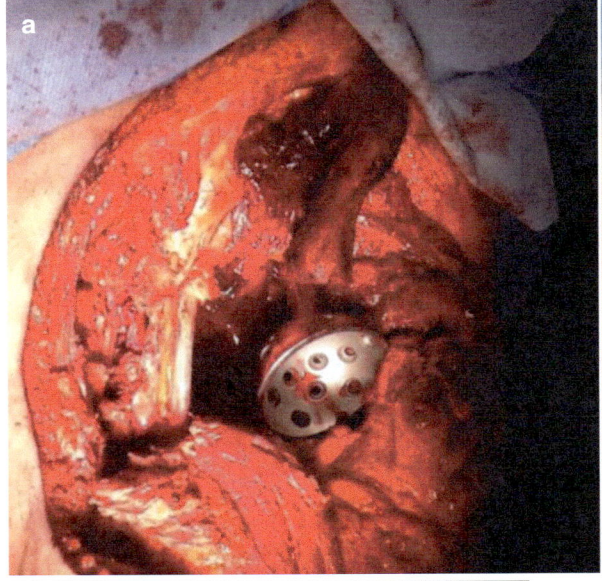
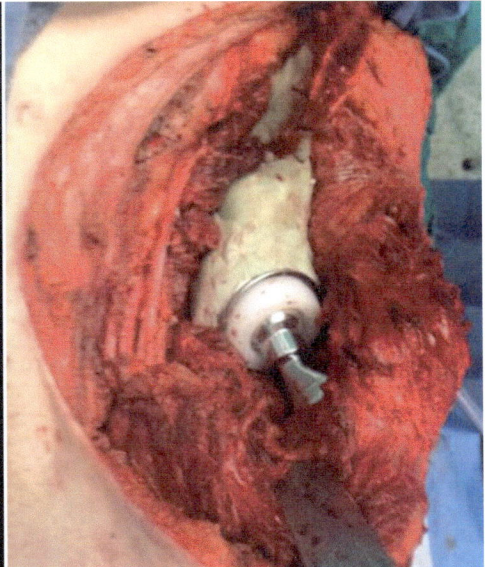
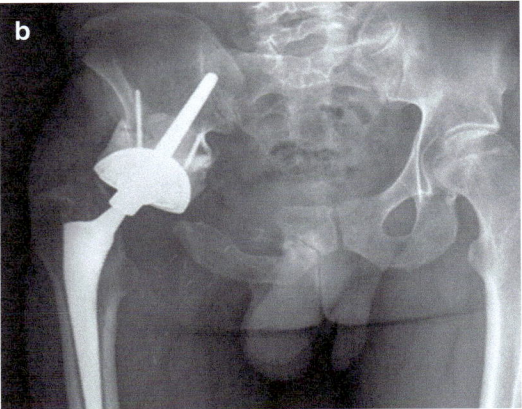

Fig. 15.4 (**a**) Intraoperative photograph, we can observe an implanted ice cream cone prosthesis with restored gap and limb length with the PMMA. Dual-mobility nonconstrained polyethylene and chrome-cobalt head were implanted to restore the joint. (**b**) AP radiographs that show the reconstruction

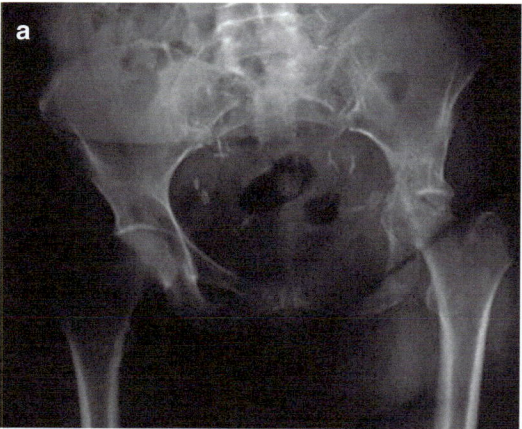

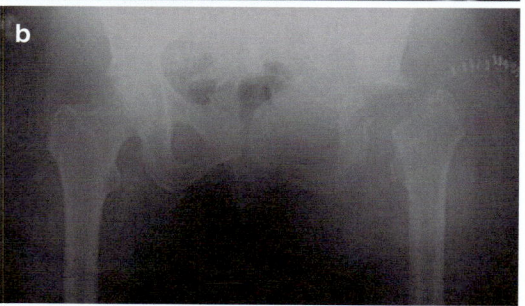

Fig. 15.5 (**a**) Plain X-rays show an acetabular protrusion of a 59-year-old female affected by bladder carcinoma and multiples metastases. She has severe left hip pain. She cannot bear any weight, and she has a pathologic fracture involving a posterior column and pubic osteolysis but poor medical condition and previous radiation therapy. Therefore, the surgical indication to relieve the pain was a resection arthroplasty. (**b**) Plain X-Rays show a resection arthroplasty of the left hip

In cases where there are no further reconstruction options available or in those patients in whom the surgical risk is high, we have to consider a resection arthroplasty (Fig. 15.5) [23]. Hindquarter amputation is the last measure reserved for cases of tumor fungating through skin, non-suppressive deep infections, or intractable pain.

15.3   Summary

We hope with time, these complicated reconstructions will be addressed more easily with more standard and predictable implant reconstruction techniques. As these resections and reconstructions involve risk of complications and blood loss, it is important to determine preoperatively if the benefits recompense the risks.

Although the reconstruction of defects in the lower limb following the resection of primary bone tumors has proved successful, the search for the optimal implant to reconstruct pelvic defects continues.

Resection of pelvic tumors is a technically demanding procedure and reconstruction demands the all-embracing use of modern surgical techniques and orthopedic implant technology [24, 25]. Several reconstructive techniques have been recommended with modest functional results and a high incidence of complications.

We must not underestimate the worth of a multidisciplinary team composed of experienced specialists devoted to the common goals of providing the best comprehensive treatment now available and helping to progress these treatment modalities in the future.

References

1. Capanna R, Campanacci DA. The treatment of metastases in the appendicular skeleton. J Bone Joint Surg Br. 2001;83(4):471–81.
2. Chow E, Harris K, Fan G, et al. Palliative radiotherapy trials for bone metastases: a systematic review. J Clin Oncol. 2007;25:1423–36.
3. Ellsworth SG, Alcorn SR, Hales RK, McNutt TR, DeWeese TL, Smith TJ. Patterns of care among patients receiving radiation therapy for bone metastases at a large academic institution. Int J Radiat Oncol Biol Phys. 2014;89(5):1100–5.
4. Rosenthal D, Callstrom MR. Critical review and state of the art in interventional oncology: benign and metastatic disease involving bone. Radiology. 2012; 262(3):765–80.
5. Lane MD, Le HB, Lee S, Young C, Heran MK, Badii M, Clarkson PW, Munk PL. Combination radiofrequency ablation and cementoplasty for palliative treatment of painful neoplastic bone metastasis: experience with 53 treated lesions in 36 patients. Skelet Radiol. 2011;40(1):25–32.
6. Toyota N, Naito A, Kakizawa H, Hieda M, Hirai N, Tachikake T, Kimura T, Fukuda H, Ito K. Radiofrequency ablation therapy combined with cementoplasty for painful bone metastases: initial experience. Cardiovasc Intervent Radiol. 2005;28(5):578–83.
7. Carrafiello G, Laganà D, Mangini M, Fontana F, Dionigi G, Boni L, Rovera F, Cuffari S, Fugazzola C.

Microwave tumors ablation: principles, clinical applications and review of preliminary experiences. Int J Surg. 2008;6(Suppl 1):S65–9.

8. Pusceddu C, Sotgia B, Fele RM, Ballicu N, Melis L. Combined microwave ablation and cementoplasty in patients with painful bone metastases at high risk of fracture. Cardiovasc Intervent Radiol. 2016; 39(1):74–80.

9. Maccauro G, Liuzza F, Scaramuzzo L, Milani A, Muratori F, Rossi B, Waide V, Logroscino G, Logroscino CA, Maffulli N. Percutaneous acetabuloplasty for metastatic acetabular lesions. BMC Musculoskelet Disord. 2008;9:66.

10. Castaneda Rodriguez WR, Callstrom MR. Effective pain palliation and prevention of fracture for axial-loading skeletal metastases using combined cryoablation and cementoplasty. Tech Vasc Interv Radiol. 2011;14(3):160–9.

11. Wunder JS, Ferguson PC, Griffin AM, Pressman A, Bell RS. Acetabular metastases: planning for reconstruction and review of results. Clin Orthop Relat Res. 2003;415S:187–97.

12. Enneking WF. The anatomic considerations in tumor surgery: pelvis. In: Enneking WF, editor. Musculoskeletal tumor surgery, vol. 2. New York: Churchill Livingstone; 1983. p. 483–529.

13. Muller D, Capanna R. The surgical treatment of pelvic bone metastases. Adv Orthop. 2015;75:1–10.

14. Piccioli A, Spinelli MS, Forsberg JA, Wedin R, Healey JH, Ippolito V, Daolio PA, Ruggieri P, Maccauro G, Gasbarrini A, Biagini R, Piana R, Fazioli F, Luzzati A, Di Martino A, Nicolosi F, Camnasio F, Rosa MA, Campanacci DA, Denaro V, Capanna R. How do we estimate survival? External validation of a tool for survival estimation in patients with metastatic bone disease-decision analysis and comparison of three international patient populations. BMC Cancer. 2015;15:424.

15. Forsberg JA, Eberhardt J, Boland PJ, Wedin R, Healey JH. Estimating survival in patients with operable skeletal metastases: an application of a Bayesian belief network. El-Deiry WS, ed. PLoS One. 2011;6(5):e19956.

16. Harrington KD. The management of acetabular insufficiency secondary to metastatic malignant disease. J Bone Joint Surg Am. 1981;4:653–64.

17. Issack PS, Kotwal SY, Lane JM. Management of metastatic bone disease of the acetabulum. J Am Acad Orthop Surg. 2013;21(11):685–95.

18. Wood TJ, Racano A, Yeung H, Farrokhyar F, Ghert M, Deheshi BM. Surgical management of bone metastases: quality of evidence and systematic review. Ann Surg Oncol. 2014;21(13):4081–9.

19. Ruggieri P, Mavrogenis AF, Angelini A, Mercuri M. Metastases of the pelvis: does resection improve survival? Orthopedics. 2011;34(7):e236–44.

20. Harrington KD. The management of acetabular insufficiency secondary to metastatic malignant disease. J Bone Joint Surg Am. 1981;63A:653–64.

21. Harrington KD. The management of acetabular insufficiency secondary to metastatic malignant disease. J Bone Joint Surg Am. 1981;63(4):653–64.

22. Sagozis P, Wedin R, Brosjö O, Bauer H. Reconstruction of metastatic acetabular defectsusing a modified Harrington procedure: good outcome after surgical treatment of 70 patients. Acta Orthop. 2015;86(6): 690–4.

23. Quinn RH. Metastatic disease to the hip and pelvis: surgical management. Tech Orthop. 2007;22(2).

24. Barrientos-Ruiz I, Ortiz-Cruz EJ, Peleteiro-Pensado M. Reconstruction after hemipelvectomy with the ice-cream cone prosthesis: what are the short-term clinical results? Clin Orthop Relat Res. 2017;475: 735–41.

25. Barrientos-Ruiz I, Ortiz-Cruz EJ, Peleteiro-Pensado M. Erratum to: reconstruction after hemipelvectomy with the ice-cream cone prosthesis: what are the short-term clinical results. Clin Orthop Relat Res. 2017;475:924.

Megaprosthesis in Metastases of the Shoulder

16

Vincenzo Denaro and Alberto Di Martino

Abstract

The purpose of treatment for patients with skeletal metastases and pathologic fractures is a singular performance that allows for functional reconstruction. The most common surgical procedure is resection of the metastatic lesion and prosthetic reconstruction. Given the recent developments of new prosthetic implants, the metastatic disease to the proximal humerus is more often treated surgically by the use of arthroplasty implants. The majority of patients will survive for a significant time after surgery, and hence a stable and pain-free limb should be the goal. When prosthesis implants are used, this allows for a good pain control, despite a poor functional outcome.

Keywords

Shoulder metastases · Megaprosthesis
Surgery · Functional outcome

16.1 Introduction

The proximal humerus is the third most common location for osteosarcoma and chondrosarcoma, the fourth most common location for giant cell tumor of bone, and the most common upper extremity location for metastatic carcinoma [1]. This can result in pain, loss of function, and pathological fracture. The restoring potential of pathologically fractured bone is low; for this reason, the necessity for operative intervention arises in many of these patients. A functional upper limb is pivotal to a patients' independence; therefore, preserving or restoring limb function is one of the goals of treatment. The increasing and often variable longevity of patients with metastatic disease coupled with higher-than-expected failure rates after internal fixation with or without intralesional treatment and radiotherapy has led to renewed interest in more aggressive local surgery through proximal humeral resection and reconstruction.

The purpose of treatment for patients with skeletal metastases and pathologic fractures is a singular performance that allows for functional reconstruction. The most common surgical procedure is resection of the metastatic lesion and prosthetic reconstruction. Alternative procedures for reconstruction after intra-articular resection of the proximal humerus comprehend osteoarticular allograft, a large-segment endoprosthesis, an arthrodesis with an intercalary allograft and/or a

V. Denaro · A. Di Martino (✉)
Department of Orthopaedics and Trauma Surgery,
University Campus Bio-Medico of Rome,
Rome, Italy
e-mail: a.dimartino@unicampus.it

© Springer International Publishing AG, part of Springer Nature 2019
V. Denaro et al. (eds.), *Management of Bone Metastases*, https://doi.org/10.1007/978-3-319-73485-9_16

vascularized fibular graft, and an allograft-prosthesis composite (APC); each has merits and demerits [2].

Compared with other anatomic regions, the proximal humerus has had encouraging functional results and implant longevity profiles after endoprosthetic reconstruction [3]. Prosthetic replacement of the shoulder in the treatment of tumors of the proximal humerus has been illustrated for the first time by Pean in 1894; the cases presented over the years since then shed light on the evolution of these implants, in terms of both design and choice of material [4]. The application of a shoulder prosthesis, after resection of the proximal humerus, initially restricted to primary neoplasms of low-grade malignancy and several benign tumors, has more recently been also enlarged to high-grade primary tumors and to isolated secondary localizations, thanks to progress made in chemotherapy and radiation treatment.

As for the selection of the type of implant, the current tendency is the using of modular prosthe-

ses that intraoperatively provide us with a wide variety of dimensions, composed by a joint component, a central part, and an intramedullary stem (Fig. 16.1), more often stabilized by cement. In terms of simplicity, adaptability, and economy, this type of prosthesis has overcome the custom made prosthesis. The use of cement in modular prostheses makes them more secure even in the long term and allows for early rehabilitation. In the context of replacement of the proximal humerus, it should be mentioned the use of prostheses coated with homologous cadaver bone transfer over which the soft tissues are reinserted, the so-called APC implants. Composite prosthesis has bone allograft coating the prosthesis, except for the articular portion. Thus, these have the advantage of reinsertion of the anatomical structures. However, these implants are rarely used in the bone metastatic patients, since usually no bony union is expected after the surgery, and this may predispose to failure.

The surgical reconstruction with arthroplasty implants must be stable during the patient's

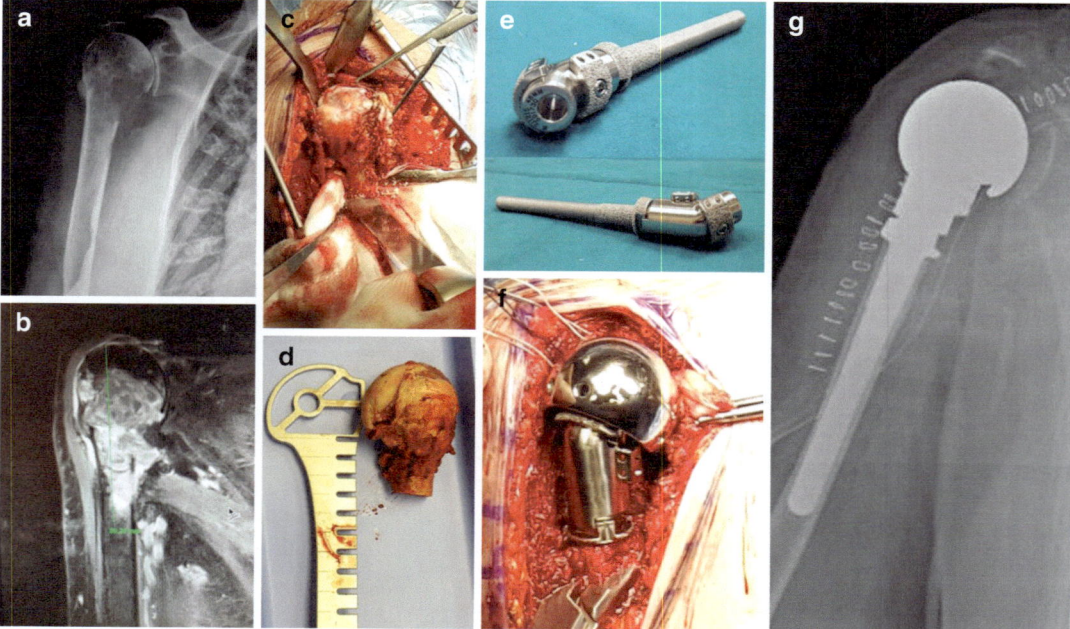

Fig. 16.1 Eighty-two-year-old patient affected by unknown malignancy (suspected for lung adenocarcinoma), presenting with a pathologic fracture sustained by a big lesion at the proxymal humerus, as confirmed by X-ray (**a**) and MRI (**b**). Surgery consisted of a proxymal humeral and tumor resection (**c**, **d**), with the implant of a modular shoulder endoprosthesis (**e**), with oversized head (**f**, **g**)

remaining lifetime. However, in recent decades, major complications like periprosthetic infections, aseptic loosening, dislocation, or subdislocation have all been described. One of the most important problems is the loss of movement in abduction between the upper limb that is often associated with subdislocation or dislocation that is prevalently superior; in fact, in so-called wide resections of the soft tissues surrounding the bone neoformation, total or subtotal resection of the deltoid muscle, of the extrarotator cuff, of the biceps muscle with its long head, is directly responsible for loss of movement. In cases where it was possible to even partially preserve these muscle structures, it is difficult to obtain stable and long-lasting reinsertion to the prosthesis itself. In order to manage these challenges, Trevira tubes-type accessory systems of biocompatible materials have been developed allowing for tubulization of the implant itself. It is then possible to directly reinsert the residual tendons to the structure [4].

16.2 Prosthetic Implants and Function

Prosthetic reconstructions have the advantages of providing immediate stabilization of the proxymal humerus and show a lower infection rate in comparison to osteoarticular allografts. However, prostheses can fail at a later stage when the surrounding stable structures become insufficient.

Compared to prosthetic reconstruction, osteoarticular allografts allow the remaining deltoid muscle and rotator tendons to be attached to the soft tissue of the allograft, which provide a better potential for maintaining shoulder stability and maximize the recovery of its function. There is no difference between the different reconstructive methods in pain relief, manual dexterity, emotional acceptance, or in posterior extension of the shoulder joint. However in cohorts of patients with either primary and metastatic tumors, APC are better than tumor prostheses in terms of forward flexion of the shoulder joint, which might be due to the functional loss of the deltoid muscles associated with tumor prosthesis. Abduction is an important function for the shoulder joint. The shoulder joint is a kind of third-class lever, with its force bearing point located between the fulcrum and the weight. Abduction varied dramatically as a function of the reconstructive procedures and site of tumors: patients treated with APC show a better abduction compared with prosthesis. Therefore, it is proposed that reconstructions following proximal humeral resections should be performed in most cases with tumor prostheses (Fig. 16.2), while in very selected patients APC can be selected to try to improve the abduction [5].

The most common surgical procedure is resection of the metastatic lesion and prosthetic reconstruction. In patients affected by metastases, treatment is aimed to palliation, and the aim of surgical margins when inserting a prostheses

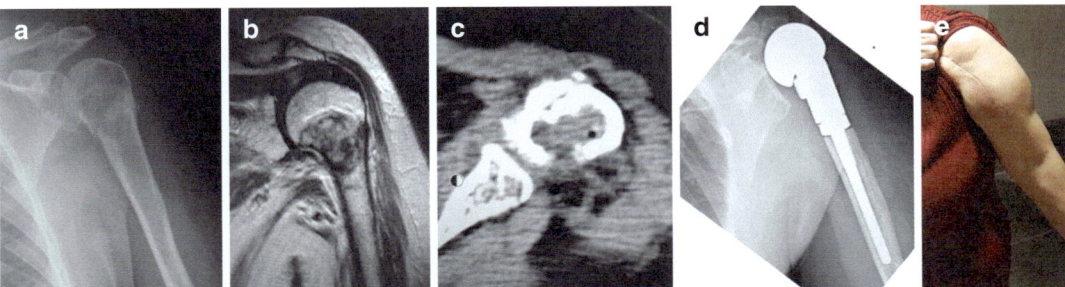

Fig. 16.2 Seventy-two-year-old patient affected by breast cancer, with a pathologic fracture at the proxymal humerus, as confirmed by X-ray (**a**), MRI (**b**), and CT scan (**c**). Surgery consisted of a proxymal humeral and tumor resection with the implant of a modular shoulder endoprosthesis with oversized head (**d**). At the 6-month follow-up, the patient is pain free, but limitation of the abduction of the shoulder is observed (**e**)

is to preserve as much bone as was reasonably possible and also to preserve and reconstruct the rotator cuff when possible. Proximal prostheses are used if there is involvement of the humeral head or insufficient healthy bone to allow proximal purchase of an intramedullary rod. As regards the ability to achieve function, if suture holes are available to reconstruct the capsule or rotator cuff to the prosthesis, then this should be done to enable greater stability at the shoulder (Fig. 16.2). If no suture holes are available, then nylon mesh/Trevira tubes fixed around the proximal part of the prosthesis can be used as a reliable anchoring site onto which capsular or rotator cuff fixation may be performed. The use of prostheses, particularly those of the more recent generation, responds to the needs to overcome the limits of loss of movement, as long as good anatomical reconstruction of the soft tissues is possible. The main problem in reconstruction with a prosthesis is the quantity of residual muscular tissue (deltoideus, extrarotators) and the stabilization system of the same to the prosthesis in order to avoid dislocation, which constitutes the main complication; this can sometimes be overcome by big-sized heads (Fig. 16.1) or by reverse shoulder arthroplasty implants when the deltoid muscle is still funcional. The distal stem of the prosthesis is in most cases fixed with polymethylmethacrylate cement at the distal medullary canal [6–9].

16.3   Clinical Results

The use of shoulder arthroplasty implants in the setting of metastatic tumors is poorly explored in literature. In particular, the available studies on the topic report on several kinds of implants and combine the clinical and functional results of shoulder tumor arthroplasty implants in both primary and metastatic tumors or for metastatic patients at all the humerus or upper limb [10]. In the systematic review by Teunis et al. [1], the authors reviewed the outcomes of patients operated on for metastases of the proximal humerus. They found that allograft-prosthesis composites and prostheses seem to have similar functional

outcome and survival rates. However, allograft (OA and APC) proximal humerus reconstructions have shown a decreased implant longevity as compared with EP reconstructions because of an increased rate of major complications requiring revision.

To determine which type of reconstruction might be most appropriate for specific patients, the functional results, postoperative complications, and implant survival of osteoarticular allograft (OA), allograft-prosthesis composite (APC), and endoprosthetic (EP) reconstructions have been compared after proximal humeral resection for the treatment of primary and metastatic bone tumors. The APC integrates the durability of an endoprosthesis and the advantages of an allograft (restored bone stock and soft-tissue attachment). However the biological reconstructions are complicated by fractures, infections, and subchondral collapse, leading to a need for implant revision or removal, and in the metastatic patient, these are not expected to undergo bone healing. Difficulties with endoprosthetic reconstruction involve consequences of surgical resection of deltoid and rotator cuff. These include proximal subluxation, instability, and a reduction in functional range of motion. The soft-tissue attachments, including the rotator cuff and joint capsule, can substitute for the deficient soft tissues of the host and can create a stable, functional construct [11]. Mid- and long-term complications, such as fracture, subchondral collapse, and infection, are however reported less frequently in prosthetic reconstructions. Conversely, glenohumeral instability is considered to be less frequent in patients with a somewhat more biological repair. However, in both OA and allograft-prosthesis composite (APC) reconstruction, instability caused by rotator cuff dysfunction is reported to be between 5 and 19% of cases compared to between 11 and 31% after endoprosthetic reconstruction (EPR): this complication may be prevented in manu cases by the use of big-sized heads.

In the study by Mayilvahanan et al. [6], they report on 5 out of 57 patients affected by metastases at the proxymal humerus. From a functional point of view, they reported the data from the overall population. They obtained maximum abduction of 45°, by scapulothoracic movement. Rotation at the shoulder was restricted to a maximum of 15° in those patients who underwent wide resections of the rotator cuff. Excellent functional outcomes were achieved in 18 patients, it was good in 25, 7 patients had a fair outcome, while the outcome in 5 patients was rated poor. The most important mechanical complication of proximal humeral endoprosthesis was a proximal subluxation of the head, painfully impinging on the subacromial arch. Such complications caused partial disability and restriction of all movements at the joint, with eventual affecton of the overall function. The authors concluded that custom mega-prosthetic replacement is an interesting therapeutic option with limited complication rates, giving a useful functional limb compared to other forms of reconstruction.

Thai et al. [7] reported a huge cohort of patients operated on for metastases at the humerus. Of these, 22 out of 96 patients were operated on for resection and implant of prosthesis at the proximal humerus. They reported 5 complications in those 22 patients, including intraoperative bleeding, myocardial infarct, stitch abscess, high-riding prosthesis, and a proximal migration of the prosthesis. From a functional point of view, three patients complained of persisting pain, and eight had restricted function; therefore they concluded that patients need to be aware that a stiff shoulder may result from surgery in this area and the main goal of treatment is pain relief.

In the manuscript by Potter et al. [3], 19 out of 49 patients were operated on for metastatic disease at the proximal humerus. They were operated on by the implant of osteoarticulat allograft in four patients, allograft-prosthesis composite in six patients, and endoprosthesis replacement in nine patients. Major complications requiring reoperation (including deep infection, symptomatic instability, fracture, and aseptic loosening) occurred in 47% of the OA group, compared with only 25% each in the APC and EP groups. In general, they recommended APC reconstruction for younger patients with primary tumors of bone, while they stated that for patients with metastatic disease, EP reconstruction is technically less

challenging and provides acceptable and reproducible results, with implant longevity likely to exceed that of the patient.

Conclusions

Reconstruction of the proximal humerus following an intra-articular resection of metastases is usually performed by the implant of an arthroplasty, which usually consists of prosthetic reconstructions, and more rarely of APC. Given the recent developments of new prosthetic implants, the metastatic disease to the proxymal humerus is more often treated surgically by the use of arthroplasty implants. The majority of patients will survive for a significant time after surgery, and hence a stable and pain-free limb should be the goal. When prosthesis implants are used, this allows for a good pain control, despite a poor functional outcome.

References

1. Teunis T, Nota SPFT. Outcome after reconstruction of the proximal humerus for tumor resection: a systematic review. Clin Orthop Relat Res. 2014;472:2245–53.
2. Wang Z, Guo Z, Li J. Functional outcomes and complications of reconstruction of the proximal humerus after intra-articular tumor resection. Orthop Surg. 2010;2(1):19–26.
3. Potter BK, Adams SC, Pitcher JD, et al. Proximal humerus reconstructions for tumors. Clin Orthop Relat Res. 2009;467:1035–41.
4. Manili M, Fredella N, Santori FS. Shoulder prosthesis in reconstruction of the scapulohumeral girdle after wide resection to treat malignant neoformation of the proximal humerus. Chir Organi Mov. 2002;87:25–33.
5. Palumbo BT, Eric R. Advances in segmental endoprosthetic reconstruction for extremity tumors: a review of contemporary designs and techniques. Cancer Control. 2011;18(3):160–70.
6. Mayilvahanan N, Paraskumar M, Sivaseelam A, Natarajan S. Custom mega-prosthetic replacement for proximal humeral tumours. Int Orthop. 2006;30:158–62.
7. Thai DM, Kitagawa Y, Choong PFM. Outcome of surgical management of bony metastases to the humerus and shoulder girdle: a retrospective analysis of 93 patients. Int Semin Surg Oncol. 2006;3:5.
8. Black AW, Szabo RM. Treatment of malignant tumors of the proximal humerus with allograft-prosthesis composite reconstruction. J Shoulder Elb Surg. 2007;16(5):526–33.

9. Puri A, Gulia A. The results of total humeral replacement following excision for primary bone tumour. J Bone Joint Surg. 2012;94:1277–81.

10. Angelini A, Mavrogenis AF, Trovarelli G, Pala E, Arbelaez P, Casanova J, Berizzi A, Ruggieri P. Extra-articular shoulder resections: outcomes of 54 patients.

J Shoulder Elb Surg. 2017;26:e337–45. https://doi.org/10.1016/j.jse.2017.04.019.

11. Abdeen A, Healey JH. Allograft-prosthesis composite reconstruction of the proximal part of the humerus. J Bone Joint Surg. 2009;91:2406–15.

New Biomaterials in Instrumentation Systems

17

R. Piana, P. Pellegrino, and S. Marone

Abstract

Metastatic tumors often cause pathologic or impending fractures. These lesions require a stable fixation that allows an early postoperative weight bearing and a durable follow-up. During years, orthopedic devices have been built up in several different materials to enhance the properties and combine elevate strength with an elastic modulus as closer as possible to the elastic modulus of bone. Carbon fiber-polyaryl-ether-ether-ketone (CF-PEEK) composite biomaterials have excellent properties in terms of mechanical strength, flexibility, and compliance, with low elastic modulus. Being these materials composite, they could be designed in order to optimize mechanical properties. Their properties of radiolucency and low interference with magnetic resonance imaging allow good follow-up of fracture healing or the evolution of the lytic lesions; low interaction levels with radiation therapies allow better planning and more effective therapies. Plates, nails, and spinal stabilization systems are available on the market to be used in all conditions where an elastic radiotransparent device is required. Even not experienced surgeons could use CF-PEEK implants with few tips. In this chapter, some cases are shown to demonstrate technical feasibility and imaging results.

Being these relatively new devices, long-term multicentric studies may be required to collect all the possible implant-related complications or failures.

Keywords

New technologies · Carbon fiber · PEEK · Reconstruction · Metastasis

17.1 Introduction

Patients with primitive and metastatic bone or soft tissue tumors are at high risk of fracture. Soft tissue tumors often require periosteal stripping and/or adjuvant therapy making pathologic fracture a real risk [1].

In long bones and spine secondary lesions, fixation should be performed to treat pathologic fractures and to perform spinal decompression. In addition, many impending fractures may require surgery before a fracture occurs. Most of the secondary lesions are not completely resolved by medical therapy, and the likelihood of the fracture site to achieve a complete callus formation is poor. Moreover, many patients need adjuvant local treatments such as radiotherapy.

Orthopedic oncology has always been a field of innovation in surgery. Innovation led to both new

R. Piana (✉) · P. Pellegrino · S. Marone
Orthopaedic Oncology and Reconstructive Surgery Unit, Città della salute e della scienza, CTO Hospital, Turin, Italy

© Springer International Publishing AG, part of Springer Nature 2019
V. Denaro et al. (eds.), *Management of Bone Metastases*, https://doi.org/10.1007/978-3-319-73485-9_17

surgical techniques and to the development of new devices. New instrumentation systems should use advanced biomaterials capable of making the surgeon's work easier, with eventual advantages for the patient. Mechanical strength, biocompatibility, ease of implantation, and costs' control are fundamental characteristics of newer surgical systems implemented into clinical practice.

One of the latest interesting innovations in orthopedic oncology is the use of composite materials. Composite materials have improved qualities in terms of lightness, strength, and radiolucency compared with traditional implants. In modern instrumentation technologies, carbon fiber-reinforced polymers are the best known and most used, being these both effective and reliable [2].

17.2 Mechanical Behavior and Biocompatibility

The great majority of pathologic fractures occur at the long bones, and these are most often managed by the use of intramedullary nailing.

Studies concerning the impact of fixation devices elasticity on fracture healing have led to controversial conclusions [3, 4]. Ideally, the fixation implant should counter bending, torsion, and shear stress sufficiently to avoid excessive mobility at the fracture site but avoiding implant breaking; at the same time, the implant should allow an adequate transmission of axial compressive forces to enhance the chances of bone healing [5]. Intramedullary nails made of titanium and steel alloys provide great stability but with a relative rigidity that bypass the fracture site with an increased stress-shielding and subsequent potential resorption of the bone [6]; in fact, cobalt-chromium and titanium alloys implants have a ten times greater elastic modulus than bone. Stress-shielding and bone resorption can be avoided by a decrease in the stiffness of the implant, with an acceleration of healing; unfortunately, too flexible implants may give poor fixation and are associated to implant failure [3, 7].

Finite element analysis has been used to study the behavior of different composite implants in comparison with traditional stainless steel and titanium alloys. In gait analysis, titanium femoral nails absorb between 70 and 74% of the axial forces during the stance phase and 91% during the swing phase [6], which could be theoretically too much to enhance healing.

In a recent study, Ben-Or et al. [8] demonstrated how the stiffness can be variated, and the subsequent micromotion of a carbon fiber composite nail in all directions could be obtained, by simply modifying the orientation of the carbon fibers. Predicting these micromovements is crucial to understand the behavior of the fixation device under specific loading conditions and determine how it is possible to stimulate callus formation. Although less used, plates may be useful in metaphyseal and epiphyseal fractures. Saidpour [9] demonstrated that carbon fiber composite plates reduced the stress-shielding effect at the fracture site when subjected to bending and torsional loads. To ensure the best healing conditions, the stiffness of the device should theoretically decrease as the bone strength increase.

In the last 30 years, more than 40 different polymers and composite materials have been tested in the trauma setting [6]. The potential advantage of composite materials consists in the possibility to change the orientation of the fibers inside the material and to modify fiber and implant shape to change mechanical properties [10]. However, tested biomaterials such as poly-l-lactide (PLLA) epoxy, polyester, poly-methyl methacrylate (PMMA), and carbon fiber-based composite suffer of some limitations [11–13]:

1. Long-term reduction in mechanical properties, sometimes before the bone healing has occurred, by the interaction with body fluids with the matrix material that may degrade the biomaterial
2. The release of fragments that can migrate into other tissues
3. Lack of ductility that does not allow to reshape the plate in the operating room as commonly performed when metal implants are used

For these reasons, manufacturers started to develop newer composite materials with improved biomechanical characteristics.

Polyaryletherketones (PAEKs) started to be commercialized in the 1980s. These consist in a family of high-temperature thermoplastic polymers. The structure of PAEKs confers stability at high temperatures, resistance to chemical and radiation damage, and the possibility to be reinforced by fibers such as carbon or glass; moreover, these possess greater strength compared to many metals. The two PAEKs used in orthopedics are poly(aryl-ether-ether-ketone) (PEEK) and poly(aryl-ether-ketone-ether-ketone-ketone) (PEKEKK).

PAEKs have a low elastic modulus that can also be modified by the addiction of carbon fibers, thus building up carbon fiber-reinforced (CFR) composite and joining different elastic modulus as shown in Table 17.1 [14].

In the late 1990s, PEEK had emerged as the leading high-performance thermoplastic candidate for replacing different metal implant components in both the orthopedic and trauma settings [15]. Carbon fiber-reinforced PEEK (CFR-PEEK) has demonstrated a high resistance to ionizing radiation, good mechanical properties, and low wear rate [15]. Moreover, Utzschneider et al. [16] studied the inflammatory response to CFR-PEEK, and ultra-high-molecular-weight polyethylene in rats' knee joints, and found a comparable inflammatory response in all the materials, suggesting that CFR-PEEK composites are a potential alternative to ultra-high-molecular-weight polyethylene in prosthetic bearing surfaces. Scotchford et al. [17] have assessed the in vitro biocompatibility of a CFR-PEEK biomaterial which showed initial osteoblast attachment and proliferation similar to titanium alloys. Brown et al. [18] examined the resistance to flexural fatigue and thermoformability of different carbon fiber-reinforced composites, including PEEK reinforced by 30% chopped PAN carbon fiber, and showed that CFR-PEEK had the highest bending fatigue resistance and toughness; it was insensitive to precondition or thermoforming, probably because of the better

compatibility between PEEK and CF. In spinal surgery, advantages of more elastic PEEK rods lay in the reduced load at the adjacent levels. In contrast with traditional rods, these permit a more physiologic load, with potential decreased risk of adjacent levels disease [19].

17.3 Radiologic Advantages

Postoperative control and routine periodic examination of the treated segment are the rule in the surgery of both primitive and metastatic tumors. However, MRI and CT artifacts from traditional titanium or stainless steel implants can obstruct the necessary postoperative surveillance imaging and make more challenging to detect recurrent disease, nonunions, and disease progression [20].

Zimel et al. [21], in a recent study, stated that CFR-PEEK intramedullary nail fixation is a superior alternative to minimize the implant artifacts on MRI or CT imaging for patients requiring long bone fixation. The imaging characteristics had been already studied in spinal surgery demonstrating to be radiolucent under every examination (X-ray, CT, MRI) [22].

Cortical bone is better seen in conventional radiographs [23] with composite implants. At the same time, CT scans show less metallic streak artifacts that limit the evaluation of the adjacent periprosthetic tissues. MRI studies can be optimized to reduce the intramedullary metal artifacts, but these are unable to eliminate the distortion immediately adjacent to the implant at the surrounding marrow space, cortex, and bone–muscle interface [24, 25].

This radiologic behavior does not involve only postoperative and long-term surveillance but above all the radiotherapy planning; in fact, Xin-Ye et al. established that a better planning of the treatment can be performed [26]. More recently an in vitro study [27] demonstrated absence of back scattering and significantly lower attenuation of carbon fiber plates and vertebral screws in comparison with traditional titanium implants. Although in vivo studies may be required to study the impact on survival and local control of disease, these features may help substantially in decreasing local complications and increase dose delivering.

Table 17.1 Elastic modulus of commonly used materials in internal fixation

Material	Elastic modulus (GPa)
PAEKs	3–4
Cortical bone	18
Titanium alloy	110
Carbon fiber (pure)	138

17.4   Surgery

Surgical techniques involving the implant of radiolucent [28] CFR-PEEK devices do not differ from the traditional metal ware. The use of radiopaque markers allows an easy implant localization in percutaneous techniques and no differences in open surgery. Standard compression or locking screws could be used on plates. Of course, the impossibility to mold the plates, as commonly occurs with stainless steel or titanium alloys implants, may decrease the indications in patients with nonconventional anatomies. Most common indications for the use of CF-PEEK nails are metastasis (lung, kidney, breast, etc.) involving humeral diaphysis (Fig. 17.1) and

metaphysis and femoral diaphysis and intertrochanteric area (Fig. 17.2). Spine surgery can be performed in a conventional fashion with CFR implants too (Figs. 17.3 and 17.4). Ultrathin titanium coatings do not affect mechanical and radiological behavior in vertebral screws.

In some cases, CF implants could be used in allograft reconstruction for primitive bone tumors (Fig. 17.5), with substantial advantages in term of MRI surveillance. Also nonmalignant diseases, such as simple bone cysts (SBC), aneurysmal bone cysts (ABC), or fibrous dysplasia, could be treated with curettage and, if required, CF-PEEK fixation. More extensive reconstruction should be performed too (Fig. 17.6), although very few cases are eligible for this surgery.

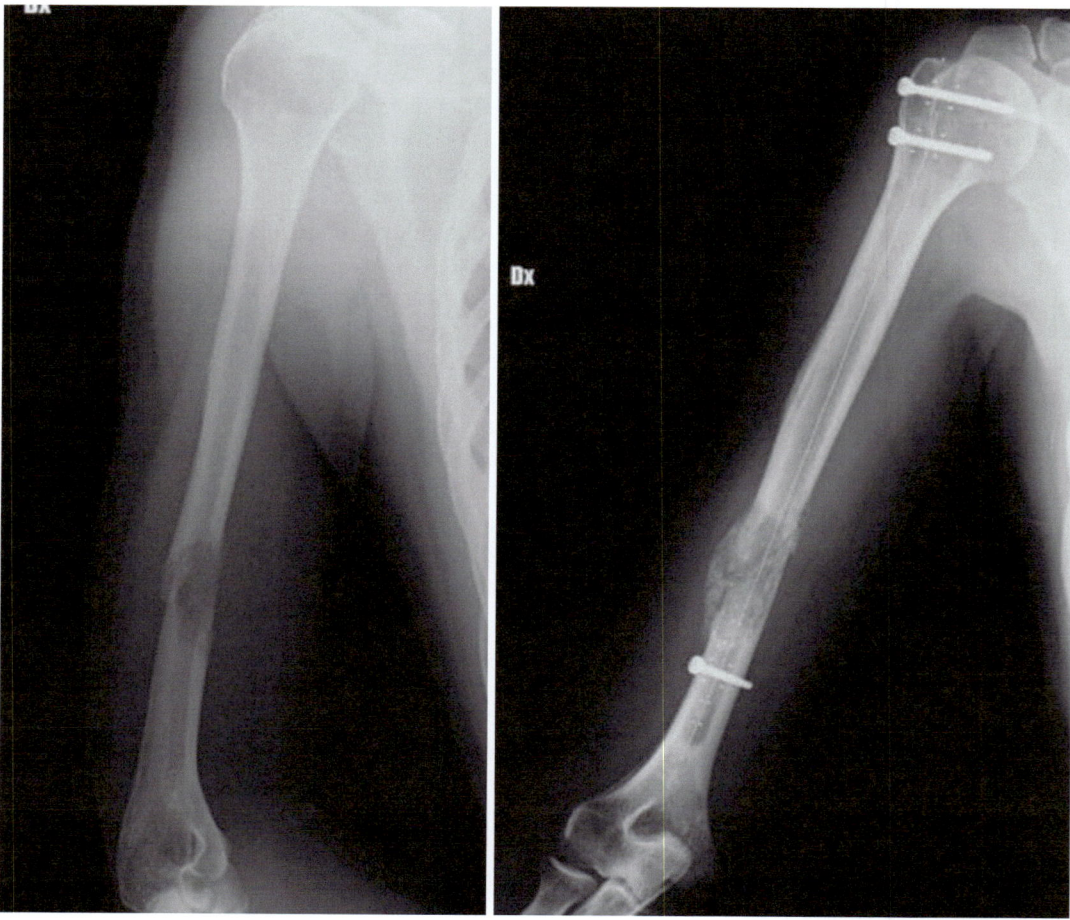

Fig. 17.1 M, 62 YY, multiple myeloma, fracture of the distal third of the right humeral shaft, surgical result at 6 months of follow-up

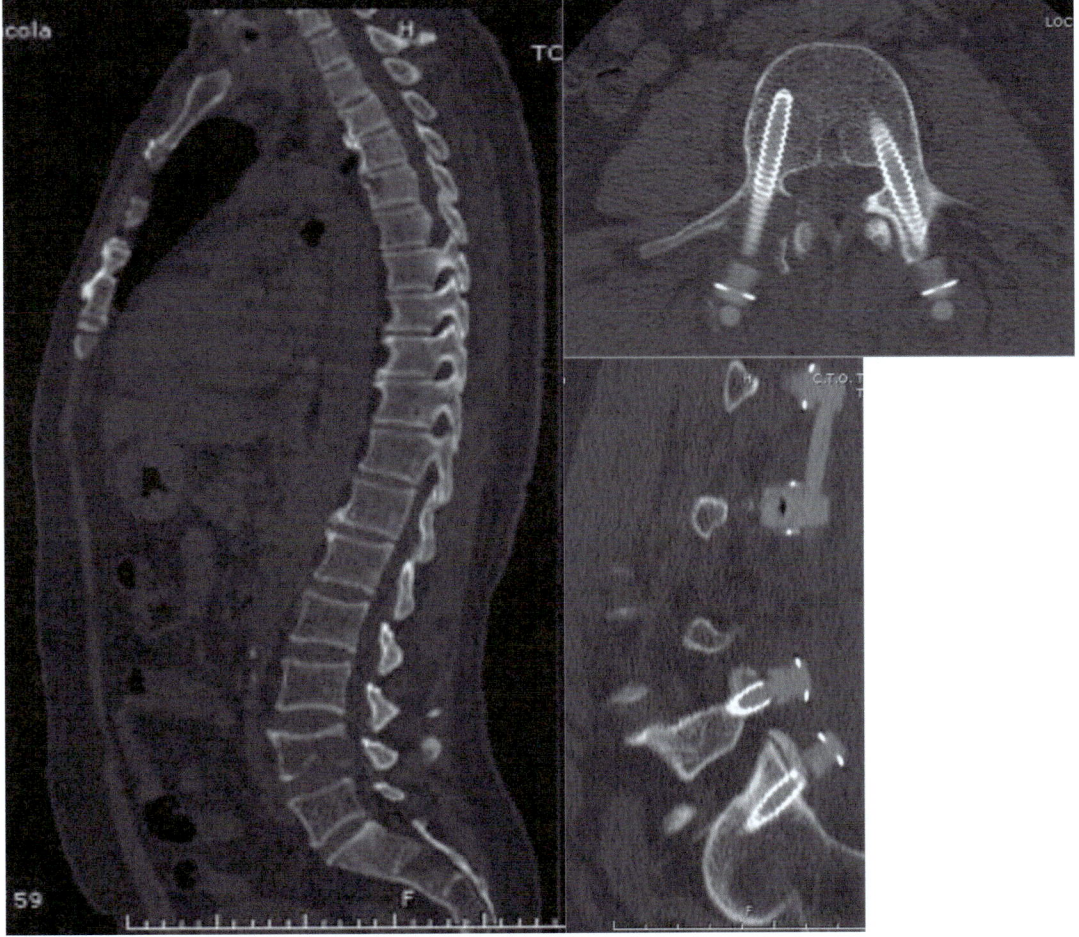

Fig. 17.2 M, 58 YY, metastatic adenocarcinoma of the lung, pathologic fracture with neurologic impairment of the fourth vertebral body: pre- and postoperative CT scan

However, despite the initial positive outcomes, multicentric studies should be performed to analyze the behavior of CF-PEEK implants in the patients with bone metastatic and observe eventual implant-related complication.

Conclusions

Carbon fiber-reinforced PEEK instrumentation systems could be routinely used in oncologic orthopedic surgery because of:

1. More physiological load sharing and lower stiffness, near to the bone values, in a situation where an excessive stress should bring to great bone resorption or implant breakage

2. Better imaging evaluation with a quite complete absence of artifacts, useful in TC and MRI imaging and in radiotherapy planning and delivering

3. No substantial differences between traditional implants in terms of surgical technique and learning curve, with early post-op weight bearing

Fig. 17.3 M, 65 YY, metastatic clear cell renal carcinoma, impending fracture of the left subtrochanteric area: postoperative image

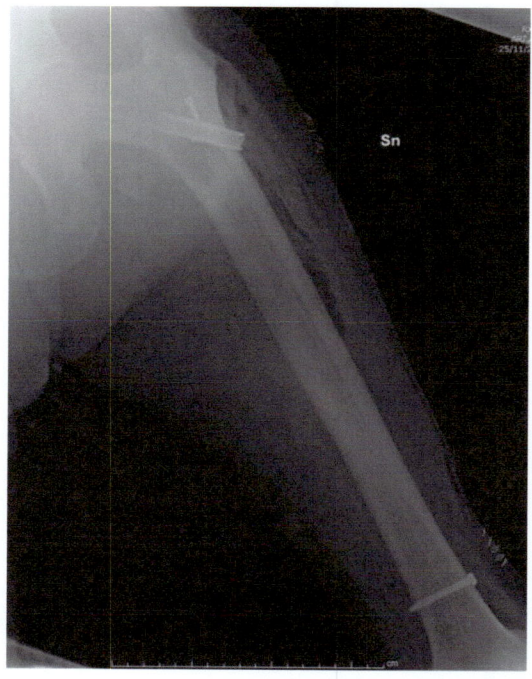

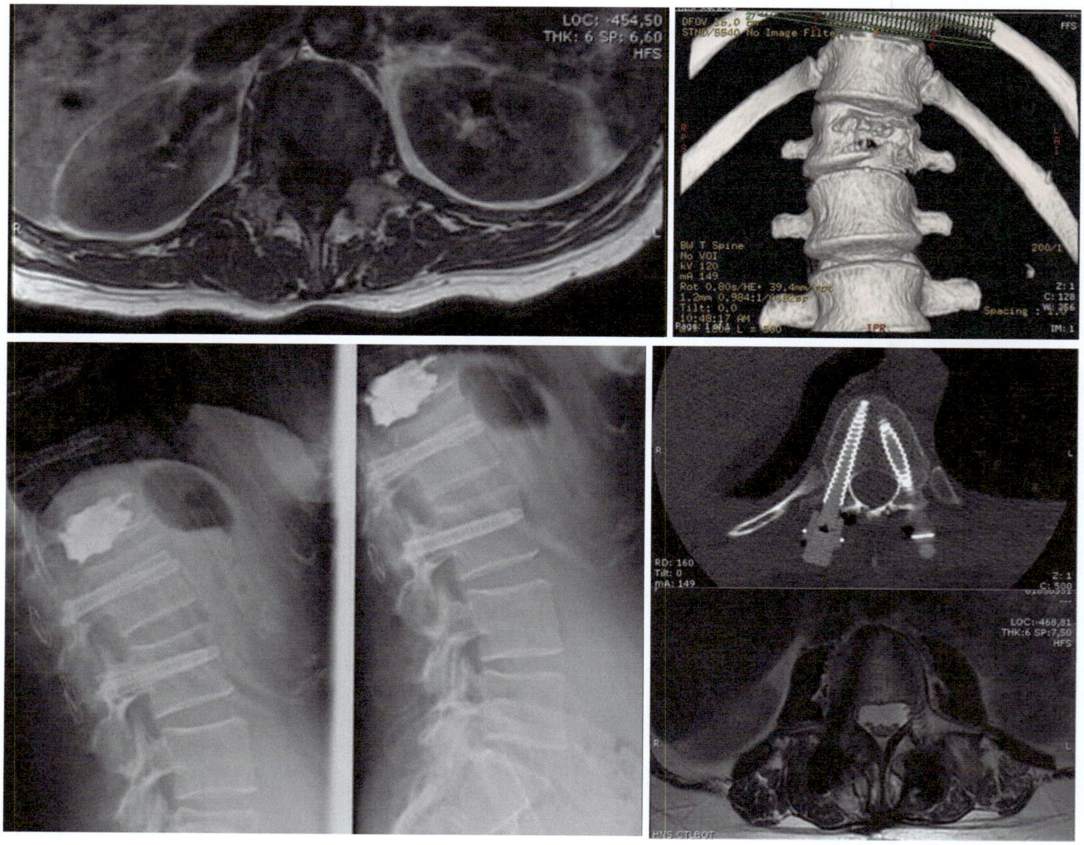

Fig. 17.4 M, 48 YY, metastatic clear cell renal carcinoma, pathologic fracture with neurologic impairment of the first vertebral body: preoperative MRI and CT reconstruction. Postoperative X-rays, CT, and MRI

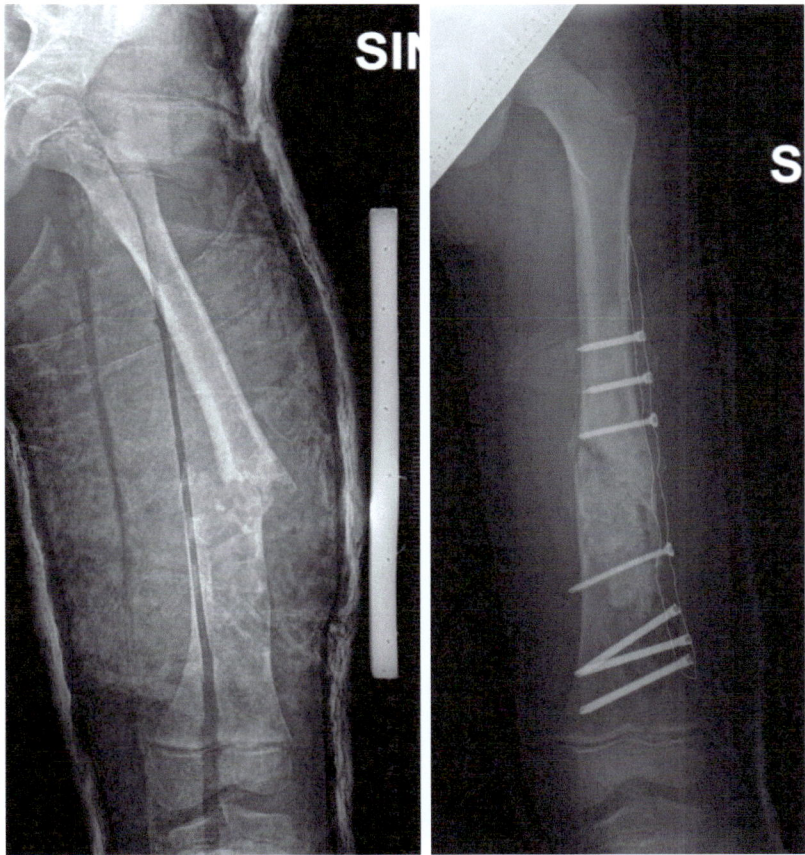

Fig. 17.5 A fractured fibrous dysplasia of the long bones in a growing child, filled with bone substitutes and fixed with a carbon fiber plate: preoperative and early postoperative (1 month) follow-up

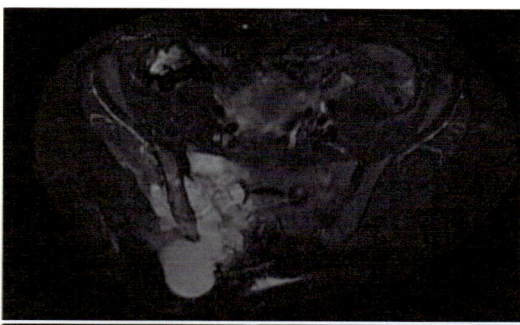

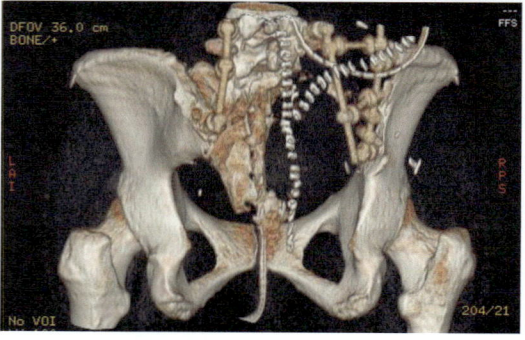

Fig. 17.6 Large chondrosarcoma involving the right hemipelvis and hemisacrum, resection and reconstruction with sacroiliac stabilization: preoperative and postoperative imaging (post-op CT scan, posterior 3-D view)

References

1. Gortzak Y, Lockwood GA, Mahendra A, Wang Y, Chung PWM, Catton CN, et al. Prediction of pathologic fracture risk of the femur after combined modality treatment of soft tissue sarcoma of the thigh. Cancer. 2010;116(6):1553–9.
2. Hillock R, Howard S, et al. Utility of carbon fiber implants in orthopedic surgery: literature review. Reconstr Rev. 2014;4(1). http://www.reconstructivereview.org/ojs/index.php/rr/article/view/55. Cited 22 Nov 2016 [Internet].
3. Epari DR, Kassi J-P, Schell H, Duda GN. Timely fracture-healing requires optimization of axial fixation stability. J Bone Joint Surg Am. 2007;89(7):1575–85.
4. Browner BD, Jupiter JB, Krettek C. Skeletal trauma: basic science, management, and reconstruction, 2-volume set. 5th ed. Philadelphia: Saunders; 2014. 2704 pp.
5. Poitout DG. Biomaterials used in orthopedics. In: Poitout DG, editor. Biomechanics and biomaterials in orthopedics. London: Springer; 2004. p. 15–20. http://link.springer.com/chapter/10.1007/978-1-4471-3774-0_2. Cited 27 Nov 2016 [Internet].
6. Cheung G, Zalzal P, Bhandari M, Spelt JK, Papini M. Finite element analysis of a femoral retrograde intramedullary nail subject to gait loading. Med Eng Phys. 2004;26(2):93–108.
7. Sha M, Guo Z, Fu J, Li J, Yuan CF, Shi L, et al. The effects of nail rigidity on fracture healing in rats with osteoporosis. Acta Orthop. 2009;80(1):135–8.
8. Ben-Or M, Shavit R, Ben-Tov T, Salai M, Steinberg EL. Control of the micromovements of a composite-material nail design: a finite element analysis. J Mech Behav Biomed Mater. 2016;54:223–8.
9. Saidpour SH. Assessment of carbon fibre composite fracture fixation plate using finite element analysis. Ann Biomed Eng. 2006;34(7):1157–63.
10. Woo SL, Lothringer KS, Akeson WH, Coutts RD, Woo YK, Simon BR, et al. Less rigid internal fixation plates: historical perspectives and new concepts. J Orthop Res. 1984;1(4):431–49.
11. Tayton K, Johnson-Nurse C, McKibbin B, Bradley J, Hastings G. The use of semi-rigid carbon-fibre-reinforced plastic plates for fixation of human fractures. Results of preliminary trials. J Bone Joint Surg Br. 1982;64(1):105–11.
12. Manninen MJ, Päivärinta U, Taurio R, Törmälä P, Suuronen R, Räihä J, et al. Polylactide screws in the fixation of olecranon osteotomies. A mechanical study in sheep. Acta Orthop Scand. 1992;63(4):437–42.
13. Suuronen R, Pohjonen T, Vasenius J, Vainionpää S. Comparison of absorbable self-reinforced multilayer poly-l-lactide and metallic plates for the fixation of mandibular body osteotomies: an experimental study in sheep. J Oral Maxillofac Surg. 1992;50(3):255–62.
14. Skinner HB. Composite technology for total hip arthroplasty. Clin Orthop. 1988;235:224–36.
15. Kurtz SM, Devine JN. PEEK biomaterials in trauma, orthopedic, and spinal implants. Biomaterials. 2007;28(32):4845–69.
16. Utzschneider S, Becker F, Grupp TM, Sievers B, Paulus A, Gottschalk O, et al. Inflammatory response against different carbon fiber-reinforced PEEK wear particles compared with UHMWPE in vivo. Acta Biomater. 2010;6(11):4296–304.
17. Scotchford CA, Garle MJ, Batchelor J, Bradley J, Grant DM. Use of a novel carbon fibre composite material for the femoral stem component of a THR system: in vitro biological assessment. Biomaterials. 2003;24(26):4871–9.
18. Brown SA, Hastings RS, Mason JJ, Moet A. Characterization of short-fibre reinforced thermoplastics for fracture fixation devices. Biomaterials. 1990;11(8):541–7.
19. Hak DJ, Mauffrey C, Seligson D, Lindeque B. Use of carbon-fiber-reinforced composite implants in orthopedic surgery. Orthopedics. 2014;37(12):825–30. Lindeque BGP, editor.
20. Koff MF, Shah P, Koch KM, Potter HG. Quantifying image distortion of orthopedic materials in magnetic resonance imaging. J Magn Reson Imaging. 2013;38(3):610–8.
21. Zimel MN, Hwang S, Riedel ER, Healey JH. Carbon fiber intramedullary nails reduce artifact

in postoperative advanced imaging. Skelet Radiol. 2015;44(9):1317–25.

22. Steinberg EL, Rath E, Shlaifer A, Chechik O, Maman E, Salai M. Carbon fiber reinforced PEEK optima— a composite material biomechanical properties and wear/debris characteristics of CF-PEEK composites for orthopedic trauma implants. J Mech Behav Biomed Mater. 2013;17:221–8.

23. Baidya KP, Ramakrishna S, Rahman M, Ritchie A. Quantitative radiographic analysis of fiber reinforced polymer composites. J Biomater Appl. 2001; 15(3):279–89.

24. Sofka CM, Potter HG, Adler RS, Pavlov H. Musculoskeletal imaging update: current applications of advanced imaging techniques to evaluate the early and long-term complications of patients with orthopedic implants. HSS J. 2006;2(1):73–7.

25. Buckwalter KA, Lin C, Ford JM. Managing postoperative artifacts on computed tomography and magnetic resonance imaging. Semin Musculoskelet Radiol. 2011;15(4):309–19.

26. Xin-ye N, Xiao-bin T, Chang-ran G, Da C. The prospect of carbon fiber implants in radiotherapy. J Appl Clin Med Phys. 2012;13(4). http://www.jacmp.org/index.php/jacmp/article/view/3821. Cited 18 Nov 2016 [Internet].

27. Nevelsky A, Borzov E, Daniel S, Bar-Deroma R. Perturbation effects of the carbon fiber-PEEK screws on radiotherapy dose distribution. J Appl Clin Med Phys. 2017;18(2):62–8.

28. Tarallo L, Mugnai R, Adani R, Zambianchi F, Catani F. A new volar plate made of carbon-fiber-reinforced polyetheretherketon for distal radius fracture: analysis of 40 cases. J Orthop Traumatol. 2014;15(4):277–83.

Infections After Surgery for MBD

18

Giulio Di Giacomo, Fabrizio Donati,
Carlo Perisano, Michele Attilio Rosa,
and Giulio Maccauro

Abstract

The life expectancy of patients with bone metastases has remarkably increased over recent years leading to higher incidence of bone metastases with major risk of pathological fractures and orthopedic treatments. Orthopedic surgery in bone metastases has a highly diversified approach and could be very invasive, requiring prosthetic implants, allograft, nails, plates or other metallic devices, vascular procedures, and plastic surgery.

Metal wear and especially megaprosthesis implantation are commonly complicated by deep infections, which are probably the most common and severe complication in orthopedic oncological surgery, considered as challenging as local relapse. The rate of infection in these treatments range from 8% to over 40%, with great variability depending on the site of replacement, age, comorbidity, resection size, and histological characteristics of primary malignant tumor involved.

Infection prevention is therefore of the utmost importance considering that, when there are poor soft tissue conditions, secondary amputation is sometimes inevitable.

Postoperative infection complications have also a heavy impact on the cost and management aspects due to hospital readmissions, extended hospitalization, the need for additional procedures, and convalescent or nursing home care.

Great interest is actually spreading about orthopedic infections in bone metastatic disease, as reflected by a great number of literature reviews, monothematic meetings, and multicenter prospective studies. According to this consideration, in this chapter we analyze all the possible actions described to prevent and treat surgical site infections following this kind of surgery, including an appropriate antibiotic prophylaxis, surgical procedures for primary and revision surgery and recent technical improvements.

G. Di Giacomo · C. Perisano · G. Maccauro
Division of Orthopedic and Traumatology, Catholic
University of the Sacred Heart, Rome, Italy
e-mail: giulio.digiacomo@email.it;
carloperisano@hotmail.it;giuliomac@tiscali.it

F. Donati (✉)
Division of Orthopedic, Bambino Gesù Children
Hospital, Rome, Italy
e-mail: fabriziodonati2@hotmail.it

M. A. Rosa
Division of Orthopedic and Traumatology, Messina
University, Messina, Italy
e-mail: marosa@unime.it

Keywords

Infection · Limb salvage surgery · Tumor
prosthesis · Antibiotic prophylaxis

18.1 Introduction

The life expectancy of patients with bone metastases has remarkably increased over recent years due to improvements in chemotherapy, radiation therapy, and other oncological treatments. It has led to a higher incidence of bone metastases with major risk of pathological fractures [1]. The rate of pathological fractures of the long bones in patients with recognized bone metastases is approximately 10% [2–5].

Orthopedic surgery in bone metastases treatment has a highly diversified approach and could be very invasive, requiring prosthetic implants, allograft, nails, plates or other metallic devices, vascular procedures, and plastic surgery [6].

Metal wear and especially megaprosthesis implantation are commonly complicated by deep infections, which are probably the most common and severe complications in orthopedic oncological surgery, considered as challenging as local relapse. The rate of infection in these treatments range from 8% to over 40%, with great variability depending on the site of surgery, age, comorbidity, resection size, and histological characteristics of primary malignant tumor involved.

Patients affected by bone metastasis are debilitated by tumor itself, chemotherapy or concomitant illness regarding other organs, and the large metal surface of the implants predispose to bacterial colonization. Infection prevention is therefore of the utmost importance considering that, when there are poor soft tissue conditions, secondary amputation is sometimes inevitable (Fig. 18.1).

Postoperative infection complications have also a heavy impact on the cost and management aspects due to hospital readmissions, extended hospitalization, the need for additional procedures (often removal and re-implantation of implanted hardware and prolonged antimicrobial therapy), and convalescent or nursing home care [7].

Great interest is actually spreading about orthopedic infections in bone metastatic disease, as reflected by a great number of literature reviews, monothematic meetings, and multicenter prospective studies [8]. It is therefore necessary to know all the possible actions used to prevent and treat surgical site infections follow-

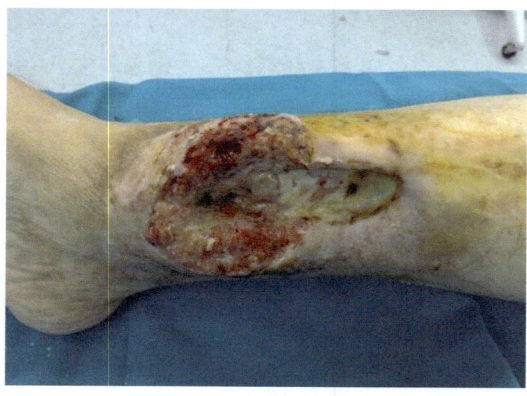

Fig. 18.1 Severe soft tissue loosening after infection following wide resection surgery and ankle tumor prosthesis reconstruction. In such condition secondary amputation is inevitable

ing this kind of surgery, including an appropriate antibiotic prophylaxis, surgical procedures for primary and revision surgery, and recent technical improvements.

18.2 Risk Factors

Several potential risk factors for postoperative site infections are well known and are connected to the kind of surgery and other performed treatments, tumor characteristics (local malignancy, histological type, depth and invasion, solitary or multiple site involvement), and also the patient's general health status.

Orthopedic surgery in metastatic bone disease treatment is highly variable, and it depends on different factors. Obviously mininvasive approach has a lower risk of infection but unfortunately is not always suitable. The prognosis is probably the main factor to be considered for an appropriate surgical indication. A patient with a life expectancy lower than 3/6 months will benefit of a less invasive treatment even if it will not restore a good function. More conservative treatments guarantee a lower risk of complications like massive blood loss, bacterial colonization, and long hospitalization that are more common in large resection and megaprosthesis implants compared to intramedullary nailing (Figs. 18.2 and 18.3).

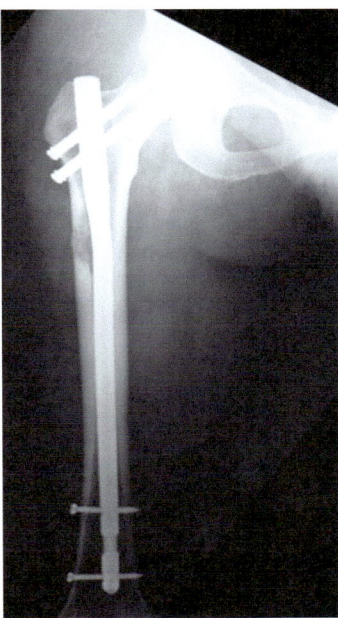

Fig. 18.2 Intramedullary nailing in a femoral impending fracture secondary to a metastatic lesion

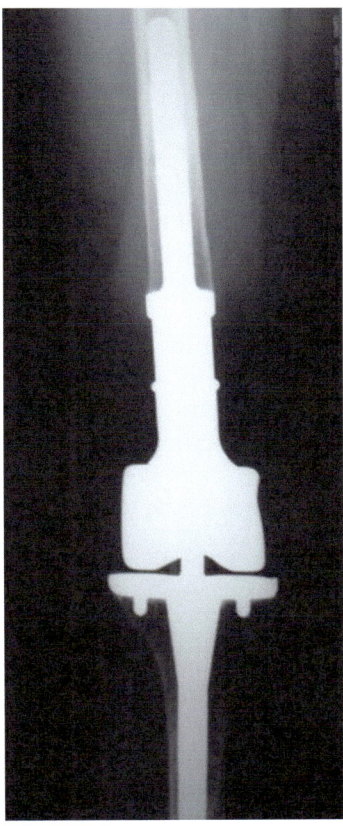

Fig. 18.3 Knee megaprosthesis after distal femur resection for a metastatic periarticular lesion. Prosthetic reconstruction allows better clinical outcome but has shown a higher risk of infection

Radiotherapy as local neoadjuvant, performed before surgery of metastatic bone disease, increases the infection risk because of tissue necrosis and a decreased blood supply and therefore to a lower immunological response. In these cases, it is not recommended to perform surgery to avoid surgical site infection and iatrogenic fractures.

Patients' immunosuppression and hyponutrition from neoadjuvant chemotherapy are other major risk factors for wound complications.

There are no demonstrations of a higher association among a specific kind of primary tumor with the risk of surgical site infection, even if a more invasive and vascularized bone metastasis could lead to higher rate of complications.

A few study analyzed the relationship between surgical site treated and the risk to develop a local infection.

Other risk factors for infections in tumor orthopedic surgery are overlapped on primary prosthetic joint surgery [4] including advanced age, obesity, diabetes mellitus, corticosteroid use, rheumatoid arthritis, previous surgery on the same joint, arthroplasty following a fracture, replaced joint (e.g., risk is greater for the knee than the hip), and perioperative surgical site complications, including hematoma and persistent surgical site drainage.

Operative risk factors include ASA classification of ≥3, operative time exceeding the 75th percentile for the procedure or exceeding 3 h, surgical site classified as contaminated or dirty, and inadequate antimicrobial prophylaxis.

18.3 Epidemiology and Diagnosis

Currently, it is difficult to avoid periprosthetic infection completely, despite the use of operating rooms with laminar airflow, systemic antibiotic treatment, and routine screening for multidrug-resistant bacteria that are becoming more and more common cause of infection.

The infection rate in limb salvage surgery following metastatic lesions ranges from 8% to more than 40% in different studies and meta-analyses, with great variability depending on several potential risk factors previously described. The infection risk is reported to be 8–35% for primary megaprostheses implants and 30–43% after revision surgery, with an average rate of 19% for lower-extremity endoprosthetic reconstruction [2, 9–11]. The infection risk for nailing in limbs' impending fracture surgery and kyphoplasty in vertebral fractures is the lowest above all the considered surgical procedures. Even an excision biopsy could lead to a devastating local infection in severely immunocompromised patients. However, it is often necessary to obtain a definitive diagnosis especially when the primary tumor is unknown.

The diagnosis of infection is essentially clinical with typical inflammation symptoms (rubor-tumor-dolor-calor). However, considering the immunological impairment of these patients, the symptoms of infection could appear with an unconventional clinical presentation (Fig. 18.4).

Fever during chemotherapy-induced neutropenia may be the only indication of a severe underlying infection, because in these cases signs and symptoms of inflammation are typically attenuated. At the same time, other hematological inflammatory parameters like CPR and ESR could be less evocative than usual.

Sometimes ultrasound examination could identify superficial or deep abscess. Total body CT scan, MRI, and body scan are commonly used to stage the tumor extension, and these could be useful also in the case of suspected infection to analyze the risk of local or systemic dissemination.

The only diagnostic examination that allows a qualitative diagnosis is a direct microbacterial examination with antibiotic susceptibility testing. It permits to identify the pathogen and to obtain information about the most appropriate antibiotic treatment.

Saprophyte bacteria of the skin are the most frequent pathogens involved in surgical site infections after surgical procedures for bone metastasis. The bacteria most commonly isolated in this cases are *S. aureus*, gram-negative bacilli, coagulase-negative staphylococci (including *S. epidermidis*), and beta-hemolytic streptococci (Table 18.1) [5, 12].

18.4 Antibiotic Prophilaxis and Antibacterial Devices

A contributing factor to surgical site infections (SSIs) in orthopedic procedures is the formation of bacterial biofilm, particularly with *S. aureus* and *S. epidermidis*, on inert surfaces of orthopedic

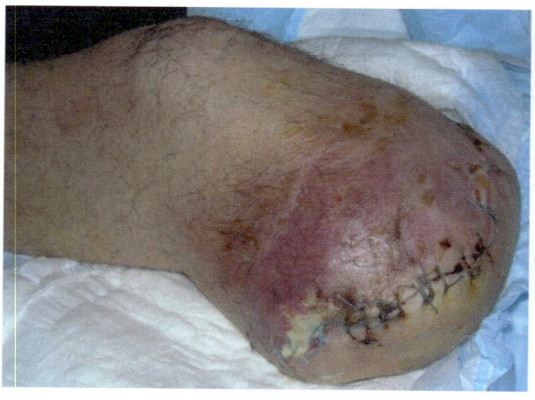
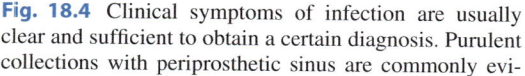
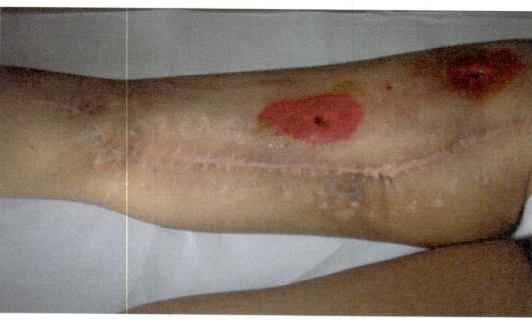

Fig. 18.4 Clinical symptoms of infection are usually clear and sufficient to obtain a certain diagnosis. Purulent collections with periprosthetic sinus are commonly evident in case of deep or superficial infection. Subclinical cases of infection must be taken in consideration and analyzed with further examinations

Table 18.1 Common bacterial pathogens affecting neutropenic patients after major orthopedic surgery

Common gram + pathogens	Common gram − pathogens
Coagulase-negative staphylococci	*Escherichia coli*
Staphylococcus aureus, including MRSA	Klebsiella species
Enterococcus species	Enterobacter species
Viridans group streptococci	*Pseudomonas aeruginosa*
Streptococcus pneumoniae	Citrobacter species
Streptococcus pyogenes	Acinetobacter species
	Stenotrophomonas maltophilia

devices. Bacterial biofilm confers antimicrobial resistance and makes antimicrobial penetration difficult [13–16].

Many options were proposed to prevent surgical infections. Surely systemic antibiotic treatments have a significant role. Many intra- and perioperative antibiotics prophylaxis regimens have been proposed [9, 17]. It is not easy to demonstrate a statistically significant supremacy of one class of antibiotics over another for antimicrobial prophylaxis in tumor orthopedic surgery, but it is mandatory to choose one among those proposed. A meta-analysis of studies found no differences in SSIs between cephalosporins with teicoplanin. Selection of a specific antibiotic prophylaxis should be based on cost, availability, and local resistance patterns according to the indication of a local infectious disease specialist considering that often each hospital have different pathogen pattern.

Literature over the last decade shows an urgent need to focus on epidemiology, early diagnosis, antimicrobial coverage for metal implants, identification of risk factors, and, most of all, on the urgent need to define guidelines for antibiotic prophylaxis [1, 3].

First-generation cephalosporins, administered from 60 to 30 min before surgery, are the agents most commonly studied and used. For patients with a beta-lactam allergy, clindamycin and vancomycin have adequate activity against the most common pathogens involved in orthopedic procedures and would be acceptable alternatives for surgery prophylaxis. Vancomycin should be included with cefazolin or used as an alternative agent for routine antimicrobial prophylaxis in institutions that have a high prevalence of MRSA surgical site infection and for patients who are known to be colonized with MRSA [18, 19].

The duration of prophylaxis in joint replacement procedures is controversial. More recent data and clinical practice guidelines do not support prophylaxis beyond 24 h [18, 20]. However, it can be reasonable to continue antimicrobial prophylaxis until all drains or catheters are removed [21].

Associated local treatment like antibiotic local washing, medicated device, or metals with antimicrobial activity is obtaining an increasing application. Among the metal with antimicrobial activity, silver has garnered much interest due to its excellent antimicrobial activity coupled with low toxicity [22]. Different medical devices exploiting the properties of silver are now available, not only in orthopedics surgery. Silver-coated tumor endoprosthesis has been introduced in medical practice almost 25 years ago initially with the aim of treating local periprosthetic infections. In literature, any severe early or late general sign of silver toxicity following silver-coated prosthesis implantation in animals or humans are described. The most important bactericidal mechanism of the silver ion is its interaction with the thiol groups of the L-cysteine residue of proteins and its inactivation of bacterial enzymatic functions [23, 24]. Other bactericidal mechanism of silver ions is the release of potassium [25], bonding to DNA [26], and generation of intracellular reactive oxygen species (ROS).

The implants of silver-coated devices are actually suggested, by some authors, as primary implants in oncologic limb salvage surgery [27–29].

The use of antimicrobial-loaded bone cement is another practice common worldwide, particularly for the prevention of infection in limb salvage surgery and megaprosthesis implants [30–33]. The results of antibiotic-loaded cements and of local antibiotic washing are widely debated. Their efficacy and their duration have been rarely statistically confirmed.

18.5 Surgical Site Infection Treatment

Surgical site infection treatment depends on patients' condition, timing, and local condition. In case of symptoms from less than 3 weeks, a stable implant, absence of sinus tract and susceptibility to antibiotics with activity against surface-adhering microorganisms, surgical treatment consists in debridement with retention of the implants combined either with antibiotics [34]. When the patient is debilitated by tumor and chemotherapy or concomitant illness or bedridden, a long-term suppressive antimicrobial treatment to control only clinical symptoms is recommended. Furthermore, permanent removal of the device or amputation is reserved for patients with high risk of reinfection and without improvement by exchange of the implant.

Otherwise, in case of high virulence bacteria, damaged soft tissue, abscess, or sinus tract, a two-stage revision with a short interval until reimplantation (2–4 weeks) is preferred, by the use of a temporary antimicrobial-impregnated bone cement spacer. When the prosthesis is colonized by microorganism resistant or difficult to treat (MRSA, enterococci, quinolone-resistant *Pseudomonas aeruginosa* and fungi), a longer interval (at least 8 weeks) is required. Two-stage procedure has the highest success outcome but has an important cost for both the patient and the surgeon [35]. This kind of surgery is usually very demanding especially in case of reintervention after wide bone resection and megaprosthesis implant. The surgeon in this case is obliged to create a reinforced custom-made spacers adapting different devices and techniques like using a metal structure (intramedullary nails, K wires, TENs, or others) covered by antibiotic-loaded cement (Fig. 18.5).

One-stage revision is still debated because it is associated to a higher risk of reinfections. In the case of intact or only slightly damaged soft tissues, in low virulent bacterial colonization, some authors propose a direct one-stage exchange of the prosthesis in the same surgical time after a wide debridement of the surgical site [36], using a prolonged antibiotic prophylaxis.

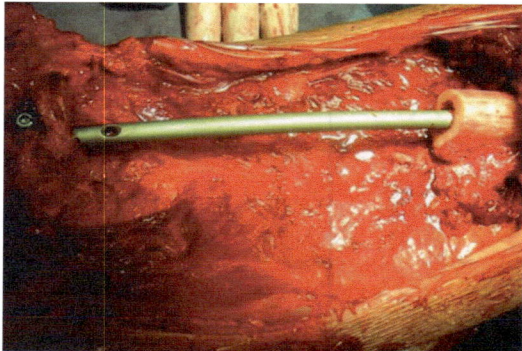
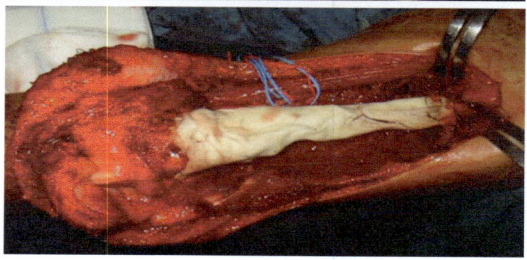

Fig. 18.5 Two-stage revision after infection of knee megaprosthesis. Custom-made spacer can be obtained using antibiotic-loaded cement reinforced by an inner metal core constituted of a common intramedullary nail

References

1. Jeys LM, Grimer RJ, Carter SR, Tillman RM. Periprosthetic infection in patients treated for an orthopaedic oncological condition. J Bone Joint Surg Am. 2005;87:842–9.
2. Capanna R, Morris HG, Campanacci D, Del Ben M, Campanacci M. Modular uncemented prosthetic reconstruction after resection of tumours of the distal femur. J Bone Joint Surg Br. 1994;76:178–86.
3. Hasan K, Racano A, Deheshi B, Farrokhyar F, Wunder J, et al. Prophylactic antibiotic regimens in tumor surgery (PARITY) survey. BMC Musculoskelet Disord. 2012;13:91.
4. Matthews PC, Berendt AR, McNally MA, et al. Diagnosis and management of prosthetic joint infection. BMJ. 2009;338:1378–83.
5. Boxma H, Broekhuizen T, Patka P, et al. Randomised controlled trial of single-dose antibiotic prophylaxis in surgical treatment of closed fractures: the Dutch trauma trial. Lancet. 1996;347:1133–7.
6. Schwartz A, Rebecca A, Smith A, Casey W, Ashman J, et al. Risk factors for significant wound complications following wide resection of extremity soft tissue sarcomas. Clin Orthop Relat Res. 2013;471:3612–7.
7. Whitehouse JD, Friedman ND, Kirkland KB, et al. The impact of surgical-site infections following orthopedic surgery at a community hospital and uni-

versity hospital: adverse quality of life, excess length of stay and extra cost. Infect Control Hosp Epidemiol. 2002;23:183–9.

8. Morii T, Morioka H, Ueda T, Araki N, Hashimoto N, et al. Deep infection in tumor endoprosthesis around the knee: a multi-institutional study by the Japanese musculoskeletal oncology group. BMC Musculoskelet Disord. 2013;14:51.

9. Racano A, Pazionis T, Farrokhyar F, Deheshi B, Ghert M. High infection rate outcomes in long-bone tumor surgery with endoprosthetic reconstruction in adults: a systematic review. Clin Orthop Relat Res. 2013;471:2017–27.

10. Shehadeh A, Noveau J, Malawer M, Henshaw R. Late complications and survival of endoprosthetic recon-struction after resection of bone tumors. Clin Orthop Relat Res. 2010;468:2885–95.

11. Mavrogenis AF, Pala E, Angelini A, Calabro T, Romagnoli C, et al. Infected prostheses after lower-extremity bone tumor resection: clinical outcomes of 100 patients. Surg Infect. 2015;16:267–75.

12. Trampuz A, Zimmerli W. Antimicrobial agents in orthopedic surgery: prophylaxis and treatment. Drugs. 2006;66:1089–105.

13. Meehan J, Jamali AA, Nguyen H. Prophylactic anti-biotics in hip and knee arthroplasty. J Bone Joint Surg Am. 2009;91:2480–90.

14. Costerton JW, Stewart PS, Greenberg EP. Bacterial biofilms: a common cause of persistent infections. Science. 1999;284:1318–22.

15. Costerton JW. Biofilm theory can guide the treatment of device-related orthopaedic infections. Clin Orthop Relat Res. 2005;437:7–11.

16. Lewis K. Riddle of biofilm resistance. Antimicrob Agents Chemother. 2001;45:999–1007.

17. Hardes J, Gebert C, Schwappach A, et al. Characteristics and outcome of infections associated with tumor endoprostheses. Arch Orthop Trauma Surg. 2006;126:289–96.

18. Antimicrobial prophylaxis for surgery. Treat Guidel Med Lett. 2009;7:47–52.

19. Mangram AJ, Horan TC, Pearson ML, et al. Guideline for prevention of surgical site infection. Infect Control Hosp Epidemiol. 1999;20:250–78.

20. Jaeger M, Maier D, Kern WV, et al. Antibiotics in trauma and orthopedic surgery—a primer of evidence-based recommendations. Injury. 2006;37:s74–80.

21. Bratzler DW, Houck PM, Richards C, et al. Use of antimicrobial prophylaxis for major surgery: base-line results from the National Surgical Infection Prevention Project. Arch Surg. 2005;140:174–82.

22. Tobin EJ, Bambauer R. Silver coating of dialysis cath-eters to reduce bacterial colonization and infection. Ther Apher Dial. 2003;7:504–9.

23. Schierholz JM, Lucas LJ, Rump A, Pulverer G. Efficacy of silver-coated medical devices. J Hosp Infect. 1998;40(4):257–62. https://doi.org/10.1016/s0195-6701(98)90301-2.

24. Kim TN, Feng QL, Kim JO, et al. Antimicrobial effects of metal ions (Ag+, Cu2+, Zn2+) in hydroxy-apatite. J Mater Sci Mater Med. 1998;9(3):129–34.

25. Tweden KS, Cameron JD, Razzouk AJ, Holmberg WR, Kelly SJ. Biocompatibility of silver-modified polyester for antimicrobial protection of prosthetic valves. J Heart Valve Dis. 1997;6(5):553–61.

26. Wan AT, Conyers RAJ, Coombs CJ, Masterton JP. Determination of silver in blood, urine, and tis-sues of volunteers and burn patients. Clin Chem. 1991;37(10):1683–7.

27. Donati F, Di Giacomo G, D'Adamio S, Ziranu A, Careri S, Rosa M, Maccauro G. Silver-coated hip megaprosthesis in oncological limb savage surgery. Biomed Res Int. 2016;2016:9079041.

28. Piccioli A, Donati F, Di Giacomo G, A Ziranu, Careri S, Spinelli MS, Giannini S, Giannicola G, Perisano C, Maccauro G. Infective complications in tumour endoprostheses implanted after patho-logical fracture of the limbs Injury 2016. https://doi.org/10.1016/j.injury.2016.07.054. Available online 25 Aug 2016.

29. Donati F, Di Giacomo G, Ziranu A, Spinelli S, Perisano C, Rosa MA, Maccauro G. Silver coated prosthesis in oncological limb salvage surgery reduce the infection rate. J Biol Regul Homeost Agents. 2015;29(4 Suppl):149–55.

30. Bourne RB. Prophylactic use of antibiotic bone cement: an emerging standard—in the affirmative. J Arthroplast. 2004;19(suppl 1):69–72.

31. Engesaeter LB, Lie SA, Espehaug B, et al. Antibiotic prophylaxis in total hip arthroplasty: effects of antibiotic prophylaxis systemically and in bone cement on the revision rate of 22,170 primary hip replacements followed 0 to 14 years in the Norwegian Arthroplasty Register. Acta Orthop Scand. 2003;74:644–51.

32. Espehaug B, Engesaeter LB, Vollset SE, et al. Antibiotic prophylaxis in total hip arthroplasty: review of 10,905 primary cemented total hip replace-ments reported to the Norwegian Arthroplasty Register, 1987 to 1995. J Bone Joint Surg Br. 1997;79:590–5.

33. Jiranek WA, Hanssen AD, Greenwald AS. Antibioticloaded bone cement for infection prophy-laxis in total joint replacement. J Bone Joint Surg Am. 2006;88(11):2487–500.

34. Zimmerli W, Trampuz A, Ochsner PE. Prosthetic-joint infections. N Engl J Med. 2004;351:1645–54.

35. Westrich GH, Salvati EA, Brause B. Postoperative infection. In: Bono JV, JC MC, Thornhill TS, Bierbaum BE, Turner RH, editors. Revision total hip arthroplasty. New York: Springer; 1999. p. 371–90.

36. Raut VV, Siney PD, Wroblewski BM. One-stage revision of infected total hip replacements with discharging sinuses. J Bone Joint Surg Br. 1994;76:721–4.

Management of Fractures and Failures Around Tumor Implants

19

Roberto Casadei, Gabriele Drago,
and Davide Donati

Abstract

As more patients with skeletal metastases live longer, many implants are at risk for mechanical failure and for tumor progression in the face of previous treatment. The causes for and treatment options available to failed cases have received some attention in the literature, but few papers suggested what surgery was the best. Failures around tumor implants can be mechanical and not mechanical. The first include dislocation, soft tissue defect, wound dehiscence, aseptic loosening, and fractures, whereas the second infections and disease progression. For all types of failure, different strategies of treatment are described.

Keywords

Complications · Mechanical failures
Infections · Disease Progression

19.1 Introduction

Improvements in the oncological management of metastatic patients have resulted in an increased population survival free of disease or with known metastases. The result has been an increased number of patients alive with skeletal metastases and the adoption of more aggressive treatment options positively impacting on patient's survival [1]. Technological developments in other fields, including material science, anesthesiology, radiographic, and new surgical techniques, have made it possible to use surgery more frequently for the treatment of these patients, with an acceptable risk of complications [2]. In literature, patients' survival is not related to the surgical treatment and to the type of implant [3].

Successful surgical treatment of bone metastases requires careful consideration of patient-specific (age, performance status, and patient anesthetist evaluation) and disease-specific variables (histotype, staging and grading, response to different therapies, pain, risk of complications, extension of the lesion) [2, 4]. The goal of treating patients with skeletal metastases is to relieve pain and to preserve function, and thus quality of life for the greatest amount of time; therefore, careful attention must be paid to each patient's estimated survival [4, 5]. Estimation of prognosis and survival is subjective. It has been shown that estimation of survival in cancer patients may be correct only in 18%, and it is underestimated in 43% of patients. Moreover, current decision-making in metastatic cancer patients needs to consider not only prognosis and survivorship but also quality of life and function [5].

From this statement, it is obvious that prognosis is a very important factor for the choice of

R. Casadei (✉) · G. Drago · D. Donati
Department of Musculoskeletal Oncology, Istituto Ortopedico Rizzoli, Bologna, Italy
e-mail: roberto.casadei@ior.it; davide.donati@ior.it

© Springer International Publishing AG, part of Springer Nature 2019
V. Denaro et al. (eds.), *Management of Bone Metastases*, https://doi.org/10.1007/978-3-319-73485-9_19

adequate surgery, and a multidisciplinary approach to bone metastases is therefore necessary. In this contest, methods to estimate life expectancy in these patients should be used whenever possible [4].

When dealing with the patient affected by a long bone metastasis, there are three different type of surgery:

1. "Radical" surgery: only in patient with a good prognosis. Patients with expected long survival that undergo en bloc/complete resection of the single bone metastasis and reconstruction with modular prosthesis, making the patient potentially disease free.
2. "Adjuvant" surgery: in patients with a fair prognosis. This treatment consists in whole metastasis removing with debulking and stabilization with nail or plate and cement which significantly decrease pain and reduce the risk of local recurrences
3. "Palliative" surgery: in patients with a severe prognosis. In these patients with poor general conditions and short survival, there is usually consensus not to treat bone lesions, but surgery is performed only to avoid complications due to bone metastases: i.e., to stabilize the bone before a fracture occurs or to decompress the spine before symptoms of spinal cord compression appear [2].

Surgery of bone metastasis should be (a) early and sometimes combined with other therapies to improve patient treatment and overall survival; (b) the most effective to avoid a second surgery (that often the patient cannot sustain); (c) planned with implants that last at least as long as the life expectancy of patient; (d) as simple as possible, to reduce the length of hospitalization; and (e) as aggressive as possible, to excise most of the bone lesion.

In this contest, surgical implants should be as solid and stable as possible to speed the functional recovery even in the case of progression of the disease. They should be able to minimize surgical-related complications while being as long as possible to stabilize the whole bone to avoid a new pathologic fracture.

Surgical procedures for bone metastases are widely chosen from intramedullary nailing (IMN), endoprosthetic reconstruction (EPR), or plating and cementation [6].

In the last years, a reduction of about 10% is observed in the overall failure rate of endoprostheses with an important reduction in the incidence of failures for each anatomic location [7, 8]. The improvement in patient survival has also resulted in patients presenting with mechanical failure of internal fixation strategies or tumor progression in the face of previous attempted stabilization [1].

The major advantages of endoprostheses are the relatively simple and quick intraoperative assembly and their immediate mechanical stability; this latter allows early weight bearing and functional recovery [9, 10], with effective and fast pain relief and longer implants survival [2, 4]. However, the use of megaprostheses has some drawbacks, such as a high risk of complications and reduced functions of the limbs due to damaged muscle attachments [2, 11]. Biologic tendinous reattachment to the metallic prosthesis is not possible and usually results in loss of strength of hip abductors and of the extensor mechanism of the knee. Allograft-prosthesis composites, used in primary malignant tumor to combine the advantages of endoprostheses with the functional improvement resulting from biologic tendinous reattachment of the hip abductors and patellar tendon due to the allograft, cannot be used in bone metastases because of the long time necessary for the allograft union and for the easy degeneration of the allograft after chemotherapy and radiotherapy [9].

Plate fixation can be acceptable only when the bone stock is adequate to secure screw fixation. Placing cement into the medullary canal gives more security to the fixation, but the potential progression of the lesions at the borders of the fixation must be considered. Plating, especially with long plates, accompanies a possibility to nerve injury at peculiar anatomical sites like in the distal humerus. Cement may also help as a local adjuvant for curettage of bone metastases with thermal damage, and it does not prevent bony healing, which might be an indirect sign that endosteal healing is not disturbed by whole bone cementing.

Intramedullary nailing (IMN) can protect a long segment of bone, and it is a simple and quick procedure with minimal morbidity [12]. However, it has been criticized because of poorer function, because the nail is inserted through rotator cuff tendon or gluteal tendons.

IMN has some advantages over EPR, including lower costs and less invasiveness [6]. IMN is convenient and effective for bone stabilization, and it is accompanied by good pain relief and early functional use of the extremity. Closed nailing allows immediate delivery of radiotherapy without the risk of wound compromise. IMN is preferred over plating due to a less contamination of the soft tissue, greater rigidity of the construct, and less damage from disease progression, but there is not an agreement about the associated use of intramedullary cement. This technique allows for immediate weight bearing in lower limbs, improved postoperative stability, and has resulted in a significant decreased incidence of subsequent fracture and other complications. However, cement within the medullary cavity together with intramedullary nails is unnecessary due to the new modern intramedullary devices with more possibilities to lock the nail, especially in the non-weight-bearing bone as humerus. However, pain relief is more rapid and more efficient when cement is used. Restoring and preserving the function gives these patients dignity and preserves the quality of life for the patients' lifespan [12]. Because of the increased survival of patients with bone metastases, complications related to failure of tumor implants that required further surgery are more and more frequent.

Many studies have investigated the prognostic factors influencing patient survival following surgical intervention for skeletal metastases, but little attention has been given to the survival of the implants used for reconstruction following resection of these metastases [1].

Studies on tumor prostheses often involve a mixture of primary sarcomas and metastases or are focused on a particular anatomic region such as the proximal femur or humerus. There are few outcome studies on the use of modular tumor prostheses in the treatment of patients with long bone metastases with regards to survival of prosthesis [5].

While many investigators have reported the outcomes of patients receiving primary metallic EPR for oncologic indications, few authors have specifically addressed the modes by which they fail [7].

Moreover, humeral implants have been less investigated compared to those of the femur; in fact, small numbers of patients limit most of the reports about surgical treatment of humeral metastases [8].

As more patients with skeletal metastases live longer, many implants are at risk for mechanical failure and for tumor progression in the face of previous stabilization. Treatment options available for failed cases have received some attention in the literature, but few papers describe the subsequent course of these patients [4].

Complications are reported to be five to ten times higher when using mega-prostheses compared to standard implants, and the overall revision rate in patients with megaprostheses of the hip is higher respect to primary total hip arthroplasty [7, 9, 13, 14].

Immunosuppressive therapy, extensile surgical dissections, longer operative time, and general patient condition can help to explain this situation [10].

In the proximal femur, endoprosthesis survival rate approximates 88% after 1 year and after 5 years. In the proximal humerus, endoprosthesis survival rate is 95% after 1 year and 76% after 5 years [5].

Some previous studies have demonstrated that in the EPR group, the rate of implant failure was lower, and overall patient survival was longer compared to the IMN group [3, 6]. However, the nail survival rate was 94.0% at 3 years; but it dropped to 62.8% at 50 months, and this device can be regarded as appropriate for a metastatic patient whose survival at 3 years is only 8.4% [6].

According to Forsberg et al., the use of EPR is useful as a salvage treatment, even at the end of life or in patients where operative time, blood loss, physiological insult, and rehabilitation requirements should be minimized. Surgeons should continue to balance the risk of perioperative complications with the benefits that are predicated on each patient's estimated life expectancy and functional goals [4].

19.2 Clinical Results

Rates of overall failure, range from 3.1 to 42% for the few patients with cancer who survive more than 1 year [4, 5]. Different failure rates are reported in literature: 6.2% [15], 10.3% [16], 11% [14], 18.3% [5], 24% [7], and 29% [9, 10, 17]. In humeral reconstruction, a failure rate of 9% at a mean time of 8 months is reported in the Wedin series [8].

Time to failure is significantly related to the anatomic location and to the mode of failure for all locations. The mean overall time for all types of failure ranges from 31 to 47 months with the shortest mean time to failure (10.9 months) observed in the distal humeral replacements and the longest (53 months) observed in proximal humeral replacements. Intervals to failure were similar for proximal tibial and distal femoral replacements [7, 10].

Major risk factors for implant failure include:

1. Preoperative radiotherapy. It is considered as an important risk factor for developing infections in immunodepressed patients with neoplastic disease, particularly after chemotherapy.
2. Wide surgical approach and the size of metal implants. These produce a significant blood loss.
3. Patient age. Usually older patients have a general status compromised from other health problems.
4. Prolonged surgical times and large soft tissue exposure. In oncologic resections these frequently occur and a higher risk of contamination is very likely.
5. High mechanical stresses on the prosthetic components. The loss of muscular insertions and the long lever arm create high bending stresses at the prosthesis-bone interface. This is considered a significant risk factor for the development of a mechanical failure.

6. Soft tissue stripping and wide excision of normal adjacent muscle and bone. These predispose to joint instability and dislocation.
7. Constrained joint prosthesis design. This substantially increases the stress between the endoprosthesis and the cement or between the endoprosthesis and the bone, with a higher incidence of loosening.
8. Tumor progression. This remains a persistent threat to endoprosthesis and limb survival [2, 7, 9].

Laitinen identified three significant factors to predict failure following resection and reconstruction: (a) previous radiotherapy combined with previous surgery, (b) intralesional excision, and (c) previous surgical intervention that is considered the most important [1]. According to Henrichs et al. [5], the most important risk factor for failure is the length of survival after operation, and this can explain the highest rate of reoperation and 60% of failures in breast cancer. Reoperations were more common in the intertrochanteric (40%) than in the subtrochanteric (33%) or in the cervical (27%) region.

Overall, the median survival in patients who underwent revision surgery was significantly higher compared with the one for patients not requiring further surgery [5, 16]. All the authors have reported a progressive reduction of the revision-free prosthetic survival rate with time:

- 92.4% at 1 year, 84.4% at 2 years, falling to 76.0% at 3 years [1]
- 92% at 3 months, 90% at 1 year, and 86% at 2 years [18]
- 75.9% at 5 years and 66.2% at 10 years [9]
- 94% after 1 year, 92% after 2 years, and 84% after 5 years [3]
- 83.1% at 1 year, 73.9% at 5 years, and 47.5% at 8 years [5]
- 68% at 5 years, 58% at 8 years [10]

In a literature review, Capanna reported an implant survival at 10 years ranging from 58 to 77% for cemented megaprostheses and from 58 to 70% for cementless megaprostheses [9].

The failure rate of primary implants (32%) was more than that of revision implants (22%), and this was almost the same of that of oncologic implants (22.6%) [10]. Implant survival rates were 80–85 and 57% in the proximal femur respectively at 5 and 8 years, whereas 66–70 and 58% in the distal femur and 49 and 36% in the proximal tibia [9, 10].

In Shehadeh series, the custom implants failed in 50% of the cases whereas modular implants in 17%. A subsequent failure was more often observed in the first type of implants compared to the second ones (32 vs 23%) [17]. The failure rate of the proximal femoral replacements was 16–20% at a median of 1.6 years, whereas that of the distal femoral replacements was 27–29.3% at a median of 1.3 years; the failure of the proximal tibial replacements was 34–42.8% at a median of 1.8 years. When the distal femoral and proximal tibial replacement are combined together, the failure rate is very high and reaches 43%.

The failure rate of the proximal, total, distal humeral replacements was, respectively, 17%, 19%, and 17% [7]. Survival of proximal humerus endoprostheses was 94.7% at 1 year and 75.8% at 5 years [5].

In the proximal femur, independently from the site, the rate of reoperation for prosthetic implants is higher compared to the osteosynthesis devices [16].

The prosthetic reconstruction outlives the metastatic patient in 92% of patients [5]. In the prosthetic group, the failure rate was higher in total arthroplasty (11%) compared to endoprostheses replacement (8%) [16].

Patients with prostheses have shown a lower mechanical failure rate and a higher rate of implant survivorship when compared to those treated with fixation [3, 8].

The failure rate of arthroplasty is lower compared to osteosynthesis both in the femur and in the humerus, being these, respectively, 6% vs 10% [8, 15, 16]. Moreover, considering bone fixation, plating has an increased failure rate (22–25%) compared to nailing (7–14%), which decreased when cement was used [8, 15, 16]. Any type of osteosynthesis has a 2-year risk of reop-

eration more than any type of endoprosthetic reconstruction: 35% vs 18%. Patients with prostheses have a rate of reoperation almost double (14 vs 8%) compared to those with reconstruction nails [16].

When the secondary reconstruction is considered, implant survival rates significantly decrease overtime: 82.6% at 1 year, 69.9% at 2 years, and 62.1% at 3 years. In patients with a previous surgical reconstruction, the rate of complications was 27%, compared to 13% for those who did not perform a revision surgery [1].

In Forsberg series, secondary failures were observed in 19% of patients, and a statistically significant difference was present among the secondary failures rate across treatment groups: EPR (7%), IMN, (45%), and plate (50%) [4]. Secondary failure occurred at a median time of 10 months from the primary surgery. Material failure was the most common cause for reoperation (88%), and the other was tumor progression (12%). Secondary failures occurred more frequently at the diaphysis (47%) followed by subtrochanteric (29%), peritrochanteric (12%), and distal femoral (12%) regions. In femoral metastases, the endoprosthetic reconstruction is more durable than other treatment methods, although few papers have reported the results of salvage treatment in this setting. Forsberg and Jacofsky pointed out the good durability of endoprosthetic reconstructions reporting 85–90% implant survivor at 5 years with salvage arthroplasty in their series [4, 19]. However, the timing of salvage surgery was relatively long for IMN compared to EPR, being, respectively, 12 vs 7 months. This makes IMN an acceptable alternative to EPR in selected patients with short life expectancies.

19.3 Failures Around Tumor Implants

According to the Dindo classification, all the fractures and failures around tumor implants are Grade IIIB, complications requiring surgical revision under general anesthesia [4, 20]. According to the classification system proposed by Henderson, failures are classified as mechanical or nonmechanical [7].

1. *Mechanical failures* include those attributable to loss of normal function of the device and/or relationships between the device components and adjacent bone and soft tissue attachments. These are divided into three types:

   Type 1: soft tissue failure, including instability, tendon rupture, or aseptic wound dehiscence

   Type 2: aseptic loosening with clinical and radiographic evidence of loosening

   Type 3: structural failure, including periprosthetic or prosthetic fracture or deficient osseous supporting structure

   According to etiology and treatment of the soft tissue modes of failure, type 1 is divided into:

   Type 1A: dislocation

   Type 1B: tendon rupture

   Type 1C: aseptic wound dehiscence [9]

2. *Nonmechanical failures* include conditions that necessitate device removal or revision that do not compromise the function of the device and its surrounding connective tissues. These are divided into two types:

   Type 4: infection requiring removal of the device

   Type 5: tumor progression with recurrence or progression of tumor and contamination of the device

In metastatic patients, bisphosphonates, besides having a synergic action with chemotherapy, are useful to reduce skeletal-related events such as type 2, type 3, and type 5 failure [15].

19.3.1 Mechanical Failure

Mechanical failures account for approximately 49–59% of all failures [7, 9, 17, 21]. Mechanical failure may occur through the implant itself, at the implant (or cement) bone interface, or through the bone (i.e., in a periprosthetic fracture);

because under loading conditions, the stresses are transmitted through the device [21].

The type of failure is related to the anatomic site. The rate of failure is the lowest for proximal femoral replacement and the highest for combined distal femoral-proximal tibial reconstruction. Endoprostheses located around the shoulder and the hip have the highest incidence of soft tissue failures, whereas the aseptic loosening is the most common type of failure in the lower extremities, especially with hinged knee prosthesis [7].

19.3.1.1 Type 1

Type 1 failures present at an average time of 26 months after surgery [22] and occur mostly at the proximal femur (33%) and at the proximal humerus (24%). These are associated with the shortest mean time to failure of 11–16 months. These were the 12% of all failures. Type 1 was the most common mode of failure with the absolute risk for all anatomic locations of 2.9% [7, 10]. However, in Laitinen series, type 1 failure occurred in only 1.1% of cases [1]. Failed primary endoprostheses requiring revision include type 1 failures in approximately 10% of cases [10].

Type 1A: Dislocation (Fig. 19.1)
Dislocation of the prosthesis occurs at an average time of 18 months and ranges from 1.5 to 25% [3, 7, 9, 14, 16, 18, 23]. Dislocations are 6% of all the complications and 8% of all the causes of revision. Only 18% of all dislocations require revision surgery [14].

In the study by Fakler et al., patients with recurrent dislocations needed conversion from hemi- to total hip arthroplasty or revision of the acetabular cup up to 25% of cases [23]. The risk of reoperation for dislocation was 4% at 1 year and 8% at 2 years, with a probability for dislocation free survival of 92% at 3 months, 91% at 1 year, and 88% at 2 years [18].

In revision surgery or in the salvage setting, the dislocation rate is generally higher even in the nonmetastatic setting, and an accurate reconstruction of the soft tissues around the prosthesis and adequate and careful aftercare treatment are mandatory [4, 9].

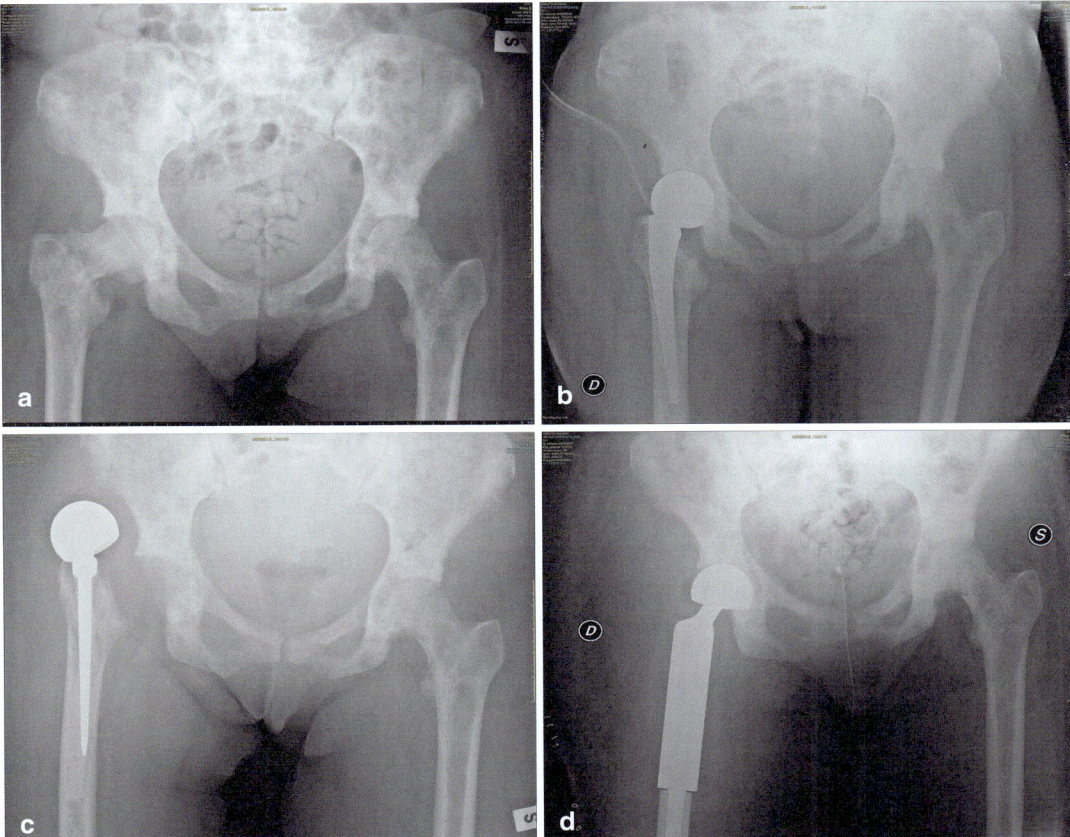

Fig. 19.1 Pathologic fracture in patients with bone metastases due to prostate cancer (**a**). Patient was treated with cemented endoprosthetic reconstruction (**b**). A dislo- cation occurred at 4 months (**c**), and therefore patient was treated with wide resection and reconstruction with bipo- lar endoprosthesis (**d**)

Choices to Avoid Dislocation

According to Thambapillary and Wedin series, the rate of dislocation was markedly reduced when bipolar implants were used as to total prox- imal femoral endoprosthesis arthroplasty (PFA), respectively, 4 vs 22% [14, 16]. The rate of dislo- cation was three times higher in the total proxi- mal femoral arthroplasty group compared to the bipolar group in Menendez series; the hemiar- throplasty design was very useful in elderly met- astatic patients with a life expectancy of less than 5 years because it allowed to maintain a lot of soft tissues around the prosthesis providing a good stability and a faster functional recovery [24]. Another factor that provides stability is an appropriate abductor repair, that can be obtained in metastatic patients by maintaining the medium

gluteus and the lateral vastus connected together in a unique wide muscular flap. Allograft- prosthesis composite, which should allow direct abductor repair to the femoral allograft, is not used in metastatic patient because of the degen- eration of the graft after chemo- and/or radiother- apy. Modular prostheses have shown good functional and long-lasting results, and the implants tend to outlive the patient [9]. Moreover, modular implants are more durable and cost- effective as to custom-made prostheses and are ready available on the shelf. Many authors have reported a limb salvage rate of over 97% and an implant survival rate at 5 years of 84% and of 82% at 10 years by using a megaprosthesis. Cemented implants are preferred to uncemented prosthesis in metastatic patients. Total hip replacement after bone resection is very similar to revision joint replacements. This surgery has a more duration and magnitude than primary total hip replacement, and so the rate of hip dislocation is higher and closer to that observed in revision total hip replacement. When treating metastatic bone disease at the hip, hemiarthroplasty is preferred to total hip replacement because it reduces the risk of hip dislocation and the risk of early reoperation in some patients [3]. Conversion of bipolar hemiarthroplasty to total proximal femoral arthroplasty, frequently performed in long-surviving patients (46%), due to later acetabular cartilage degeneration is rarely necessary in the bone metastases patient [3, 14].

Management of Dislocation

The majority of dislocations are treated by closed reduction, and these patients usually are fare very well [4, 11]. When the conservative treatment is not associated with good results and recurrent dislocation recurs, a revision of the prosthesis is mandatory. Usually, bipolar is changed to total hip arthroplasty combined with an artificial ligament fixed to the sovracetabular region to maintain the prosthesis suspended and to stabilize the implant to reduce the dislocating moment. When dislocation occurs in arthroplasty, the cup and the head can be changed with a dual mobility cup and also a different offset is chosen. The risk of dislocation in patients with oncologic prostheses can be reduced fixing a Trevira's mesh around the prosthesis and on the other side around the acetabular ring with intraosseous stitches. These synthetic devices allow for a strong adhesion of the soft tissues on the prosthesis but carry a higher risk of late infections. Using regular or long-stemmed revision femoral components with preservation of the greater trochanter with improvement of the hip joint stability can explain the low failure rate. Preservation and repair of the hip capsule as well as applying a bipolar head whenever possible is recommended to improve safety and reduce the higher dislocation risk of proximal femoral replacements. If preservation of the capsule is not possible, attachment tubes for soft tissue reconstruction or tripolar cups might help in reducing the risk of dislocation.

The dislocation must be prevented as more as possible in order to obtain a real advantage over intramedullary nailing in patients with expected longer survival [23].

Type 1B: Tendon Rupture

A tendon rupture occurs at an average time of 58 months, in approximately 2.5% of patients. It occurs at the extensor apparatus at the knee when megaprostheses are implanted after tumor resection, but this complication can be observed only in metastatic patients with a long survival [9]. In 6% a symptomatic patellofemoral impingement was treated with patellar replacement, debridement, synovectomy, and hemiarthroplasty [25].

When an endoprosthesis was used in polyaxial joints such as proximal humeral and proximal femoral ones, soft tissue failures following prosthetic replacement account for 29% of all the failures, while hinge prostheses used for uniaxial joints like the elbow and knee have soft tissue failures in only 5.7% [7].

Management of Soft Tissue Failure

The use of LARS® ligament is a safe and effective choice to enhance prosthetic reconstructions, providing good muscles reattachment and improving joint stability after reconstruction following tumor resection. Combined with modular prosthetic reconstruction of the proximal tibia or proximal femur, Ligament Advanced Reinforcement System (LARS®) reconstruction of the knee extensor apparatus or strengthening of the gluteus muscles is often necessary.

LARS® can be available as a band or a tube with similar functional results. Extensor mechanism reconstruction by LARS® shows good function and satisfactory implant survival after primary reconstruction of the extensor mechanism after proximal tibia resection. The same results have been obtained after excision of the gluteus muscles in proximal femur resection. The median survival of LARS® implanted primarily was better than in the case of secondary implantation. An extremely low risk of mechanical rupture or infection of LARS® was reported in the literature, and the estimated 5-year survival of this device was 92% [26, 27].

Type 1C: Aseptic Wound Dehiscence

Aseptic wound dehiscence occurs earlier at an average time of 6 months after surgery and ranges from 2 to 23% of patients [2, 5, 9, 28].

Management of the Aseptic Wound Dehiscence

Sometimes wound infections solve by intravenous antibiotic therapy without surgical intervention (4.5%), but more often (57%) they needed operative wound revision without prosthetic replacement [2, 7, 12, 25]. In Capanna series [9], type 1C complications often required surgical debridement (10%), and it was combined with a plastic surgery procedure in 30% of cases. Operative wound revision consists of clearing from the granulation tissue, irrigating with a disinfectant solution, and sometimes with local therapy implanting sponge containing antibiotic. Usually, intraoperative evaluations are culture-negative, and the wounds heal without further complications [2].

Resection of musculoskeletal tumors may result in large soft tissue defects that cannot be closed primarily and require prolonged dressing changes and complex surgical interventions for wound coverage. The use of vacuum-assisted wound closure facilitates wound healing and primary wound closure in patients who have large soft tissue defects after resection of a musculoskeletal tumor. This system causes a reduction of the defect in size with a viable granulation tissue extended for 25% of the surface. This allows primary closure in 30% of cases, primary closure with skin grafting in 61%, and healing by secondary intention in 9% of patients [29].

19.3.1.2 Type 2: Aseptic Loosening

In patients with tumor prostheses, the rate of aseptic loosening reported in literature is very different, being 1% [2], 3% [9], 5% [10], 7% [5], 17% [14], 19% [7], and 23% [13].

By a literature revision, aseptic loosening:

1. Appears later. It occurs at an average time ranging from 35 months to 76 months, and therefore it is rarely observed in metastatic patients [7, 9, 10].

2. Is more frequent in cementless implants (2–15%) whereas only 0–8% in cemented prostheses.
3. Is less common in rotating hinge system at the knee [9].
4. Is more frequent in prostheses implanted in hinged joints than in polyaxial articulations [7].
5. Is more common in lower extremity prostheses compared to all upper extremity prostheses.
6. Is more frequent in revision reconstructions (6%) compared to primary implants (4%) but after a longer time (3 vs 2.6 years) [10].
7. Is more common in oncologic prostheses than in total arthroplasty for osteoarthritis [28].

Management of Aseptic Loosening

Many cases of aseptic loosening have asymptomatic radiographic findings, and therefore these do not require revision surgery. Conversely, in the case of radiographic signs and symptoms of instability as severe load-related pain, a prosthesis replacement is mandatory [2, 5, 21].

19.3.1.3 Type 3: Structural Failure
(Fig. 19.2)

(a) Prosthesis Breakage and (b) Periprosthetic Fracture.

The main classification systems used for periprosthetic fractures, the Vancouver for the proximal femur and the Rorabeck for the distal femur, take into account three parameters: site of the fracture, stem stability, and bone quality. However, these are not much useful in endoprosthesis fractures after bone tumor removal because of the different biomechanics of the implants, for lack of consideration of the cause of the fracture, and for the lack of the evaluation of the functional status of the patient. Healey highlighted the need for a new classification for fractures in megaprostheses [30]. Moreover, Gebhart and Shumelinsky suggested to divide fractures basing on fracture location, status of the bone, and prosthetic stem interface [31]. Wright and Colfield described a classification of periprosthetic fractures to guide the treatment of the humerus fracture in standard shoulder replacement [32]. In

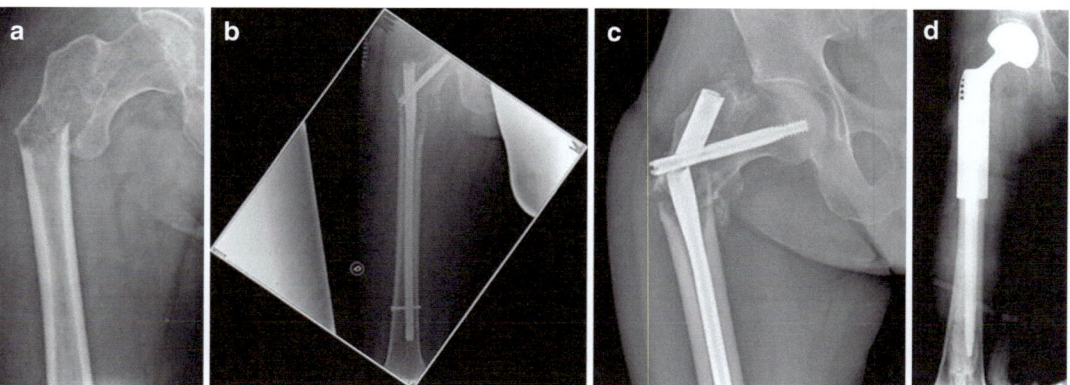

Fig. 19.2 Pathologic fracture in femoral metastasis due to breast cancer (**a**). Patient was treated with preventive locked nail and radiotherapy (**b**). At 8 months, a nail breaking occurred (**c**), and a resection of the proximal femur and reconstruction with a modular prosthesis was necessary (**d**)

this system, fractures are classified into three different types according to fracture level in relation to the stem: type A, fracture located at the tip and extending more than 1/3 of the length of the stem; type B, fractures centered at the tip, but with extension less than 1/3 of the length of the stem; and type C, located distal to the tip, with extension to the distal humeral metaphysis. In 1999, Worlan published a classification also taking into consideration the stability of the implant and suggested a different treatment accordingly [33, 34]. The unified classification system for periprosthetic fractures is more frequently used [35].

Type A is a fracture of an apophysis or protuberance of bone.

Type B involves the bed supporting or adjacent to an implant (B1, the implant is still well fixed; B2, the implant is loose; B3, the implant is loose and the bone bed is of poor quality).

Type C involves a fracture which is in the bone containing the implant but distant from the bed of the implant.

Type D is a fracture affecting one bone which supports two replacements.

Type E involves two bones supporting one replacement.

Type F is a fracture involving a joint surface which is not resurfaced or replaced but is directly articulating with an implant [21].

Type 3 failures occur from 7.1 to 17% of the implants [1, 7, 9]. It occurs at an average time of 50 months from the first surgery and more frequently occurs at the distal humerus 33% and distal femur 23%, whereas it is lower for proximal humeral and total femoral replacements [7, 9].

Prosthesis Breakage

Breakage of the prosthesis accounted for 22% of all failures and for 72% of all type 3 failures in Capanna study [9], whereas it is observed in 20% of cases in Wedin series [16]. In the literature, the average incidence of prosthetic component breakage was 4.5%, ranging between 0 and 7.7% [25] without significant differences among different sites [9].

In Tanaka and Fakler studies, 4% and 17% of intramedullary nails broke through their proximal parts at a mean time, respectively, of 21 and 4 months [6, 23]. Pattern of breakage at the proximal part of the IM rod was similar in all patients and fracture occurred in the subtrochanteric area. In the rare cases where acetabular fractures occurred after falling down of the patient, an arthroplasty was implanted [2].

Periprosthetic Fracture

Periprosthetic fractures around standard hip and knee replacements have been widely studied, and their management is now fairly routine, whereas few papers have reported the treatment of periprosthetic fractures around tumor endoprostheses [21].

Periprosthetic fractures at the lower limb ranges from 1 to 22%, whereas these are rare at the upper limbs, ranging from 0.5 to 3% in shoulder hemiarthroplasty [33].

A periprosthetic fracture is 6–7% of all failures and 18% of all type 3 failures [9, 16, 25]. In Thambapillary series, periprosthetic fractures occurred in 3% of all the revised patients, and 50% of these were treated surgically [14]. In Wedin study, endoprosthetic replacements showed a periprosthetic fracture rate of 3.7% which is comparable with that of periprosthetic non-pathological fractures after revision surgery (2.4%) [16]. A fracture was more frequent (19%) in implant without cement than in those with cement (11%).

In Barut series, 66% of fractures occurred after the first prosthesis implantation, 22% after the first revision, 6% after the second one, and 6% after the third revision surgery [21]. The median time between implantation of the last prosthesis and the occurrence of the fracture approximated 38 months. Ninety per cent of patients reported falling from height, while 10% had stress fractures. According to the UCS classification, these fractures were classified as B1 in 11%, B2 in 6%, C in 67%, and F in 16% of cases. Half of fractures occurred on the side of the resected bone, 33% on the opposite side, and 17% at the patella. Periprosthetic fractures around tumor endoprostheses are different from that around standard implants, being the former more frequently type C, whereas the latter are type B [21, 33].

The revision rates for all patients for any reason after surgery for fractures were 27% at 5 years and 55% at 10 years, respectively, and these rates increase to 32 and 67% for operated patients. The cumulative probability of revision only for mechanical reasons after surgery of the periprosthetic fracture was 8% at 5 years and 20% at 10 years. The median time from the treatment of the fracture for mechanical reason to the revision was 76 months [21].

In Henrichs study, 4% of patients had a periprosthetic fracture at 2.5 years after implantation of proximal humerus endoprosthesis [5]. In the humerus, failures were more frequent in complete fractures compared to patients treated for impending fractures (11% vs 4%), and nonunion and stress fracture were, respectively, 35% and 20% of all failures. This may suggest that prophylactic surgery is useful to decrease the incidence of fracture and so the reoperation rate [8].

The use of cement as a fixation material did not prevent the fracture from healing, and it is associated to better functional results at 6 months. However, after 6 months, the functional scores did not differ anymore [12].

Management of Periprosthetic Tumor Fractures

After infection and aseptic loosening, periprosthetic fracture is the third most common complication leading to revision. Often in literature, fracture rates are included in a long series of possible complications without the report of periprosthetic fractures alone and with no detailed treatment recommendations. Moreover, there is currently no consensus about which should be the standard management for periprosthetic fractures in this patients' population.

Intramedullary nailing has a higher rate of complications requiring reoperation (26%) than endoprosthesic replacement in the treatment of pathologic fractures at the proximal femur (18%) [11]. The rate of fracture union is considerably less than 50% for breast and renal carcinoma or even absent for lung carcinoma. Patients treated with intramedullary nails have a significantly higher complication rate in actual pathologic fractures than in impending fractures. Postoperative radiotherapy on impending fractures may cause a pathologic fracture in only 13% because weight bearing induces stress to osteosynthetic devices and the risk of failure is conspicuously lower [23].

When intramedullary nail breakage occurs, conversion to a tumor prosthesis is preferred even if this procedure has a more risk of infection [6, 23, 25].

When periprosthetic fractures are combined with tumor progression or infection, treatment options should be those related to these more significant complications [33].

Surgical options usually include fixation with a plate or, more rarely, with intramedullary nail, in combination with adjuvants such as bone cement, or revision with conventional endoprostheses or modular tumor endoprostheses [5].

In tumor patients, many biomechanical factors including stress shielding, poor bone quality, fibrosis, thinning of the cortical bone, and subsequent bone reabsorption at the interface between the bone or cement and the prosthetic stem increase the risk of fracture. Other factors are the absence of osteointegration at the bone-implant interface, bone devascularization after reaming and cement heating, the lack of hypertrophy of the loaded bone, and the increase of stress bypass of the host bone around a stiff intramedullary stem.

The quality and quantity of bone stock, as well as the quality of soft tissues, should be carefully evaluated before planning the management of periprosthetic fractures around tumor endoprostheses. Bone stock may be scarce, bone quality may be deteriorated after radiation therapy, and the soft tissues have sometimes been severely traumatized. The treatment of periprosthetic fractures may be nonsurgical or surgical with conservative or revision options [33]. Fracture healing with no surgical treatment can be possible in 11% of cases and only in fractures that occur in peripheral sites like the ankle [21]. The treatment of periprosthetic fractures around tumor endoprostheses may be different from that of conventional joint replacements due to patient's general conditions and implant characteristics. Surgery is more aggressive in patients with bone tumor than in those with conventional joint disease. Moreover, metastatic patients often cannot undergo another surgery due to progression of the disease. In tumor megaprostheses, the bone available for

fixation is often limited, and a high rate of complications is frequently observed after revision surgery [21].

Based on the timing, periprosthetic fractures should be considered as fractures occurred during the surgery or as late complications, and each requires a different surgical approach. Intraoperative fractures can result from a technical error, whereas early or late postoperative fractures may be related to trauma or being combined with loosening, infection, or disease progression. An eccentric reaming and cortical perforation of the shaft increase the risk of an intraoperative periprosthetic fracture. Moreover, cementless stem, revision surgery, and potential mismatch between the bow of the femur and the bow of the stem, which is accentuated when a long revision stem is used, should be avoided. When an intraoperative fracture occurs, it can be treated by a plate or with a bigger size and longer cemented prosthesis. Rarely, in not dislocated postoperative fractures, a spontaneous healing can be obtained, after cast immobilization and weight-bearing proscription. When a patient has a poor performance status, a limited life expectancy, or severe comorbidities, no surgery is indicated. If the periprosthetic fracture is combined with stem breakage or with stem mobilization, revision of the implant with another prosthesis is mandatory. However, when the prosthesis remains stable, plate and wiring/screw fixation or cast immobilization is useful to fracture healing, but often these procedures could not be indicated in metastatic patients because of the low rate of bone healing, the high risk of postoperative infection, and the potential complications.

The optimal option would be a less invasive surgical procedure, above all in patients with poor prognosis and in those with low functional requests. In some cases, surgical difficulty is due to the lack of bone of good quality for a stable fixation when a long resection is performed and when the fracture is distal to the stem; therefore, in some cases arthrodesis is still an option, mainly at the knee, because of their acceptable impact on the segmental function. When a plate is used for a periprosthetic fracture fixation, with monocortical screws at the level of the stem and bicortical screws in bone segments at the extremity of the stem, it can provide adequate resistance to stresses and allow fracture healing [33].

Management of Fractures at the Upper Limb
Most of the fractures at the upper limbs are intraoperative, and these represent the 20% of all the complications associated with shoulder arthroplasty. Shoulder prosthetic implants after bone tumor resection are less frequent, and periprosthetic fractures are even more rare. If the length of the stem bridges the fracture, and the tip of the prosthesis extends beyond the most distal fracture site, the prosthesis is stable, and cast immobilization is often sufficient to heal. Sometimes an open anatomic reduction and internal fixation can be performed using wires, screw fixation, or angular stable plating that gives excellent results using a monocortical fixation at the stem region to obtain stability of the fracture site. On the contrary, revision prosthesis with bigger and longer stem is necessary. When glenoid bone stock is preserved, even with pre-existent rotator cuff dysfunction, a revision shoulder reverse arthroplasty can improve the function of the shoulder.

Patients with distal humeral fractures have more risk of failure of the fixation device or the prosthetic implant. According to Wedin et al. [8], plating of the distal humeral fractures have a high rate of failure, and therefore a modular tumor prosthesis might be a better choice in carefully selected patients. In Bickels series, a reoperation/revision rate of 9% was observed after the surgical resection of humeral metastases [36]. The humerus is a non-weight-bearing bone and compared to a weight-bearing bone, such as the femur, the rate of failure should be lower; however, the distal humerus shows poor results with a failure rate of 33%. The plate failures are caused by stress fractures, poor initial fixation, and nonunion. The overall rate of reoperation averages 6% in the prosthetic and 10% in the osteosynthesis group. A reoperation rate of 17% has been observed in the modular tumor prostheses. The

indication for this type of prosthesis was a proximal diaphyseal or metaphyseal lesion with significant cortical destruction not amenable by osteosynthesis [8]. Nailing and plating are the most frequent methods used to treat diaphyseal fractures, due to the lower rate of secondary failure, respectively, 7% vs 22% [8]. Many authors prefer to treat pathologic fractures with plate or nail and cement. Bone cement is used in 83% of plate fixations, but only in 30% of cases with nails. According to the Wedin et al. [8], by using nail and cement, the failure rate of diaphyseal fractures is 6% compared to 3% in patients with nailing alone.

However, there is not an agreement on cement using combined to nail due to the different results about pain relief, functional outcome, and rate of complications in patients with bone metastasis.

19.3.2 Nonmechanical Failure

Nonmechanical failures rate range from 41 to 51% [7, 9].

19.3.2.1 Type 4: Infection (Fig. 19.3)
The absolute risk of type 4 failure for all anatomic locations approximates 8.4% [7]. Infections are 5% of all complications and 17% of all causes of revision [14].

Infection remains the most common type of failure for endoprostheses and has a significant effect on the ultimate patient outcome. The infection rate of primary endoprostheses is reported from 2 to 20% and increases to 43% after revision surgery [1, 3, 9, 16, 18, 23, 37]. In oncologic patients, the risk of infection is increased due to the length of procedures, extensive surgical dissections, limited soft tissue coverage, and immune compromising treatments [10]. Furthermore, the high mortality of the patients also reduces the probability that a late infection with low virulent bacteria would become a clinical problem [3].

Different revision rates are reported in literature to control infection: 23% [1], 37% [14], 38% [17], 67% [5], and 89% [9]. At the same way, different percentages of secondary amputations are reported: 10% [9], 25% [18], and 75% [1].

In patients with previous surgery, the incidence of infection was higher compared to those undergoing primary prosthetic implants [1, 13, 17].

According to Henderson et al., proximal tibia was the most frequent side of type 4 failure (45%), whereas proximal femur the most rare (only 18%). These data were confirmed by Kostuj but not by Capanna, who found that proximal femur was the less common side of type 4 failure, whereas the most frequent site for infection was the distal femur (14%) [9, 13].

The same rate of infection was observed in cemented and cementless stems, whereas infection rate in non-silver-coated prostheses (13%) was higher than that in silver-coated prostheses (4%) [5, 9]. In Hardes study, the infection rate was substantially reduced from 17.6% in the titanium to 5.9% in the silver group [38]. In the titanium group, 38.5% of patients had to undergo amputation due to persistent infection, whereas in patients with silver-coated prosthesis amputation was not necessary. Therefore, the use of silver-coated prostheses can reduce the infection rate in the medium term, and less aggressive treatment of infection are necessary in these patients [38] However, Kostuj reported silver-coated implants had a more incidence of infection (83%) compared to titanium implants (20%) and chrome-cobalt implants (15%) [13].

Type 4 failures occurred significantly more often in hinged prostheses than in polyaxial prostheses [7].

The time of occurrence of infection ranged from 1 to 70 months with different mean time: 3 months [18], 16 months [9, 37], and 47 months [7]; 47% of septic complications occurred after 1 year from surgery [9].

The causative microorganisms found in the tissue cultures were *coagulase-negative staphylococci* (60%), *S. aureus* (20%), *Enterococcus species* (13%), *Pseudomonas aeruginosa* (6%), *Actinobacter baumanii* (3%), *Proteus mirabilis* (3%), and *Streptococcus pyogenes* (3%). In 20% of patients, a polymicrobial infection was found. An acute infection was present in 80% of patients and a low-grade infection in 20%. A sinus tract communicating with the prosthesis was present in 20% of patients. Prior infection and wound disorders are considered significant risk factors for deep infection, and in 33% of patients, the soft tissue situation was classified as poor [7, 13].

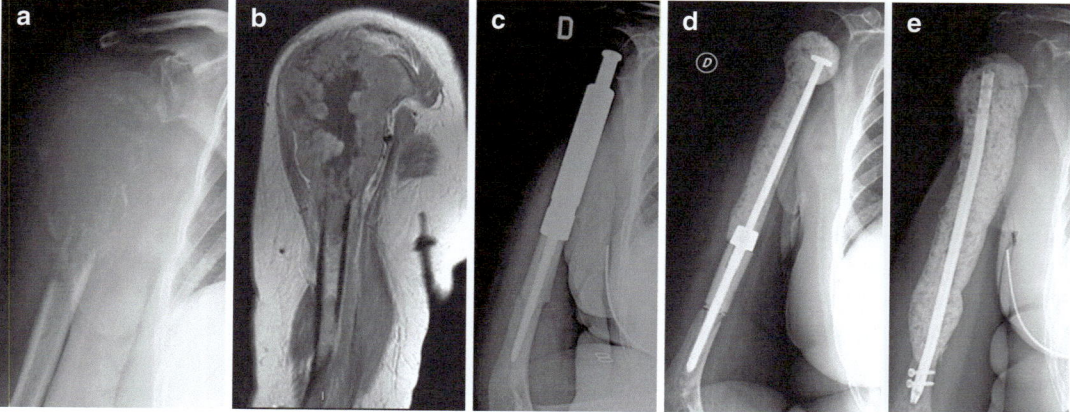

Fig. 19.3 Humeral metastases due to kidney cancer (**a**, **b**). Patient was treated with resection and modular prosthesis (**c**), but at 3 months an infection occurred. Patient was treated with replacement of the prosthetic body with a cement spacer combined with antibiotic therapy (**d**). After 3 months Cement and stem of the prosthesis were removed and a new cement spacer with rod was implanted because infection values were high again (**e**). When infection values returned normal, a new modular prosthesis was implanted

Management of Infections

Infection is the most common complication in tumor prostheses. Although infection is a severe complication, which may not only require further revision surgery, prolonged hospitalization, antibiotic treatment, and rehabilitation, but also exposes patient to significant further risks such as amputation or compromised overall survival due to interference with radio- or chemotherapy.

Superficial and low-grade perioperative infections can be treated conservatively with antibiotic suppression, and local delivery of antibiotics is important to mitigate the risk of infection in these patients [4].

However, treatment of deep infections is often difficult and time consuming, with a high rate of reoperations. Repeated reoperations and intravenous antibiotic treatment are unable to adequately treat these infections, so that secondary amputation often remain the only solutions available, with a rate ranging from 19 to 46% of cases [28, 37]. Furthermore, when acute polymicrobial infection occurs, additional surgical intervention is necessary, and when application of chemotherapy and radiation therapy is performed a higher risk of failed limb salvage is observed [37].

When an early infection occurs due to superinfected seroma or hematoma, debridement with prosthesis retention and one-stage reimplantation without the changing of stems combined with adequate antibiotic therapy for any months can be successful [28].

In a late low-grade infection, an intravenous antibiotic therapy can avoid a revision surgery, but if inflammatory parameters rise, prosthesis removal and cement spacer implantation should be done [14, 37].

One-stage revision surgery cannot be recommended when late high-grade infection appears because one-stage revision is useful only from the first days after the onset of symptoms to first month. When a late high-grade infection occurs, a two-stage revision with reimplanation of the prosthesis should be intended [14, 37].

If this procedure is not possible, only an arthrodesis or an amputation can be performed. The most important factor to make possible a limb salvage surgery is the soft tissue condition to allow a sufficient coverage; otherwise, the risk of reinfection is increased, and an amputation is mandatory. A prosthesis reimplantation can be suggested at a minimum of 4–6 weeks after inflammatory parameters remain normal. During adjuvant chemotherapy, a reimplantation should be avoided because of a higher risk of reinfection in the immuno-compromised patient.

All the procedures useful to prevent infection should be applied to avoid these difficult surgical treatments. Prevention of this complication is of particular importance for patients undergoing tumor resection and endoprosthetic replacement for impending or pathologic fractures secondary to metastatic bone disease, to preserve mobility and independence for the longest time possible, and to spare them the drastic reduction in quality of life, invariably associated with prosthetic infection. Though the high infection rates (25%), the higher reinfection rates (43%), and the high incidence of amputation (35%), most experts in musculoskeletal infectious diseases considered excessively long perioperative antibiotic prophylaxis as an error even if certain conditions clearly benefit from pre-emptive therapy with administration of antibiotics over several days. Therefore, standard guidelines for routine antibiotic prophylaxis should not be applied by most orthopedic oncologists to metastatic patients undergoing limb-preserving surgery [18, 39].

After a two-stage revision, an amputation due to a reinfection occurs in 10% [9], 17% [28], and 27% [13], but in Shehade series, this can be observed up to 66% of cases [17]. When a prosthesis is used in failed internal fixation, infection rate increases to 10% [19] or 15% [1]. In this group of patients, amputation after infection reaches up to 75% [1]. In 46.7% of cases with deep infections, a recurrent or persisting infection was observed. The recurrent infections were observed from 21 to 49 months after the two-stage revisions [13].

19.3.2.2 Type 5: Tumor Progression

According to the classification by Alvi and Damron [15], the progression of the disease is divided into:

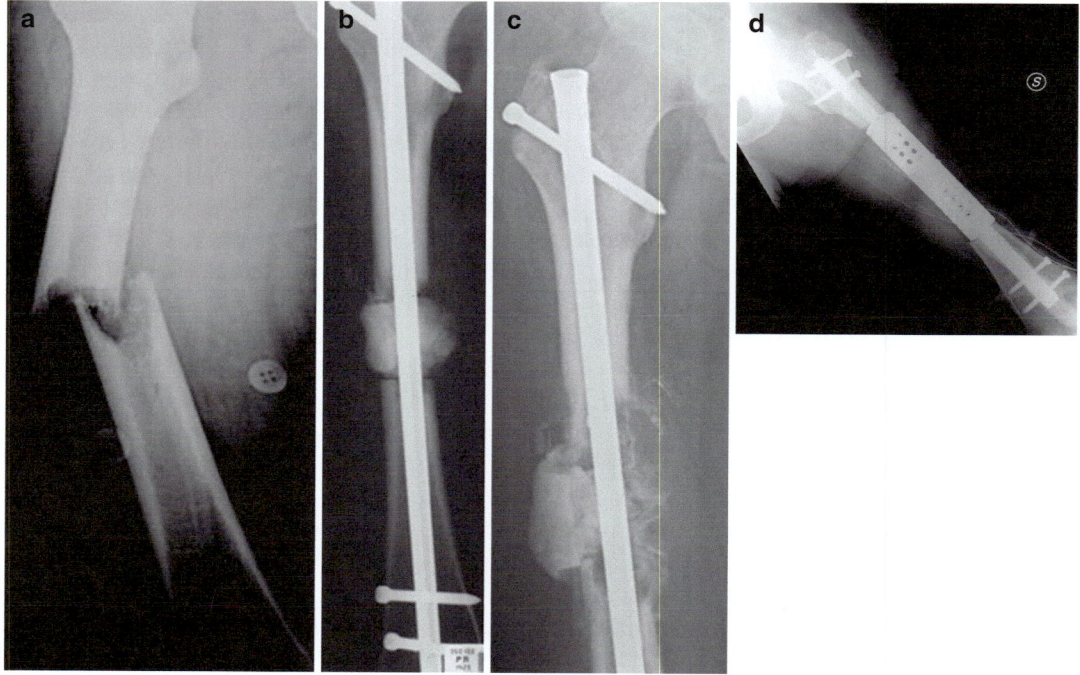

Fig. 19.4 Pathologic fracture of the femur in patient with metastasis due to breast cancer (**a**). Patient was treated with curettage and cement, and femur was stabilized with locked nail (**b**). A local progression of the disease occurred at 6 months in spite of systemic therapy (**c**). Patient was treated with wide resection of the femur and reconstruction with diaphyseal prosthesis (**d**)

Type I: local progression of the originally identified main lesion (Fig. 19.4)

Type II: local progression of originally identified, discretely separate lesions (lesions that were not the primary source of concern)

Type III: occurrence of an entirely new, previously unrecognized lesion (Fig. 19.5)

Type 5 failure due to disease progression has a different rate according different types of series reported in literature: 3.7% [1]. 5% [9], 5% [8]. 6% [2]. 7% [10]. 8% [14]. 11% [15]. 11% [5]. 17% [7]. and 20% [16].

Tumor progression failure is more frequent in distal humerus (33%) and proximal femur (25%) replacement, whereas it is less common in total femoral replacement (2.6%). The absolute risks of failure for all anatomic locations approximates 4.3% [7].

The time of local relapse is different in reported studies and ranges from 9 to 46 months [7, 9, 16].

In 13% of cases, the disease progression occurs at the femur and in 4% at the humerus. 72% were type I and occurred at a mean 10 months: 18%, all with myeloma, were type II and occurred at a mean time of 20 months. Only 9% of patients experienced type III progression at 24 months after surgery [15].

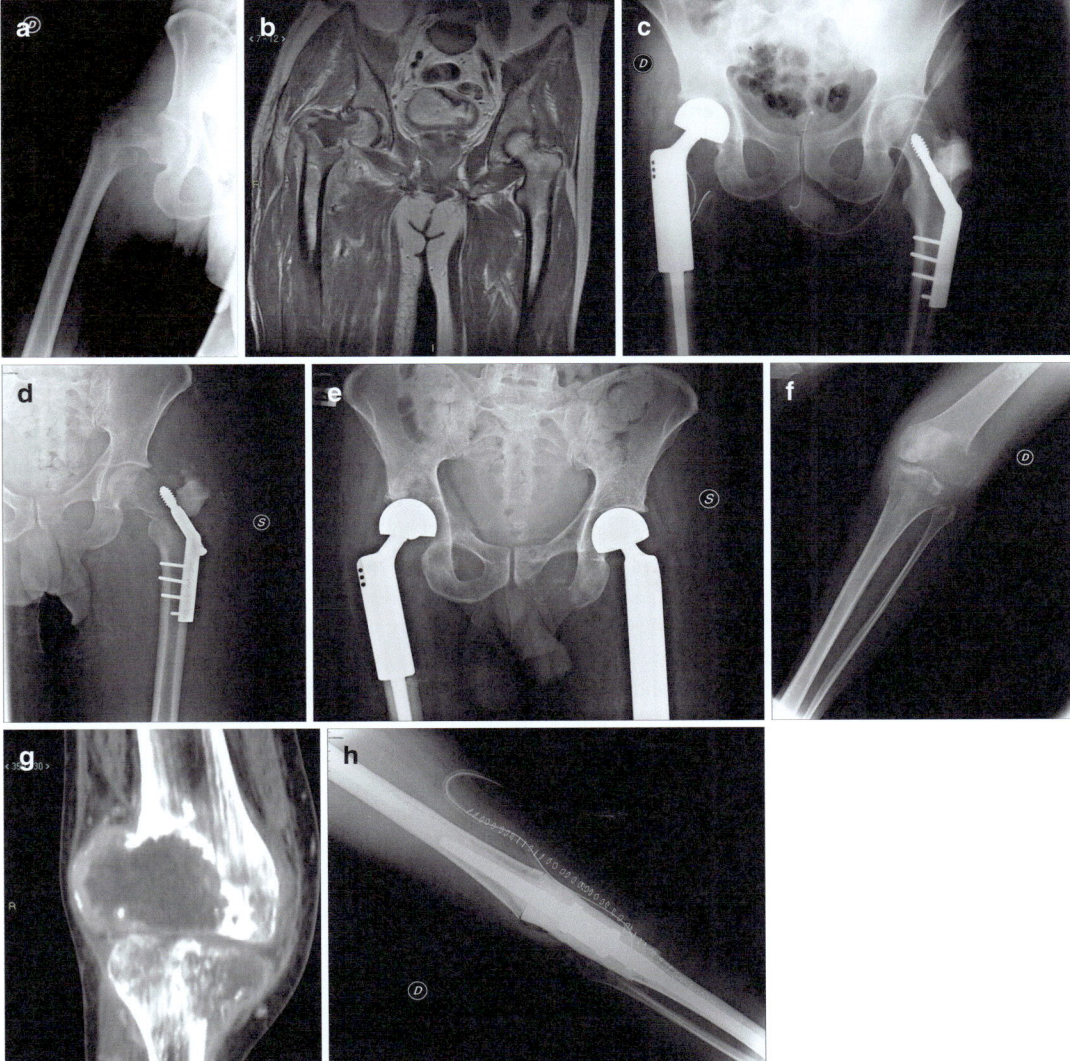

Fig. 19.5 Pathologic fracture in bone metastasis due to kidney cancer (**a**). MRI showed the lesion in the right femur and a second lesion in the trochanteric area of the left femur (**b**). In a first time, patient was treated with wide resection and reconstruction of the right femur with modular prosthesis and in a second time with curettage and plate with cement in the left femur (**c**). However, after 3 months, a pathologic fracture and loosening of the implant due to disease progression occurred (**d**). Patient was treated with another wide resection and prosthesis (**e**). At 6 months, a new bone metastasis of the left distal femur and proximal tibia was observed at x-rays and CT-scan (**f**, **g**). Patient was treated with a resection of the knee and reconstruction with prosthetic arthrodesis (**h**)

Tumor progression failures occurred more often after primary tumor resection (4.7%) than after treatment of metastatic disease (2.2%). This significant difference in tumor progression failures is likely due to the relatively shorter survival of the patients with metastatic disease.

There were no significant differences in tumor progression when the joint type or extremity were considered, and between cemented and non-cemented endoprostheses.

Disease progression is the most frequent cause of an amputation in metastatic patients. Therefore, all possible recommendations to prevent disease progression in various anatomic sites should be realized [7].

In Henrichs study, the incidence of local recurrence was more frequent in metastases from renal cell carcinoma [5]. Obviously, the mean survival rate is lower in patients with local recurrence (22 months) compared to those without disease progression (37 months). Resection of metastases and reconstruction with modular tumor endoprostheses allows better oncological and functional outcomes in selected patients, whereas an incomplete or absent excision of metastatic lesions is associated with inadequate relief of pain and higher rates of local tumor progression [2, 5].

A resection of long bone metastases and replacement is suggested for large destructive solitary metastases when primary cancer type responds to treatment and is excised with a curative intent [5]. In Henrichs series, modular tumor endoprostheses were a successful option also in patients with multiple metastases [5], seen the high survival rate observed even in patients with multiple metastases (28 months for early-onset multiple metastases, 39 months for late-onset multiple metastases in patients with a good prognosis). Patients with late single metastasis have the best survival: 91% at 1 year, and 29% at 5 years. In these cases, a curative surgical approach is indicated, and in 92% of the metastatic patients, the reconstruction outlives the patient. After a wide resection, the recurrence rate was 13.6%, and after marginal or intralesional resection it was 33.3%. Mean event-free survival in solitary metastasis with wide resection was 41.0 months, and after intralesional resection, it was 29.2 months. However, Henrichs did not observe a statistically significant difference in survival between wide and marginal resections, even though it was suggested that tumor-wide resection could increase the survival [5]. In type 5 failures, a second operation is necessary

in 22% of cases; in 13%, tumor progression occurred in patients with previous surgical interventions [5, 14] with the need for component revision in 25%, and major revision in 50% of the patients [1].

Management of Disease Progression

The oncologic consultation is important to consider chemotherapy, hormonal treatment, antiangiogenic agents, and immunotherapy when appropriate. Bisphosphonates also should be considered for those patients that have the indications [5, 15].

Usually, preoperative radiotherapy has a negative effect when a subsequent reconstruction is performed in those patients that already had surgery. The appropriate therapy in those with previous instrumentation and radiotherapy therefore remains unclear, and so the use of postoperative radiotherapy is often reduced even if in other series it showed to reduce the hardware failure rate and reoperation, probably by limiting the disease progression [1, 15]. However, more often disease progression occurs despite perioperative radiotherapy to the implanted region in metastatic patients.

A short instrumentation in the affected long bone would be difficult to recommend owing to disease progression. However, the most frequent disease progression is due to the extension of the main initial lesion and not to another distant new bone metastasis, even though a prophylactic stabilization of the entire bone with longer than standard implants can be indicated due to the high disease progression rate (11%), with 6% of implant revision. A resection and prosthetic reconstruction is preferred more commonly in kidney and myeloma bone lesions to avoid type 5 failure that frequently occurs in these histotypes [15].

Due to contamination of canal after nailing of bone metastases, tumor progression is more frequent because of intralesional surgery. Revision reconstruction due to tumoral progression should be considered a palliative intervention aimed at pain relief or preservation of function when another type of fixation is performed or a curative surgery aimed at tumor excision when a prosthetic reconstruction is performed [1].

In Lee series, patients treated with arthroplasty for proximal femoral metastases showed a lower rate of surgical revision for disease progression (3%) compared to intramedullary nail fixation (41%) [40]. Therefore, patients who undergo intralesional surgery are at high risk of reoperation for type 5 failure.

Type I progression could be treated with internal fixation or arthroplasty, whereas type II progression could be treated initially by using appropriately sized longer devices based on preoperative templating, designed to cover the affected areas without necessarily protecting the entire bone or by routine prophylactic protection of the entire bone. Finally, type III progression could be treated adequately by longer fixation implants stabilizing the entire bone or by modular megaprostheses with long stems [15].

In the study by Alvi et al., 54% of the patients underwent reoperation: 36% in type I, 9% in type II, and 9% in type III progression [15].

Sometimes, a massive local recurrence of the neoplasm occurs early, and no surgery can be performed because of the bad performance status of the patient. Other patients could be referred for palliation radiotherapy, which temporarily results in a disease stabilization confirmed by the radiological examination [2].

Conclusions

The determination of the cause of failure is the key to address the strategy of patient management. Prostheses dislocation can be treated conservatively, but usually a revision of the prosthesis is necessary. Soft tissue defect can be reinforced with Lars or Trevira's mesh. Surgical wound dehiscence usually recovers with medications and antibiotic therapy, and sometimes a VAC therapy is necessary for a secondary closure. In all symptomatic asepting loosenings, a revision of the prosthesis is mandatory. Osteosynthesis and endoprosthetic reconstruction are equally safe methods to treat fractures around the implants. Patient survival is not influenced by type of surgery or choice of implant. Patients with good performance status and with preoperatively ambulatory capacity might benefit from primary endoprosthetic reconstruction due to longer implant durability. Infection is the most common cause of periprosthetic implant failure. In these patients, a two-staged procedure with antibiotic-coated spacer insertion and prolonged IV antibiotic therapy is recommended. Once the infection is resolved, a bigger megaprosthesis, with or without silver coating, can be implanted, or alternatively an arthrodesis can be performed.

If tumor recurrence/progression is the cause of the implant failure, the assessment of the operability and the estimation of the survival are crucial to determine the strategy of treatment. If the patient can undergo surgery, another megaprosthesis should be used; if it is possible or alternatively, joint arthrodesis is another option. Amputation should be taken into consideration only when the above-mentioned techniques cannot be used.

Disclosure Each author certified that he or she has no commercial associations (e.g., consultancies, stock ownership, equity interest, patent/licensing arrangements, etc.) that might pose a conflict of interest in connection with the submitted article.

References

1. Laitinen M, Parry M, Ratasvuori M, Wedin R, Albergo JI, Jeys L, et al. Survival and complications of skeletal reconstructions after surgical treatment of bony metastatic renal cell carcinoma. Eur J Surg Oncol. 2015;41(7):886–92.
2. Guzik G. Results of the treatment of bone metastases with modular prosthetic replacement—analysis of 67 patients. J Orthop Surg. 2016;11:20.
3. Sørensen MS, Gregersen KG, Grum-Schwensen T, Hovgaard D, Petersen MM. Patient and implant survival following joint replacement because of metastatic bone disease. Acta Orthop. 2013;84(3): 301–6.

4. Forsberg JA, Wedin R, Bauer H. Which implant is best after failed treatment for pathologic femur fractures? Clin Orthop. 2013;471(3):735–40.
5. Henrichs M-P, Krebs J, Gosheger G, Streitbuerger A, Nottrott M, Sauer T, et al. Modular tumor endoprostheses in surgical palliation of long-bone metastases: a reduction in tumor burden and a durable reconstruction. World J Surg Oncol. 2014;12:330.
6. Tanaka T, Imanishi J, Charoenlap C, Choong PFM. Intramedullary nailing has sufficient durability for metastatic femoral fractures. World J Surg Oncol. 2016;14:80.
7. Henderson ER, Groundland JS, Pala E, Dennis JA, Wooten R, Cheong D, et al. Failure mode classification for tumor endoprostheses: retrospective review of five institutions and a literature review. J Bone Joint Surg Am. 2011;93(5):418–29.
8. Wedin R, Hansen BH, Laitinen M, Trovik C, Zaikova O, Bergh P, et al. Complications and survival after surgical treatment of 214 metastatic lesions of the humerus. J Shoulder Elbow Surg. 2012;21(8):1049–55.
9. Capanna R, Scoccianti G, Frenos F, Vilardi A, Beltrami G, Campanacci DA. What was the survival of megaprostheses in lower limb reconstructions after tumor resections? Clin Orthop. 2015;473(3):820–30.
10. Pala E, Henderson ER, Calabrò T, Angelini A, Abati CN, Trovarelli G, et al. Survival of current production tumor endoprostheses: complications, functional results, and a comparative statistical analysis. J Surg Oncol. 2013;108(6):403–8.
11. Steensma M, Boland PJ, Morris CD, Athanasian E, Healey JH. Endoprosthetic treatment is more durable for pathologic proximal femur fractures. Clin Orthop. 2012;470(3):920–6.
12. Laitinen M, Nieminen J, Pakarinen T-K. Treatment of pathological humerus shaft fractures with intramedullary nails with or without cement fixation. Arch Orthop Trauma Surg. 2011;131(4):503–8.
13. Kostuj T, Streit R, Baums MH, Schaper K, Meurer A. Midterm outcome after mega-prosthesis implanted in patients with bony defects in cases of revision compared to patients with malignant tumors. J Arthroplast. 2015;30(9):1592–6.
14. Thambapillary S, Dimitriou R, Makridis KG, Fragkakis EM, Bobak P, Giannoudis PV. Implant longevity, complications and functional outcome following proximal femoral arthroplasty for musculoskeletal tumors: a systematic review. J Arthroplast. 2013;28(8):1381–5.
15. Alvi HM, Damron TA. Prophylactic stabilization for bone metastases, myeloma, or lymphoma: do we need to protect the entire bone? Clin Orthop. 2013;471(3):706–14.
16. Wedin R, Bauer HCF. Surgical treatment of skeletal metastatic lesions of the proximal femur: endoprosthesis or reconstruction nail? J Bone Joint Surg Br. 2005;87(12):1653–7.

17. Shehadeh A, Noveau J, Malawer M, Henshaw R. Late complications and survival of endoprosthetic reconstruction after resection of bone tumors. Clin Orthop. 2010;468(11):2885–95.
18. Hettwer WH, Horstmann PF, Hovgaard TB, Grum-Scwensen TA, Petersen MM. Low infection rate after tumor hip arthroplasty for metastatic bone disease in a cohort treated with extended antibiotic prophylaxis. Adv Orthop. 2015;2015:428986.
19. Jacofsky DJ, Haidukewych GJ, Zhang H, Sim FH. Complications and results of arthroplasty for salvage of failed treatment of malignant pathologic fractures of the hip. Clin Orthop. 2004;427:52–6.
20. Dindo D, Demartines N, Clavien P-A. Classification of surgical complications: a new proposal with evaluation in a cohort of 6336 patients and results of a survey. Ann Surg. 2004;240(2):205–13.
21. Barut N, Anract P, Babinet A, Biau D. Peri-prosthetic fractures around tumor endoprostheses: a retrospective analysis of eighteen cases. Int Orthop. 2015;39(9):1851–6.
22. Capanna R, Campanacci DA. The treatment of metastases in the appendicular skeleton. J Bone Joint Surg Br. 2001;83(4):471–81.
23. Fakler JK, Hase F, Böhme J, Josten C. Safety aspects in surgical treatment of pathological fractures of the proximal femur—modular endoprosthetic replacement vs. intramedullary nailing. Patient Saf Surg. 2013;7(1):37.
24. Menendez LR, Ahlmann ER, Kermani C, Gotha H. Endoprosthetic reconstruction for neoplasms of the proximal femur. Clin Orthop. 2006;450:46–51.
25. Houdek MT, Wagner ER, Wilke BK, Wyles CC, Taunton MJ, Sim FH. Long term outcomes of cemented endoprosthetic reconstruction for periarticular tumors of the distal femur. Knee. 2016;23(1):167–72.
26. Hobusch GM, Funovics PT, Hourscht C, Domayer SE, Puchner SE, Dominkus M, et al. LARS® band and tube for extensor mechanism reconstructions in proximal tibial modular endoprostheses after bone tumors. Knee. 2016;23(5):905–10.
27. Stavropoulos NA, Sawan H, Dandachli F, Turcotte RE. Use of ligament advanced reinforcement system tube in stabilization of proximal humeral endoprostheses. World J Orthop. 2016;7(4):265–71.
28. Houdek MT, Wagner ER, Wilke BK, Wyles CC, Taunton MJ, Sim FH. Late complications and long-term outcomes following aseptic revision of a hip arthroplasty performed for oncological resection. Hip Int. 2015;25(5):428–34.
29. Bickels J, Kollender Y, Wittig JC, Cohen N, Meller I, Malawer MM. Vacuum-assisted wound closure after resection of musculoskeletal tumors. Clin Orthop. 2005;441:346–50.
30. Healey JH, Morris CD, Athanasian EA, Boland PJ. Compress knee arthroplasty has 80% 10-year survivorship and novel forms of bone failure. Clin Orthop. 2013;471(3):774–83.

31. Gebhart M, Shumelinsky F. Management of periprosthetic fractures in patients treated with a megaprosthesis for malignant bone tumours around the knee. Acta Orthop Belg. 2012;78(4):558–63.

32. Wright TW, Cofield RH. Humeral fractures after shoulder arthroplasty. J Bone Joint Surg Am. 1995;77(9):1340–6.

33. Piccioli A, Rossi B, Sacchetti FM, Spinelli MS, Di Martino A. Fractures in bone tumour prosthesis. Int Orthop. 2015;39(10):1981–7.

34. Worland RL, Kim DY, Arredondo J. Periprosthetic humeral fractures: management and classification. J Shoulder Elb Surg. 1999;8(6):590–4.

35. Duncan CP, Haddad FS. The Unified Classification System (UCS): improving our understanding of periprosthetic fractures. Bone Joint J. 2014;96-B(6):713–6.

36. Bickels J, Kollender Y, Wittig JC, Meller I, Malawer MM. Function after resection of humeral metastases: analysis of 59 consecutive patients. Clin Orthop. 2005;437:201–8.

37. Hardes J, Gebert C, Schwappach A, Ahrens H, Streitburger A, Winkelmann W, et al. Characteristics and outcome of infections associated with tumor endoprostheses. Arch Orthop Trauma Surg. 2006;126(5):289–96.

38. Hardes J, von Eiff C, Streitbuerger A, Balke M, Budny T, Henrichs MP, et al. Reduction of periprosthetic infection with silver-coated megaprostheses in patients with bone sarcoma. J Surg Oncol. 2010;101(5):389–95.

39. Racano A, Pazionis T, Farrokhyar F, Deheshi B, Ghert M. High infection rate outcomes in long-bone tumor surgery with endoprosthetic reconstruction in adults: a systematic review. Clin Orthop. 2013;471(6):2017–27.

40. Lee SH, Kim HS, Park YB, Rhie TY, Lee HK. Prosthetic reconstruction for tumours of the distal tibia and fibula. J Bone Joint Surg Br. 1999;81(5):803–7.

Stop, Think, Stage, Then Act

20

J. J. Willeumier, C. W. P .G. van der Wal, R. J. P. van der Wal, P. D. S. Dijkstra, and M. A. J. van de Sande

Abstract

The treatment of pathologic fractures should be the final stage of a concise pathway including diagnostics, imaging, and survival prediction. If the treatment of a pathologic fracture is rushed, this can lead to severe and needless complications. Several important pitfalls should be avoided:

– The cause of a pathologic fracture or the origin of a solitary lesion should be known. Without a final diagnosis, a new solitary lesion should always be regarded as primary tumour.
– One should be cautious of a spontaneous fracture or of a fracture after minimal trauma, since there can be an underlying pathology.
– It is important to realise that a pathologic fracture does not heal like a traumatic fracture. This must be considered when deciding on the treatment strategy.
– Pain is not a firm prognostic factor for the risk of an impending fracture. More than one lesion can be present in a bone, so complete imaging is essential.
– The treatment strategy should depend in great part on the expected survival. The aim of the treatment should be to give the patient a stable limb in a single operation. The extent of the surgery and the implant should thus be in balance with the expected survival, preventing overtreatment and unnecessary complications.

Therefore, it is important to "stop, think, stage, then act".

Keywords

Bone metastasis · Pathologic fracture · Primary bone tumour · Diagnostics · Biopsy · Imaging · Survival

When treating patients with impending or pathologic fractures, there are several pitfalls to be aware of and to avoid. These pitfalls will be discussed in this chapter, accompanied with clinical examples and recommendations on how to prevent such complications. In general, if one adheres to a simple motto, many complications can be avoided. The motto is *stop*, *think*, *stage*,

J. J. Willeumier (✉) · C. W. P .G. van der Wal · R. J. P. van der Wal · P. D. S. Dijkstra · M. A. J. van de Sande
Department of Orthopaedic Surgery,
Leiden University Medical Center,
Leiden, The Netherlands
e-mail: j.j.willeumier@lumc.nl;
majvandesande@lumc.nl

then act. A pathologic fracture is not an emergency, and there is no need to rush the treatment of pathologic fractures; prior to their management, thorough diagnostics, staging, and treatment planning should be performed.

20.1 A New Solitary Lesion Is a Primary Bone Tumour Until the Contrary Is Proven

A bone lesion with unknown aetiology should be regarded as a primary bone tumour until proven otherwise. Adhering to this rule prevents us from erroneously regarding a primary bone tumour as a metastatic lesion and treating it consequently. Curative treatment of a primary bone tumour starts with the diagnostics and a biopsy and is often found impossible after surgical treatment of a pathological fracture [1–3]. All intra-lesional fixations will lead to further dissemination of tumour cells, and extensive salvage surgery and often amputations, in case of unsalvageable limbs, are required, as illustrated by Case 1. In worse cases, resection of the primary tumour is not even an option anymore due to its widespread dissemination.

Note: It is easy to prevent inadvertent fixation, if the origin of the lesion is determined before any action is undertaken.

When a patient presents with a bone lesion, there often are three scenarios:

1. The patient is known for metastatic bone disease.

2. The patient is known for a malignancy but not with metastatic (bone) disease.

3. The patient is not known for malignancy.

In the first case, the lesion is generally not solitary since previous bone metastases have been diagnosed, and an additional histological confirmation of the current lesion is not indicated as such. Note that a biopsy might still be warranted if the lesion is not characteristic of the established primary tumour [4].

In the case of a solitary lesion, shown in the two other cases, a definitive diagnosis should be established prior to any treatment. Even in patients with a known primary malignancy, the possibility of a second primary tumour should not be ignored. Although the incidence of a bone tumour as second primary is low, it is not uncommon [5]. Case 2 describes why it is important to stop and think before acting, even in patients with known malignant disease.

Adequate imaging of the lesion and of the chest, abdomen and pelvis (in patients without history of cancer), and laboratory analyses provide relevant information that will identify the origin of the lesion in approximately 85% of the patients [6]. Core needle biopsies are the final step to provide a conclusive diagnosis of metastatic disease. Depending on the location, these can be obtained by an open or percutaneous approach, or CT-guided, according to the principles of musculoskeletal tumour biopsy [7]. The biopsy tract will require total excision if the diagnosis is a primary tumour, without compromising limb salvage, so the biopsy should be carefully planned and performed by, or after consultation with, a specialist oncology orthopaedic surgeon. Biopsies through the posterior gluteal flap, quadriceps muscles, and neurovascular structures should be avoided, and only one compartment should be affected [8]. Just like treating an undiagnosed bone lesion as bone metastasis, the random placement of a biopsy needle can cause unnecessary problems and is a pitfall that can be prevented by stopping and thinking before acting.

The above diagnostic steps are widely recognised and included in the Dutch, British, and American guidelines for the diagnostics and treatment of pathologic fractures [9–11].

20.2 A Fracture After a Low Impact Trauma Is Suspicious

It is essential to be alert for the signs of a pathologic fracture because failure to recognize the pathological origin of a fracture will lead to wrong treatments and poor outcomes. A pathologic fracture is a fracture occurring without adequate trauma due to lack of local bone strength or to a systemic disease. Examples of low impact or inadequate traumata are falls from standing height or less, torsional movements (e.g. turning in bed), collisions with objects during normal activities (e.g. bumping into table). Normal, healthy bone should be able to sustain such low-impact traumas without fractures. When a patient presents without adequate trauma to explain a fracture in the long bones, especially if the patient is >40 year old, a metastasis is the most common diagnosis. Differential diagnoses are osteoporosis, multiple myeloma, and a primary malignant bone tumour. In patients with metastases, fractures develop in approximately 10–15% of the patients, in most cases without any preceding (low impact) trauma [12]. X-rays of metastatic lesions commonly show well-defined lytic lesions with a narrow zone of transition, although blastic lesions also occur. Especially permeative lesions with cortical weakening without clear destruction on radiographs can be misread. In addition, fractures are commonly transverse.

20.3 A Pathologic Fracture Is Not a Normal Fracture

Pathologic fractures due to metastases should not be regarded as normal, traumatic fractures. While traumatic fractures occur in healthy bone that will be able to regenerate and heal, the disease process in the bone of a pathologic fracture hinders normal bone remineralisation. The mechanisms responsible for metastatic lesions fractures are based on the imbalance between bone resorption and formation. In healthy adults, weight-bearing bones are in a constant state of remodelling to adjust for functional demands or to repair micro-fractures that appear as a part of normal activity. This remodelling occurs as a result of a coupled activity of osteoclasts resorbing bone and osteoblasts laying down new bone [13]. In bone metastases, this coupled process has become distorted. Depending on the stimulation of osteoclasts and osteoblasts, lytic or blastic lesions may develop. In osteolytic lesions, tumour-derived parathyroid hormone-related peptide (PTHrP) leads to increased osteoclast activation [14], while overstimulation of the formation of osteoblasts leads to osteoblastic lesions [13].

Fracture-healing rates depend on the type of primary tumour and are reported to range from 44% for kidney tumours, approximate 37% for breast cancer, and up to 0% for lung cancer [15]. A life expectancy of more than 6 months is the most positive factor predicting fracture healing [15]. Even when the bone healing is possible, it is often delayed [7]. This has implications, and we should amend our treatment strategies accordingly; a rigid stabilisation of the pathologic fractures should be pursued perioperatively. A conservative treatment with closed reduction and cast immobilisation is regarded as obsolete because of the minimal fracture healing that is expected. Only in specific patients, for example, in those with a very short expected survival, extensive comorbidities, or metastases in non-weight-bearing bones, the conservative treatment should be considered. Bone-ingrowth/press-fit prostheses are generally not recommended because the residual metastatic disease, after intra-lesional resections, will cause a rapid loosening and failure of the implant. Additionally, bone-ingrowth/press-fit prostheses require a period of non-weight-bearing for osseointegration, while immediate weight-bearing is one of the primary aims of surgical treatment [3]. Also when using plates for internal fixation, the plate should be long enough to withstand the torsional forces of muscles on a fractured bone, as illustrated by Case 3.

20.4 Pain Is a Doubtful Indicator for an Impending Fracture

Fracture prediction is one of the most difficult and debatable aspects of the treatment of bone metastases. Multiple studies have described prognostic factors for fracturing: size, cortex breakthrough, circumferential involvement, lesion type, anatomic location, and pain [16, 17]. Although all prognostic factors are subject to considerable debate, pain calls for resistance, and one should be cautious in making decisions depending on it. Pain has been reported in only one study as a prognostic factor, but this study and its corresponding score are commonly referred to [16]. Several authors have reported that pain is not a reliable sign, because of its subjectivity (i.e. suppressed by the use of pain-killers for other indications) [18, 19] and uncoupled relation to the size of the lesion [20, 21]. Dijkstra et al. found that pain in general was not related to the occurrence of a fracture, but that increasing pain in the short-term period before fracture was related to the event [21]. The latter might correspond to current thoughts on the role of functional pain, e.g. pain during weight-bearing, but there are no studies reporting on the relation between functional pain and fractures.

Pain alone, in a small lesion without fracture risk, should never be a solitary indication for surgical treatment. Only if the pain is nonresponsive to radiotherapy, surgery should be considered. Additionally, pain should never be a reason to hasten the diagnostics and staging process. Pain medication, ranging from paracetamol and non-steroidal anti-inflammatory drugs to opioids, can reduce pain in most patients [22].

20.5   Bone Metastasis Often Implies Extensive Disease

Imaging of the entire affected long bone before surgical treatment is essential. If one bone metastasis is present, it can be expected that multiple metastases are present, often located within the same bone. The majority of patients present with more than one bone metastasis, while 2% presents with a solitary bone metastasis [23]. Hasty treatment decisions without considering whether other lesions are present can lead to insufficient stabilisation of the affected bone and possibly the need for further stabilisation in a second stage. Knowledge of metastases in other long bones than the bone requiring treatment is also advisable, to detect whether there are other lesions in need of treatment and to give adequate post-operative and rehabilitation instructions. This can be obtained with X-rays of both humeri and femurs, and with a whole body bone scan or PET-CT. A complete overview of the extent of bone disease can improve the care of patients, for example, by simultaneous treatments, and can prevent unexpected events in the recovery, e.g. when using crutches to mobilise with an unknown large lesion in the humerus.

When stabilising an actual or impending fracture, the region of the lesion is the primary region of interest. Additionally, knowledge obtained with whole-bone X-rays should be taken into account when deciding on the method of stabilisation. When treating impending fractures with an intramedullary nail, prophylactic stabilisation of the entire long bone is considered the standard of care [24]. Also if fractures of the shaft or distal femur are treated with intramedullary nails, it is advisable to prophylactically stabilise the femur neck with a cephalomedullary nail. When treating the lesion of interest (e.g. the proximal femur) with prosthesis, it is less straightforward to stabilise the entire femur because that implies far more extensive surgery. In all cases, the extent of the (prophylactic) surgery should weigh against the risk of developing another metastasis in need of treatment. As metastases develop more commonly in the proximal part of the bone than the distal part, prophylactic stabilisation of the proximal femur is more common.

20.6   "Once in a Lifetime" Palliative Surgery: The Need for Survival Prediction

The surgical stabilisation should be durable for the remaining lifetime of a patient, while the recovery and rehabilitation time should not exceed the life expectancy or be too demanding in the light of the expected survival [25]. This sounds very logical, but it is one of the most difficult aspects of the surgical treatment of bone metastases. It encompasses survival prediction on one hand and prediction of the longevity of an implant and disease progression on the other hand. Nonetheless, the aim of tailored treatment should be to suffice for the remaining lifetime, without the need of revision surgery because the implant failed or the fixation was insufficient. This puts an extra burden on patients and will significantly influence their quality of life. In patients who are in the last phase of life, all should be done to avoid unnecessary (extensive) operations. Adequate prediction of the remaining lifetime before deciding on the treatment strategy is thus required for each individual patient. To aid physicians in this prediction, several prognostic models have been developed as discussed in chapter 4. A simple, straightforward model to use is a model that requires only three variables: the clinical profile, which is based on the primary tumour; the Karnofsky performance score; and the presence or absence of visceral and/or brain metastases, as developed by Willeumier et al. [26]. This leads to four different categories which correlate with a median survival and survival rates at 1, 3, 6, 12, and 24 months (Fig. 20.1). The categories are further grouped into four clinically relevant categories (A–D) which correlate with a survival of >12 months, 6–12 months, 3–6 months, and <3 months, respectively. These results are subsequently used when determining the treatment strategy. The impact of expected survival is especially large in patients with proximal femur metastases and in patients with solitary bone metastases. In general, proximal femur metastases are treated with intramedullary nails

or with (endo)prosthetic reconstructions. The choice between the two strategies is based on the amount of bone stock of the femur head, but more importantly on the expected survival. Although 1-year implant survival rates are difficult to analyse due to the extreme influence of the competing risk of death and they have not been reported in literature, the survival of a standard cephalomedullary nail (without adjuvant cement) can be expected to be 1–2 years. This is due to the load-sharing characteristics of the intramedullary nail, the fact that a pathologic fracture generally does not heal, and the risk of lysis over time. If a patient is expected to live longer, an intramedullary nail is thus not the optimal solution, as failure of the implant might require revision surgery, as illustrated by Case 4. Likewise, patients with solitary lesions of kidney and thyroid cancer can be expected to have a long survival, especially if adequately treated with en bloc resection [27]. En bloc resection and prosthetic reconstruction should also be considered if the location of the lesion, in combination with the expected survival of the patient, does not ideally lend for internal fixation with an intramedullary nail or a plate, as Case 5 illustrates.

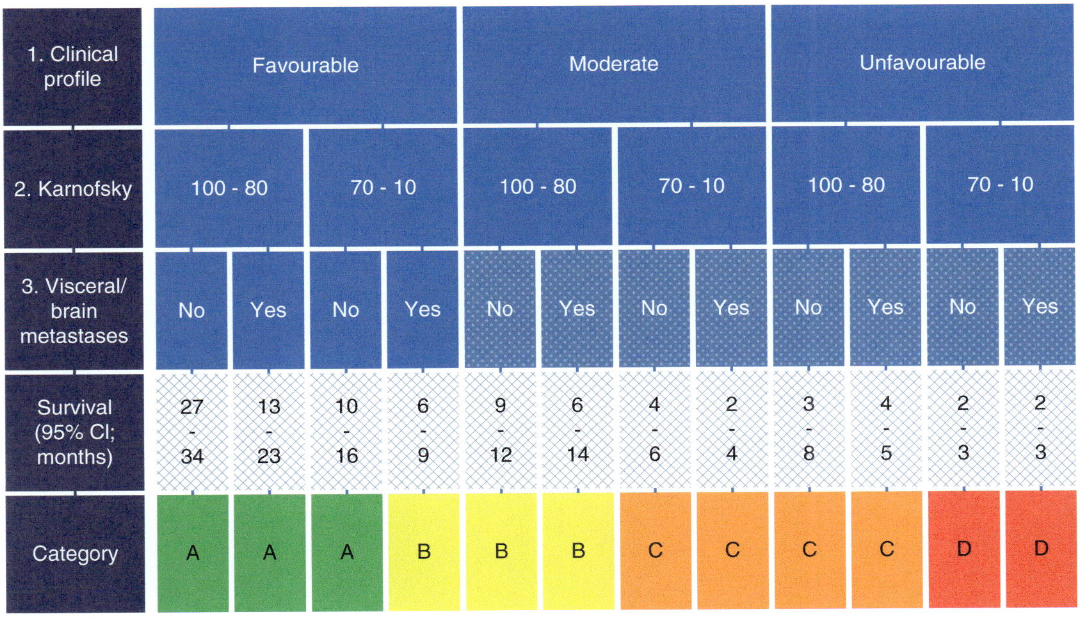

1. Clinical profile	Favourable				Moderate				Unfavourable			
2. Karnofsky	100 - 80		70 - 10		100 - 80		70 - 10		100 - 80		70 - 10	
3. Visceral/ brain metastases	No	Yes	No	Yes	No	Yes	No	Yes	No	Yes	No	Yes
Survival (95% CI; months)	27 - 34	13 - 23	10 - 16	6 - 9	9 - 12	6 - 14	4 - 6	2 - 4	3 - 8	4 - 5	2 - 3	2 - 3
Category	A	A	A	B	B	B	C	C	C	C	D	D

Fig. 20.1 Flowchart for stratification of patients with long bone metastases

Case 1

A 69-year-old lady with no relevant medical history was seen a week after she felt a sudden sharp pain in the left groin area after taking a step in the kitchen. X-ray showed a sub-trochanteric pathologic fracture (Fig. 20.2a), and subsequently an MRI was performed. Two radiologists reviewed the MRI and concluded the fracture was based on a fibrous dysplasia lesion. No other diagnostics were performed, and the fracture was stabilised with a lateral femoral nail with two screws in the neck (Fig. 20.2b). Iliac crest harvested autologous bone graft was used to fill the cavity of the lesion. The patient was instructed to refrain from weight-bearing for 6 weeks and was discharged in overall good condition. Results from pathology however showed a grade II chondrosarcoma after which patient was referred to a tertiary referral centre for orthopaedic oncology. Due to the fact that there was possible contamination of the entire femur with the grade II chondrosarcoma, making a curative resection difficult, and the good overall health of the patient, it was discussed with the patient to follow a "watch and wait" strategy. Three months

later, the patient presented with a large tumour mass in the soft tissue around the left hip causing pain and immobility. A proximal femur resection was then performed during which the intramedullary nail was removed and alcohol was used as adjuvant for the intramedullary cavity. Peroperatively, it was clear that the tumour had progressed further distally. A modular bipolar proximal femur endoprosthesis with a stem length of 22 cm was placed (Fig. 20.2c). Ten months post-operatively, the patient was able to function sufficiently and without pain in the hip, although the distal femur and knee were getting increasingly painful. Imaging showed recurrence of the chondrosarcoma in the distal femur and lung nodules suspect for metastases. Unfortunately, the only remaining surgical option would be an ex-articulation of the hip. Together with the patient, it was decided to follow a palliative line with radiotherapy (20 Gy) to decrease the pain, although this did not have the desired effect. This left only pain medication to relieve the pain. Three years after her presentation with a painful hip, patient passed away due to progressive disease.

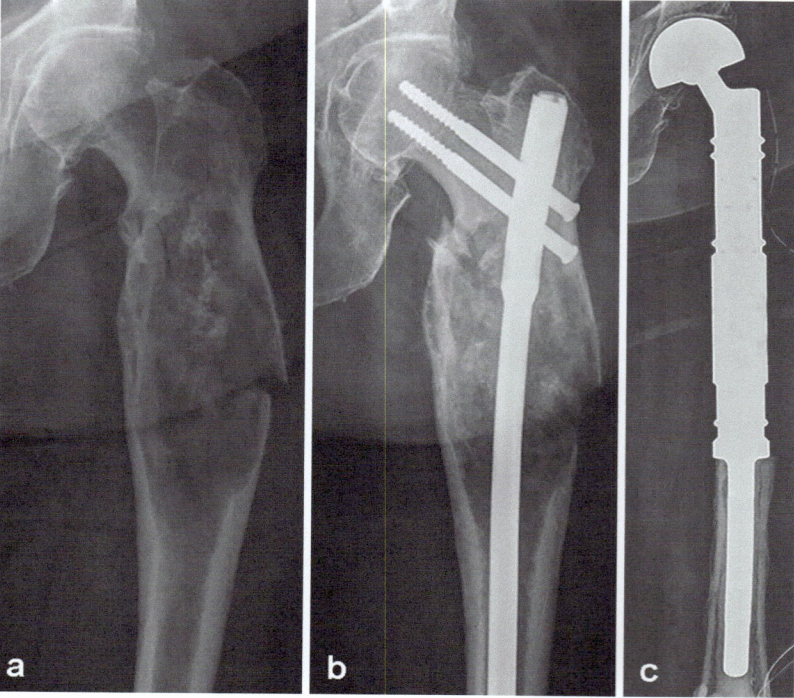

Fig. 20.2 Initial "whoops" treatment of a proximal femur pathologic fracture due to a primary tumour, requiring subsequent resection and reconstruction with a modular tumour prosthesis

In this case, a biopsy should have been performed beside the conventional (X-ray) and additional imaging of the lesion (MRI or CT). This would have given the patient a chance at a curative resection of a primary chondrosarcoma.

Case 2

A 72-year-old man with coloncarcinoma in the past was admitted to the hospital with an impending fracture of the left distal femur (Fig. 20.3a). The bone scan was suspect for a solitary bone metastasis. With the working-diagnosis of an impending fracture due to bone metastasis, the femur was prophylactically stabilised with an intramedullary nail (Fig. 20.3b), and a perioperative biopsy was taken. Pathological analysis showed no malignant cells; however, more extensive histopathology tests showed a telangiectatic

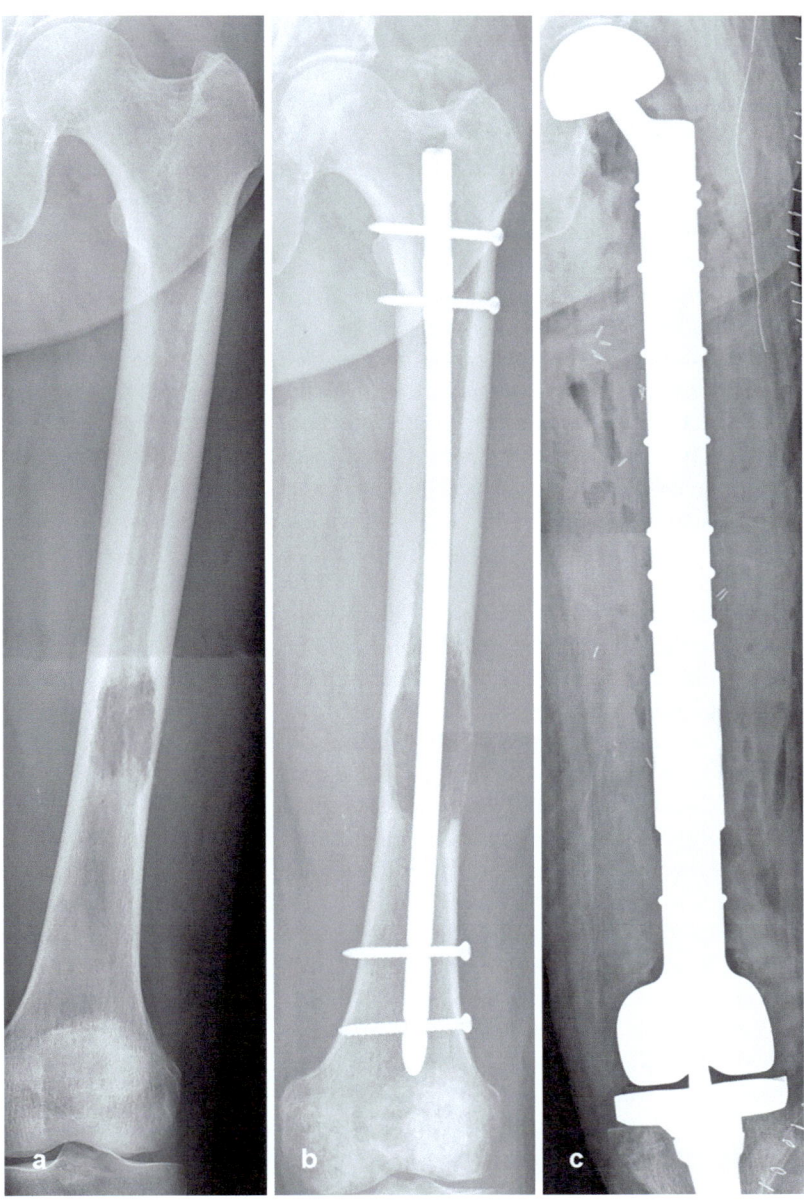

Fig. 20.3 Initial "whoops" treatment of an impending pathologic fracture of the femur shaft due to a second primary tumour, requiring total femur resection and reconstruction

osteosarcoma. There was thus a second primary tumour without metastases. Treatment included preoperative chemotherapy (adriamycine; three cycles) followed by an en bloc resection of the entire femur and reconstruction with a total femur endoprosthesis (Fig. 20.3c). Resection margins were clear and chemotherapy was continued. Unfortunately, within a month, two complications occurred: an infected prosthesis with *Staphylococcus aureus* and luxation. Both were treated accordingly. The patient was discharged from the hospital 2 months after presentation with suppression therapy of the infected prostheses and is still alive 6 years after "whoops" surgery and en bloc resection.

This is an example of a patient with a known malignancy and a second primary tumour. This case stresses the need of a biopsy in patients without diagnosed metastatic bone disease. Due to too quick surgical fixation, treatment of the bone tumour required very extensive surgery. This, and the fact that two operations were needed within short time, will have contributed to the chance of a periprosthetic joint infection. Fortunately, because the entire femur was resected, an oncologic good outcome was achieved.

Case 3

A 74-year-old man with a curatively treated carcinoma of the larynx in the past presented with a pneumonia and a painful left arm. CT scan of the thorax showed a large lung tumour.

X-ray of the arm showed a lytic lesion in the distal third of the humerus with such involvement of the cortex that a fracture was impending (Fig. 20.4a). Therefore, prophylactic stabilisation was performed with a small fragment (five hole) Locking Compression Plate (LCP) after curettage, phenolisation (alcohol), and cementplasty of the lesion (Fig. 20.4b). The patient was instructed that the arm could be used as normal (unless limited by pain), and post-operative radiotherapy was initiated. Three weeks later, however, the arm was increasingly painful, and the patient felt more movement within the arm. The plate appeared to have broken out, and an actual fracture of the humerus was present

(Fig. 20.4c). During revision surgery, the two proximal screws were entirely loose, and extensive tumour tissue was visible. Refixation was performed with a large LCP (12 holes) and four proximal locking screws and four distal screws with adjuvant cement in the fracture cavity (Fig. 20.4d). Two months after the first LCP, the patient passed away.

Case 4

A 64-year-old woman with a history of breast cancer successfully treated 15 years earlier presented at the emergency department with a painful left hip after a light fall several weeks before. A pertrochanteric fracture was diagnosed and regarded as pathologic due to her medical history and the minimal trauma. A bone scan showed multiple other metastatic localisations in the costae and spinal column, but no other lesions in the left femur. To stabilise the fracture, a long gamma nail was placed (Fig. 20.5a). Post-operatively full weight-bearing was allowed, and adjuvant radiotherapy (24Gy in 6 fractions) was administered. A year-and-a-half later, the patient presented again with a painful and shortened leg: the gamma nail was fractured at the height of the neck screw, and there was a dislocation of the fracture parts (Fig. 20.5b). A new gamma nail was placed with cement around the neck screw (Fig. 20.5c). Six months later, the patient remained painful, and the CT scan showed a subtrochanteric pseudoarthrosis with lysis around the neck screw and collapse of the cranial part of the femoral head. To prevent further lysis and collapse, cement augmentation around the neck screw was performed. Two months later, however, progressive migration of the neck screw through the femoral head was observed (Fig. 20.5d). It was decided to remove the gamma nail and place a proximal femoral endoprosthesis (Fig. 20.5e). This was complicated by a deep venous thrombosis 6 weeks post-operatively, which was treated accordingly. The patient was able to mobilise with the proximal femur prosthesis during the remaining 4 years of her life.

In this case, an adequate estimation of the expected survival could possibly have spared her several operations. At the initial diagnosis of the

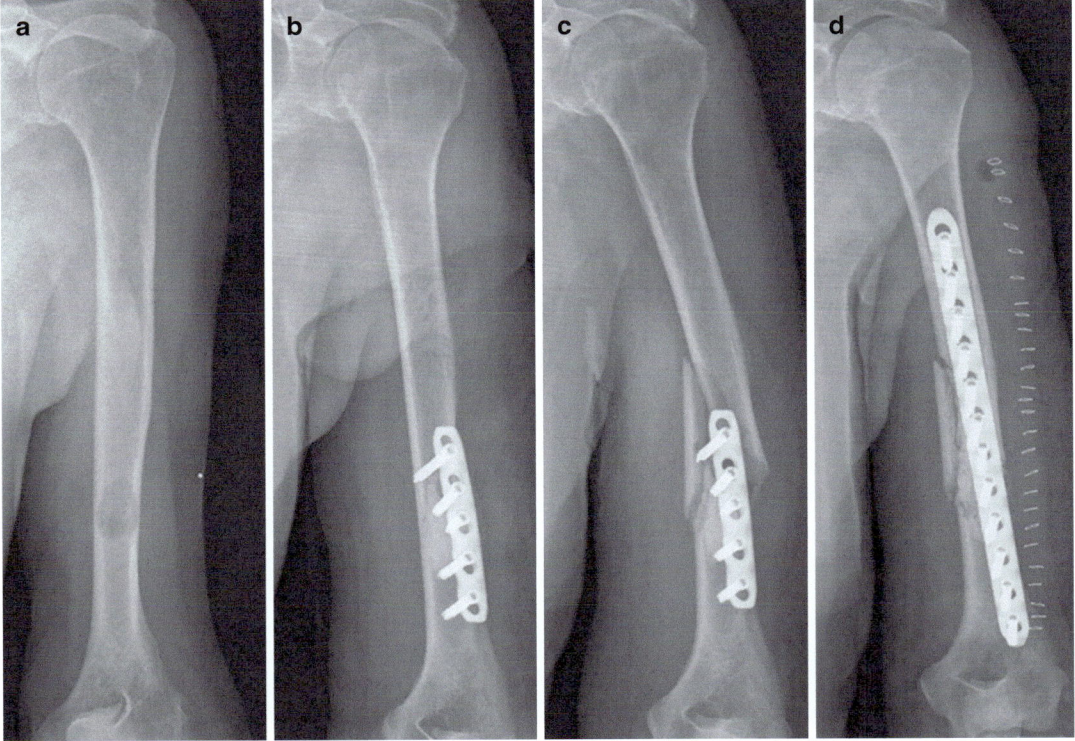

Fig. 20.4 Failed initial plate fixation of an impending pathologic fracture of the distal humerus, revised with a longer plate and cement augmentation

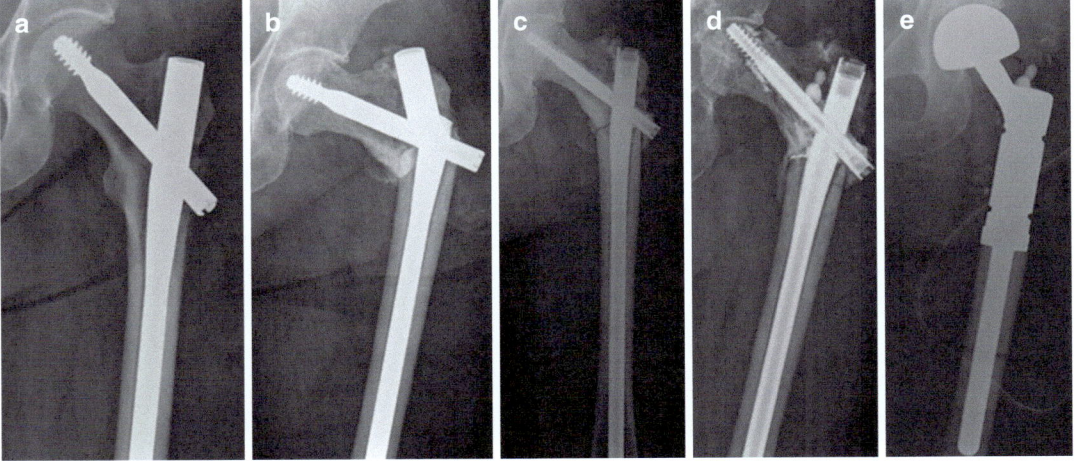

Fig. 20.5 Failed intramedullary nail 1.5 years after stabilisation of a pathologic fracture of the proximal femur, initially treated with a new nail and cement augmentation, but eventually requiring resection and revision with a modular tumour prosthesis

metastasis, there was a patient in good health, without visceral and/or brain metastases, with a primary breast cancer. All prognostic models would expect a survival of more than 1 year, and therefore this patient could have been treated with a prosthesis primarily.

Case 5

A 45-year-old woman with a clear medical history presented at the emergency department with a painful left leg, unable to bear weight. Her complaints had started directly after turning in bed. Additionally, she mentioned that she had been having some complaints at the knee for the previous couple of months, she had been tired, and she was losing weight unintendingly. The X-ray showed a transverse distal femur fracture and a directly performed CT-thorax/abdomen which showed a large tumour in the kidney, without signs of visceral metastases (Fig. 20.6a). A biopsy of the lesion with the pathologic fracture was performed and confirmed the diagnosis of a metastasis from the clear cell carcinoma. A bone scan showed there were numerous other lesions in the pelvis and the other long bones, among others in the right femur. Subsequently a stabili-

sation of the distal femur fracture was performed with a plate osteosynthesis without cement (Fig. 20.6b). Post-operative radiotherapy (20Gy in 5 fractions) was administered. A maximum load of 25 kg was set for the left leg, so the patient could only mobilise with crutches. The patient also started with a tyrosine kinase inhibitor (pazopanib). Over the following 5 months, pathologic fractures of the right humerus and right femur occurred which were treated accordingly, but these significantly affected the ambulatory ability of the patient. The left knee had also remained painful despite optimal pain medication. Further imaging of the knee showed that there was no consolidation of the transverse fracture, that there were also vertical fractures, and that the plate was not completely adjacent to the bone (Fig. 20.6c). To improve the quality of life of the patient (i.e. pain reduction and possibility for better mobilisation), it was decided to revise the insufficient plate osteosynthesis of the left femur. A distal femur resection was performed, and modular tumour knee prosthesis was implanted (Fig. 20.6d).

This case is an example in which a primary en bloc resection and prosthetic reconstruction

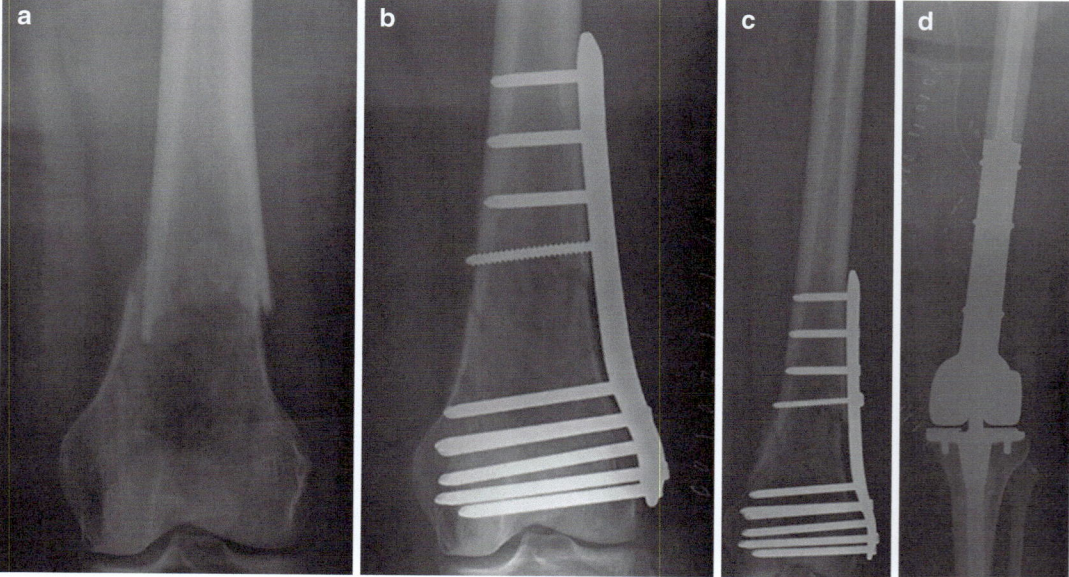

Fig. 20.6 A pathologic distal femur fracture, treated initially with a plate osteosynthesis but requiring revision to a modular distal femur prosthesis

should have been considered. The location of the fracture, in combination with the presence of multiple other bone lesions which could impair the rehabilitation, and the expected medium-term survival of the patient were signs that a plate fixation could be insufficient. Keeping in mind that a stabilisation of a pathologic fracture should be "once in a lifetime" and that the aim of the surgery is to maintain quality of life (i.e. being able to mobilise), a more durable option as primary stabilisation would have been preferable. Generally, such en bloc resections and reconstructions are performed in tertiary orthopaedic oncology centres, so patients should be referred if a more straightforward stabilisation is expected to be insufficient.

Conclusions

These cases illustrate the importance of stopping, thinking, and staging before acting. Patients with pathologic fractures do not require emergency stabilisation, and it cannot be stressed enough that a diagnosis of the lesion should be present before any surgical intervention. The next step is to decide on the adequate surgical modality for a fracture that (unlike traumatic fractures) has minimal healing tendencies. In this decision, accurate survival estimation is the most important factor besides location, fracture type, and patient preference, because a stabilisation should be "once and for all", while the recovery should be in proportion with the expected survival.

References

1. Scolaro JA, Lackman RD. Surgical management of metastatic long bone fractures: principles and techniques. J Am Acad Orthop Surg. 2014;22(2):90–100.
2. Adams SC, Potter BK, Pitcher DJ, Temple HT. Office-based core needle biopsy of bone and soft tissue malignancies: an accurate alternative to open biopsy with infrequent complications. Clin Orthop Relat Res. 2010;468(10):2774–80.
3. Biermann JS, Holt GE, Lewis VO, Schwartz HS, Yaszemski MJ. Metastatic bone disease: diagnosis, evaluation, and treatment. J Bone Joint Surg Am. 2009;91(6):1518–30.
4. Quinn RH, Randall RL, Benevenia J, Berven SH, Raskin KA. Contemporary management of metastatic bone disease: tips and tools of the trade for general practitioners. Instr Course Lect. 2014;63:431–41.
5. Jacofsky DJ, Haidukewych GJ. Management of pathologic fractures of the proximal femur: state of the art. J Orthop Trauma. 2004;18(7):459–69.
6. Rougraff B, Kneisl J, Simon M. Skeletal metastases of unknown origin. A prospective study of a diagnostic strategy. J Bone Joint Surg Am. 1993;75(9):1276–81.
7. Ruggieri P, Mavrogenis AF, Casadei R, Errani C, Angelini A, Calabro T, et al. Protocol of surgical treatment of long bone pathological fractures. Injury. 2010;41(11):1161–7.
8. Bryson DJ, Wicks L, Ashford RU. The investigation and management of suspected malignant pathological fractures: a review for the general orthopaedic surgeon. Injury. 2015;46(10):1891–9.
9. British Orthopaedic Oncology Society, British Orthopaedic Society. Metastatic bone disease: a guide to good practise 2015. http://www.boos.org.uk/wp-content/uploads/2016/03/BOOS-MBD-2016-BOA.pdf.
10. Oncoline. Richtlijn botmetastasen 2010. http://www.oncoline.nl/botmetastasen. Updated 15 June 2010.
11. American Academy of Orthopedic Surgeons. OrthoInfo: metastatic bone disease 2011. http://orthoinfo.aaos.org/PDFs/A00093.pdf. Updated Oct 2011.
12. Saad F, Lipton A, Cook R, Chen YM, Smith M, Coleman R. Pathologic fractures correlate with reduced survival in patients with malignant bone disease. Cancer. 2007;110(8):1860–7.
13. Roodman GD. Mechanisms of bone metastasis. Discov Med. 2004;4(22):144–8.
14. Weilbaecher KN, Guise TA, McCauley LK. Cancer to bone: a fatal attraction. Nat Rev Cancer. 2011;11(6):411–25.
15. Gainor BJ, Buchert P. Fracture healing in metastatic bone disease. Clin Orthop Relat Res. 1983;178:297–302.
16. Mirels H. Metastatic disease in long bones. A proposed scoring system for diagnosing impending pathologic fractures. Clin Orthop Relat Res. 1989;249:256–64.
17. van der Linden YM, Kroon HM, Dijkstra SPDS, Lok JJ, Noordijk EM, Leer JWH, et al. Simple radiographic parameter predicts fracturing in metastatic femoral bone lesions: results from a randomised trial. Radiother Oncol. 2003;69(1):21–31.
18. Hipp JA, Springfield DS, Hayes WC. Predicting pathologic fracture risk in the management of metastatic bone defects. Clin Orthop Relat Res. 1995;312:120–35.
19. Van der Linden Y, Dijkstra P, Kroon H, Lok J, Noordijk E, Leer J, et al. Comparative analysis of risk factors for pathological fracture with femoral metastases. J Bone Joint Surg Br. 2004;86(4):566–73.
20. Hoskin P. Scientific and clinical aspects of radiotherapy in the relief of bone pain. Cancer Surv. 1987;7(1):69–86.

21. Dijkstra PDS, Oudkerk M, Wiggers T. Prediction of pathological subtrochanteric fractures due to metastatic lesions. Arch Orthop Trauma Surg. 1997;116(4):221–4.

22. Kane CM, Hoskin P, Bennett MI. Cancer induced bone pain. BMJ. 2015;350:h315.

23. Hosaka S, Katagiri H, Honda Y, Wasa J, Murata H, Takahashi M. Clinical outcome for patients of solitary bone only metastasis. J Orthop Sci. 2016; 21(2):226–9.

24. Leopold SS. Editor's spotlight/take 5: prophylactic stabilization for bone metastases, myeloma, or lymphoma: do we need to protect the entire bone? Clin Orthop Relat Res. 2013;471(3):703–5. https://doi.org/10.1007/s11999-012-2656-1.

25. Willeumier JJ, van der Linden YM, van de Sande MAJ, Dijkstra PDS. Treatment of pathological fractures of the long bones. EFORT Open Rev. 2016;1(5):136–45.

26. Willeumier JJ, van der Linden YM, van der Wal CWPG, Jutte PC, van der Velden JM, Smolle MA, van der Zwaal P, Koper P, Akri L, de Pree I, Leithner A, Fiocco M, Dijkstra PDS. An easy-to-use prognostic model for survival estimation for patients with symptomatic long bone metastases. J Bone Jt Surg. 2018;100(3):196–204.

27. Ratasvuori M, Wedin R, Hansen BH, Keller J, Trovik C, Zaikova O, et al. Prognostic role of en-bloc resection and late onset of bone metastasis in patients with bone-seeking carcinomas of the kidney, breast, lung, and prostate: SSG study on 672 operated skeletal metastases. J Surg Oncol. 2014;110:360–5

Common Pitfalls in the Management of Skeletal Metastases

21

Carol D. Morris and Maria Silvia Spinelli

Abstract

The surgical management of patients with skeletal metastases presents a unique set of challenges. The potential clinical scenarios and associated complications are endless. This chapter will review some of the common hazards encountered when treating patients with impending and complete pathologic fractures. Specifically, the pitfalls around assumptions about metastatic status and life expectancy will be highlighted. In addition, intraoperative decision-making related to the underlying primary disease and associated complications will be emphasized.

Keywords

Pathologic fracture · Bone cement implantation syndrome · Life expectancy · Skeletal metastases

C. D. Morris (✉)
Division of Orthopaedic Oncology, Department of Orthopaedic Surgery, The Johns Hopkins University, Baltimore, MD, USA
e-mail: cmorri61@jhmi.edu

M. S. Spinelli
"Fatebene Fratelli" Hospital–Isola Tiberina, Rome, Italy

21.1 Introduction

A pitfall is an unapparent source of trouble or danger that often leads to unexpected difficulties and a negative result. The treatment of patients with metastatic disease involves many potential pitfalls, many of which are based on the physician's bias (intentional and unintentional) in treating patients with "palliative" intent. Palliative care is an evolving concept in patients with skeletal metastases. The advances in systemic therapies for carcinoma are slowly turning skeletal metastases into a chronic disease for many patients. In some instances, metastatic cancer to bone should be given consideration similar to that of primary sarcomas of bone. In other instances, the palliative aims are straightforward, and the associated benefits are short-lived. Each patient requires an evaluation that maximizes the chances of achieving desired expectations and expected outcomes of surgery while minimizing morbidity. This chapter highlights some of the common pitfalls that lead to suboptimal outcomes when treating patients with skeletal metastases.

21.2 Diagnostic Assumptions

Diagnostic accuracy is essential. If a patient's metastatic status has not been confirmed, it should not be assumed. Many neoplastic and nonneoplastic conditions have overlapping symptoms and imaging characteristics. If a bone metastasis presents as the first evidence of metastatic disease, that metastasis should be biopsied. This is particularly true for patients with impending pathologic fractures in whom surgery is being considered and in patients who present with an isolated bone lesion. Although metastatic disease is the most common clinical scenario in older patients (>40 years) with bone lesions, primary bone sarcomas, of which chondrosarcoma is the most common, must be considered. Although metastatic disease is obvious in patients who present with multiple bony lesions, establishing a primary diagnosis is important to guide systemic treatment if applicable. For patients with an isolated bone lesion, a work-up for an unknown primary cause should be undertaken [1]. Although the approach should be individualized, the work-up commonly includes a computed tomography scan of the chest, abdomen, and pelvis; a whole-body bone scan; and blood and urine chemistry profiles. If such a work-up fails to establish a primary carcinoma, the patient should be treated as though a primary bone sarcoma is the cause, and

a biopsy via a limb-sparing approach should be performed.

A common pitfall is to assume that a history of cancer, whether remote or recent, is responsible for a new skeletal lesion. Figure 21.1a shows a lytic lesion in a 50-year-old woman with a history of breast cancer. A cephalomedullary nail was placed to prevent an impending pathologic fracture from presumed metastatic disease (Fig. 21.1b). The final pathologic analysis showed an osteosarcoma of bone. Disease treatment after intramedullary nailing is now challenging, and options are limited because of contamination of the buttock for nail entry and involvement of the entire femoral canal during reaming (Fig. 21.1c). Such scenarios are common and often result in proximal amputations to achieve adequate local control. In addition, the act of reaming theoretically forces tumor emboli into the circulation and lungs. Adams et al. [2] reported on eight patients with primary bone sarcomas who underwent intramedullary nailing for presumed metastatic carcinoma. Six patients required amputation for tumor control. The recommended approach is to establish a diagnosis before surgical treatment.

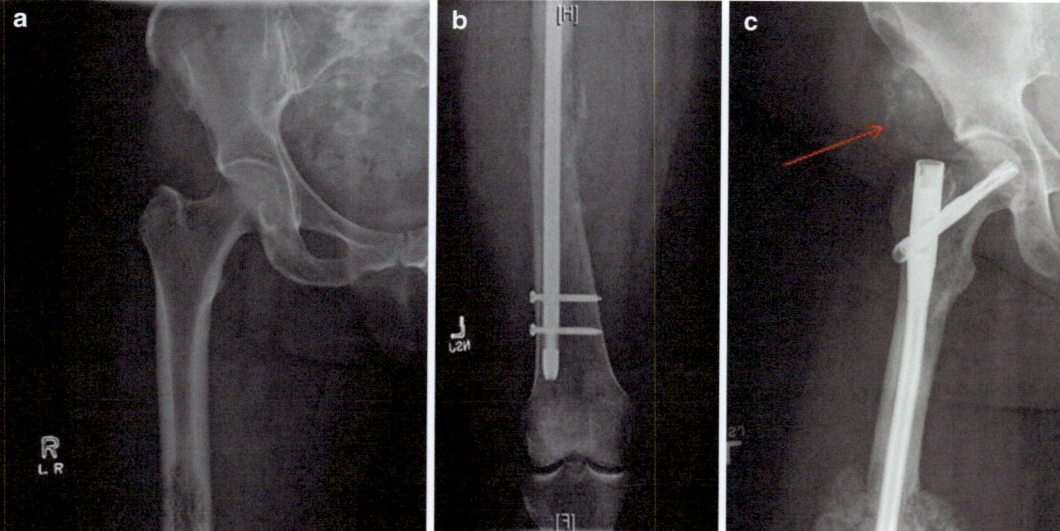

Fig. 21.1 (**a**) Anteroposterior radiograph of an impending pathologic fracture in a 50-year-old woman. (**b**) Radiograph after intramedullary nailing of the femur. Final diagnosis was osteosarcoma. (**c**) Radiograph of the buttock showing that it is now contaminated with tumor (*arrow*), as is the soft-tissue envelope around the femur and the distal femur from medullary instrumentation

Another scenario in which presuming metastatic status can be detrimental is when a patient with pathologic fracture has a history of cancer but now has a new primary cancer. Studies have shown that adult and pediatric cancer survivors are at increased risk of developing a second primary cancer compared with the general population [3, 4]. Failure to perform a biopsy can lead to a delay in diagnosis and can subject the patient to ineffective systemic or local treatment.

If a patient's metastatic status has been documented by previous skeletal or visceral biopsy, a new biopsy is not required. When diagnostic tissue is required, a needle or curettage specimen is preferred as an alternative to reaming. The importance of establishing the correct diagnosis before treatment of a skeletal lesion, whether surgical or nonsurgical, cannot be overstated.

There are instances in which a final diagnosis cannot be rendered in a timely manner. Patients who present with pathologic fractures often require immobilization to obtain the necessary diagnostic work-ups. Figure 21.2a shows a transverse femur fracture of a patient who had experienced a low-energy fall. The history and fracture pattern are representative of a pathologic fracture. The next step in treatment would be to rule out a primary cancer, usually by computed tomography of the chest, abdomen, and pelvis. A frozen section analysis during open biopsy of the fracture does not yield a definitive diagnosis and requires further investigation. In these circumstances, a limited form of fixation such as a short plate provides temporary fracture immobilization and contains contamination (Fig. 21.2b). One cannot be faulted for staging procedures in the face of diagnostic uncertainty.

21.3   Estimating Life Expectancy

Attempts to quantify survival estimates for patients with past and impending pathologic fractures have been rigorously studied [5, 6]. It is clear from the research that prognosis is difficult to predict. Multiple factors have been correlated

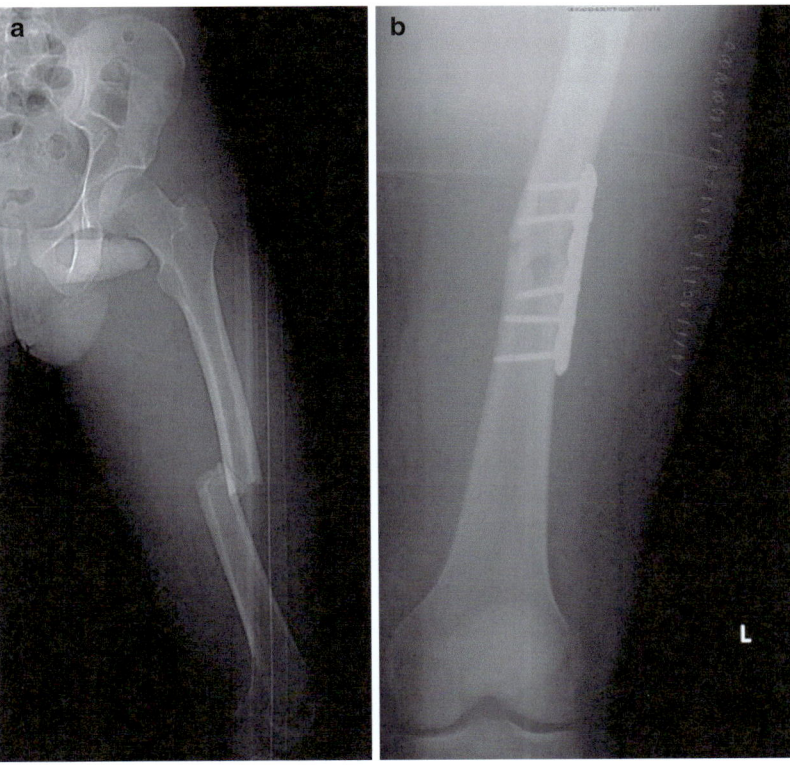

Fig. 21.2 (**a**) Conventional radiograph of a transverse pathologic femur fracture. (**b**) Conventional radiograph showing a short plate that allows for bone stabilization with minimal surrounding contamination until a final diagnosis can be rendered

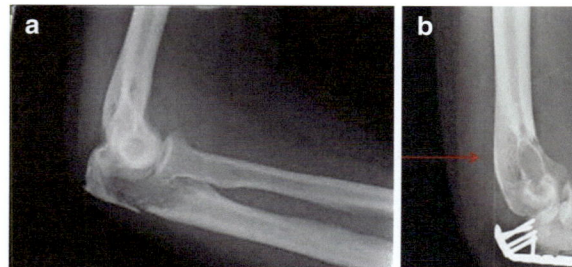
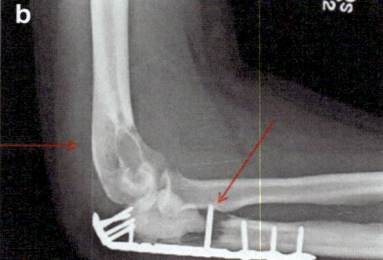
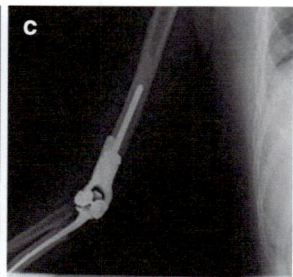

Fig. 21.3 (**a**) Conventional radiograph of a 57-year-old man with a painful proximal ulnar metastasis from thyroid cancer. (**b**) Conventional radiograph of the elbow showing local disease progression (*arrows*) 6 months later requir- ing revision of the implant. (**c**) Conventional radiograph taken 2 years after the original surgery. The patient contin- ues to experience adequate disease control and good function

with life expectancy, including primary diagno- sis, the presence of visceral metastases, hemoglo- bin, age, and performance status [7]. Chapter 4 ("Survival Estimation in Patients with Metastatic Bone Disease") presents a scientific summary of the rationale and efficacy of survival estimation tools. The more accurate the prediction, the more likely the patient's and surgeon's expectations will overlap. Under- and overtreatment are unde- sirable outcomes.

Perhaps the most common treatment dilemma involves the proximal femur, which is the most common site of long bone metastases. Although most surgeons agree that pathologic fractures of the femoral neck are best treated with arthro- plasty, the treatment of peritrochanteric fractures is more controversial [8, 9]. Life expectancy is an important consideration when choosing an implant, which also depends on other factors, including response to systemic therapies. Various factors must be considered when choosing inter- nal fixation for fractures of the proximal femur, including radiosensitivity of the primary disease and surgeon expertise. Patients whose life expec- tancy is short might be best treated with palliative care, including pain management and radiation, rather than surgery. Patients with intermediate life expectancy are likely to benefit from devices that splint the bone such as intramedullary implants or plate-and-screw constructs. Patients with long life expectancy may be best served with implants that replace bone such as arthro- plasty or megaprostheses.

Consider the case of a 57-year-old man with a history of thyroid carcinoma who presents with minimal visceral disease and a proximal ulnar metastasis (Fig. 21.3a). The fracture is treated with internal fixation and cement augmentation. The patient continues to experience good disease control systemically but experiences local dis- ease progression. The device ultimately fails (Fig. 21.3b). A more accurate survival estimation might have guided the surgeon to choose a more durable reconstruction method (Fig. 21.3c).

21.4   Disease-Specific Treatment

Not all bone metastases behave the same. For example, myeloma is radiosensitive, whereas renal cancer is historically radioresistant. Prostate cancer may be hormone sensitive, whereas certain breast cancers may be hormone refractory. Knowledge of biologic behavior of the underlying disease aids physicians in deter- mining how much internal fixation is adequate. This is especially important for cases of periar- ticular disease, in which the choice of implant depends on the expected biologic behavior and perceived treatment sensitivity even during the short term. Consider the lytic lesion in the peritrochanteric or subtrochanteric femur shown in Fig. 21.4a. The implant choice depends on the biologic behavior of the primary cancer and its sensitivity to available adjuvant treatment. If the lesion represented is a plasmocytoma (myeloma),

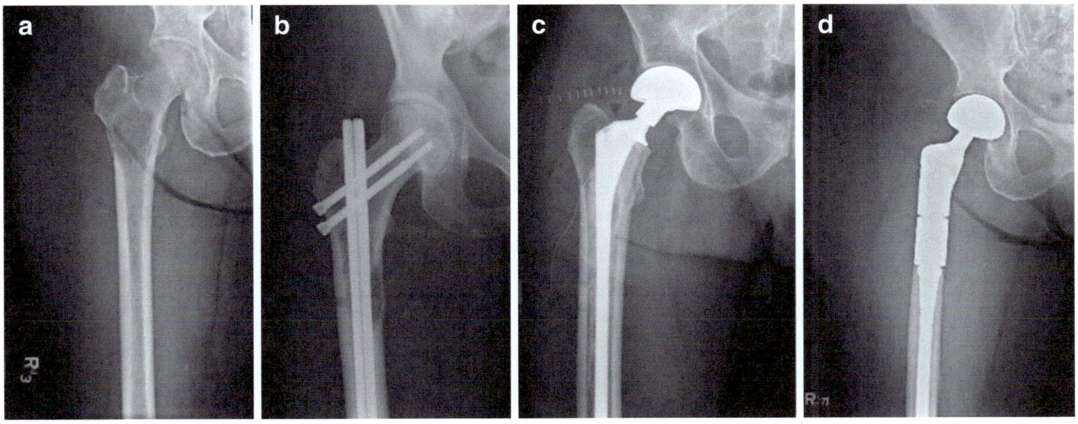

Fig. 21.4 (**a**) Conventional radiograph of the proximal femur showing a lytic lesion in the proximal femur at risk for pathologic fracture. (**b**) Treatment of a proximal femur lesion with a cephalomedullary nail as might be performed for myeloma. (**c**) Treatment of an impending pathologic proximal femur fracture with long-stemmed cemented hemiarthroplasty as might be performed for metastatic breast cancer. (**d**) Excision and reconstruction of a proximal femur metastasis as might be performed for metastatic renal cancer

a cephalomedullary nail is an excellent fixation choice (Fig. 21.4b). The procedure is moderately invasive with predictable outcomes, and long-term survival of the implant is likely given to the radiosensitivity of the tumor. If the disease is breast cancer, a hemiarthroplasty might be considered (Fig. 21.4c) because bone regeneration is less certain and radiosensitivity varies. If the primary diagnosis is renal cancer, resection and proximal femur replacement should be considered (Fig. 21.4d). Renal cancer is often radioresistant, and systemic treatment has had a tremendously positive effect on life expectancy. This tenet holds true throughout the skeleton (e.g., proximal humerus, distal femur, proximal tibia). For lesions with uncertain biologic behavior or when the treating surgeon lacks megaprosthetic expertise, steps can be taken to increase the longevity of the internal fixation device through the liberal use of adjuvants (e.g., liquid nitrogen, argon beam coagulation) and cement augmentation. These supplements are also beneficial for anatomic locations such as the distal tibia, in which reconstruction options are limited.

Renal cancer and melanoma deserve special mention. Many new systemic treatment options for these diseases have had considerable success at increasing life expectancy, which has resulted in an increase not only in the number of patients with metastases but also in the number of patients experiencing mechanical failure of fixation devices. Laitinen et al. [10] reported on 253 patients who underwent surgery for renal cell carcinoma metastasis to bone. A significant proportion (55%) had bone as the only site of distant disease, and 39% had a solitary skeletal metastasis. The risk of surgical failure was greatest in those treated with internal fixation and radiation. When implant failure occurred in this group, the incidence of amputation was high. The authors concluded that, when reasonable, resection and endoprosthetic replacement should be considered. Lin et al. [11] reported on 295 patients with oligometastatic disease in renal cell carcinoma. Although they could not prove a survival advantage of wide excision compared with intralesional curettage, they noted that local control was more challenging in the patients who were treated intralesionally. A similar finding has been noted in metastatic melanoma. Krygier et al. [12] reported on 37 patients with metastatic melanoma to bone. The osseous metastases in this series were locally aggressive with high local recurrence in patients treated with internal fixation and radiation. Two patients ultimately required amputation for symptomatic disease control. Metastasectomy with reconstruction appears to offer superior disease control in some patients with metastatic renal cancer or melanoma to bone. Although the rehabilitation after reconstruction for metastasectomy may be prolonged, the long-term benefits appear to be favorable. Appropriate patient selection is critical to successful outcomes.

Finally, recent advancements in the systemic treatment of renal cancer have incorporated vascular endothelial growth factor inhibitors as frontline treatment. These humanized monoclonal antibodies selectively bind vascular endothelial growth factor receptors, thereby inhibiting tumor growth by preventing endothelial cells from creating vascular channels. Although these antiangiogenic effects are desirable for tumor control, they have potential negative effects on wound healing. The first-generation compounds required patients to cease treatment for weeks. Current research is contradictory regarding the timing of surgery in patients taking these medications [13]. When treating patients who are taking these antiangiogenic agents (or any systemic agent that may compromise wound healing), the timing of surgery must be considered carefully. In some instances, it may be beneficial to pre-emptively treat bones at risk before initiating lengthy treatment courses to avoid a break in systemic therapy or postoperative wound complications.

21.5 Operative Considerations

21.5.1 Adequate Fixation

There is a delicate balance between under- and overtreating osseous metastases. The goal is to provide a durable construct that allows immediate weight-bearing and that will last the patient's lifetime while requiring minimal postoperative rehabilitation. "One bone, one operation" is a common mantra for surgeons who treat skeletal metastases. When planning reconstructions, physicians should consider the likelihood of disease progression and unlikely fracture healing (Fig. 21.4a–d). For example, a 65-year-old man has a symptomatic acetabular lesion from metastatic prostate cancer as seen in Fig. 21.5a. The

patient was treated with cemented total hip arthroplasty (Fig. 21.5b). His disease progressed, leading to failure of the acetabular component (Fig. 21.5c). Anticipation of disease progression would likely have directed alternative acetabular fixation such as a protrusion cage or rebar construct (Fig. 21.5d), thereby transferring the force of weight-bearing to intact areas of the bone [14, 15].

The proximal femur is a common site of instrumentation failure after treatment for metastatic disease, with 50% of lesions occurring in the femoral neck, 30% in the subtrochanteric area, and 20% in the intertrochanteric area [16]. For peritrochanteric lesions, internal fixation devices are likely to fail in the setting of disease progression (Fig. 21.6). Revision of failed internal fixation devices is challenging. Steensma et al. [17] reported on 298 patients with metastatic disease to the proximal femur treated with nailing or endoprosthetic reconstruction. The endoprosthetic group experienced fewer implant failures and revisions compared with the group treated with nailing or internal fixation. When internal fixation is chosen instead of endoprosthetic reconstruction, curettage of disease before nail placement and debulking of associated soft-tissue masses can increase implant longevity [18]. Augmentation with cement to bridge cortical defects that are unlikely to heal also improves implant durability. Patients in whom the disease cannot be resected completely should be evaluated by a radiation oncologist. The addition of postoperative radiation is associated with a decreased rate of revision surgery [19].

21.5.2 Bone Cement Implantation Syndrome

Long-stemmed femoral components commonly used for treating metastatic disease in the femur have drawbacks. Intraoperative cardiopulmonary complications secondary to the systemic effects of cement have been well-described. Bone cement implantation syndrome (BCIS) describes a complex of sudden physiologic changes that occur within seconds to minutes of cement

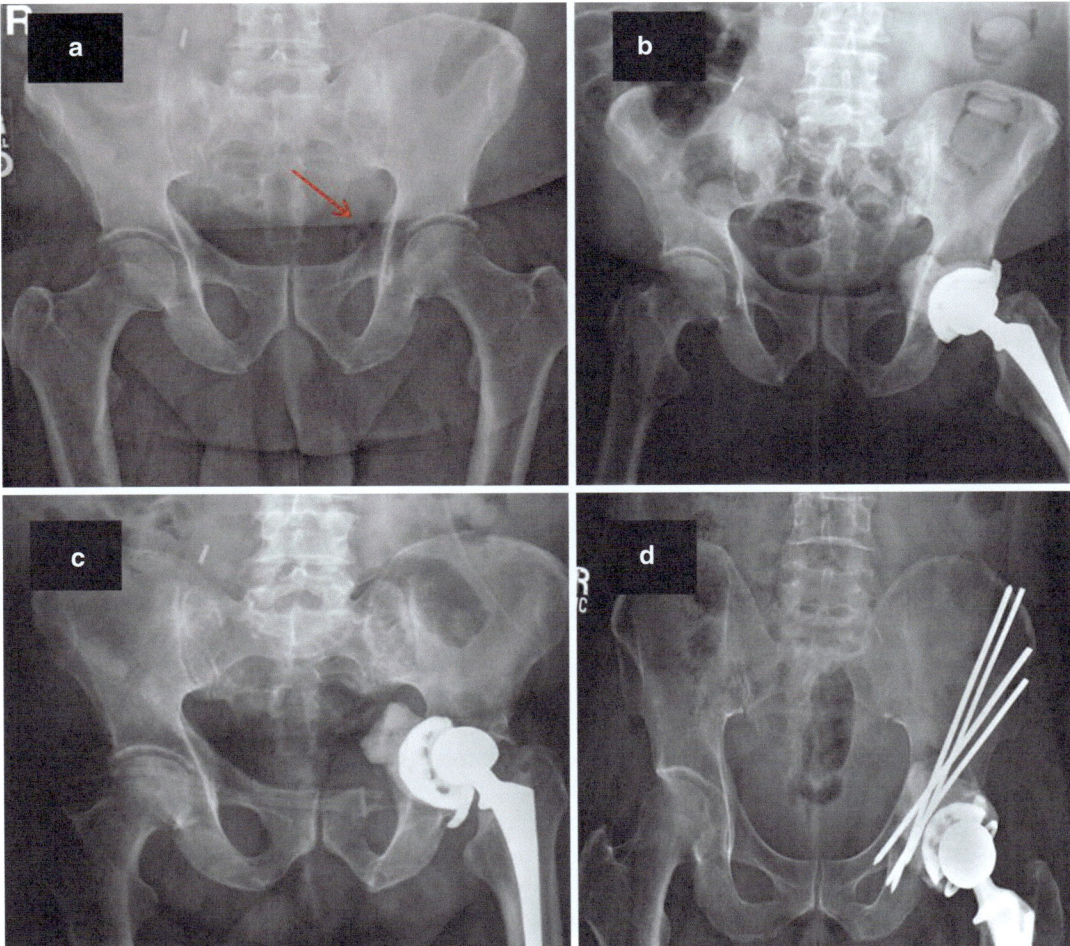

Fig. 21.5 (**a**) Conventional radiograph of the pelvis in a 65-year-old man with metastatic prostate cancer. The *arrow* indicates a symptomatic lytic lesion in the acetabulum. (**b**) The patient has undergone reconstruction with a cemented total hip replacement. (**c**) The acetabular component ultimately fails. (**d**) Revision to a more durable construct allows for immediate, full weight-bearing and is designed to last the patient's lifetime

implantation: polymerization of cement leads to intramedullary hypertension; residual monomer acts as a vasodilator; fat, marrow elements, and cement particles are pushed into the circulation; and the complement system is activated. These actions lead to hemodynamic instability, which can lead to hypotension, hypoxia, bronchoconstriction, arrhythmia, and ultimately death. Patterson et al. [20] described 7 cases of BCIS. In their series, four patients died during surgery. The authors associated BCIS with long-stemmed implants and the use of >2 bags of cement. Xing et al. [21] questioned whether long-stemmed implants were necessary for the treatment of proximal femur metastases. In their series of 203 patients, revision rates were the same for short-stemmed and long-stemmed (>25 cm) components. Patients in the long-stemmed group experienced twice as many cardiopulmonary complications, including death. This led the group to suggest that the benefits of long femoral stems did not outweigh the risks associated with their use. When using long-stemmed femoral components, precautions can minimize the burden of embolic complications. Before cementing, communication with the anesthesia team is

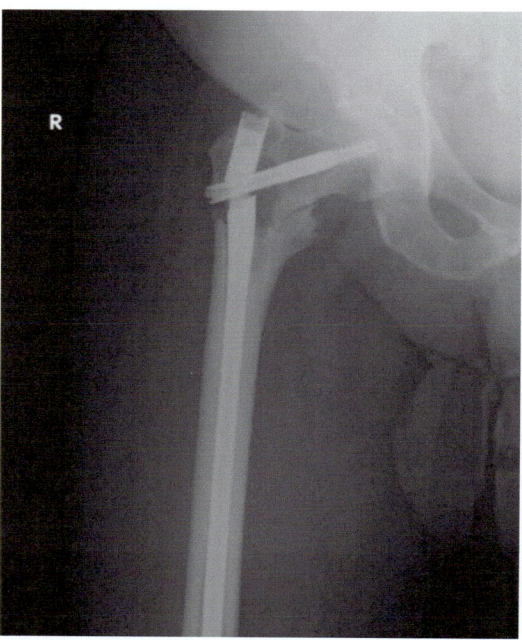

Fig. 21.6 Radiograph of the proximal femur showing implant fracture in the setting of metastatic lung cancer

paramount. Volume repletion with blood products should be performed such that the systolic blood pressure is adequate to withstand a sudden hypotensive episode. Because emboli affect the ability to oxygenate by blocking blood flow and gas exchange in the lungs, increasing the percentage of inhaled oxygen allows for a margin of safety if an embolism occurs. Placement of a vent hole within the femoral diaphysis, using, for example, a one-fourth-inch drill bit, has been described to decrease the embolic load. Collectively, these measures appear to decrease the severity of BCIS and the associated rate of deaths. Patients with severe underlying pulmonary disease are likely best treated with shorter stems or with noncemented components.

21.5.3 Beware of Other Bones at Risk

Patients with metastatic disease often have more than one long bone at risk of fracture. A physical survey of all long bones should be undertaken during the preoperative evaluation. Limbs for which the patient reports a history of discomfort or those that are painful to palpation on physical examination should be evaluated with conventional radiographs. Even mild patient-reported discomfort warrants additional attention with at least a thorough physical examination because patients with advanced cancer are often taking narcotic medications that may mask a pathologic process. When additional sites of clinically relevant disease are located, the surgeon must decide whether surgery would be beneficial. Consideration of the rehabilitation plan influences the decision. For example, a patient with an impending hip fracture will need to bear weight through the upper extremities during rehabilitation. If the patient has a humeral lesion at risk of fracture, consideration should be given to fixing the humerus prophylactically to maximize the lower extremity mobility goals and prevent a subsequent pathologic fracture. In addition, the entire surgical team needs to be cognizant of other bones at risk of fracture to prevent inadvertent injury during patient positioning and other preparation activities.

Moon et al. [22] reported their experience of simultaneous nailing of two or more pathologic fractures during a single surgical encounter. Two of 16 patients experienced a fatal cardiopulmonary complication. The authors concluded that the risk of simultaneous nailing was no greater than that of unilateral nailing. Patient selection remains crucial to achieve acceptable morbidity profiles.

21.6 Summary

Although the surgical principles of treating skeletal metastases are often straightforward, incorporating all the nuances of treatment takes considerable thought. Always biopsy the first metastasis when metastatic status has not been confirmed. With the number of prediction tools available, genuine attempts should be made to predict life expectancy. Consider disease biology in surgical planning because it will guide the most appropriate implant choice. Finally, expect the unexpected in the operating room. Be prepared to change quickly from plan A to plan B or C.

References

1. Rougraff BT. Evaluation of the patient with carcinoma of unknown origin metastatic to bone. Clin Orthop. 2003;415(Suppl):S105–9. https://doi.org/10.1097/01.blo.0000093049.96273.e3.

2. Adams SC, Potter BK, Mahmood Z, Pitcher JD, Temple HT. Consequences and prevention of inadvertent internal fixation of primary osseous sarcomas. Clin Orthop. 2009;467(2):519–25. https://doi.org/10.1007/s11999-008-0546-3.

3. Kebudi R, Ozdemir GN. Secondary neoplasms in children treated for cancer. Curr Pediatr Rev. 2017;13:34–41. PMID: 27848891.

4. Moitry M, Velten M, Tretarre B, Bara S, Daubisse-Marliac L, Lapotre-Ledoux B, et al. Development of a model to predict the 10-year cumulative risk of second primary cancer among cancer survivors. Cancer Epidemiol. 2017;47:35–41. https://doi.org/10.1016/j.canep.2017.01.001.

5. Forsberg JA, Eberhardt J, Boland PJ, Wedin R, Healey JH. Estimating survival in patients with operable skeletal metastases: an application of a Bayesian belief network. PLoS One. 2011;6(5):e19956. https://doi.org/10.1371/journal.pone.0019956.

6. Piccioli A, Spinelli MS, Forsberg JA, Wedin R, Healey JH, Ippolito V, et al. How do we estimate survival? External validation of a tool for survival estimation in patients with metastatic bone disease-decision analysis and comparison of three international patient populations. BMC Cancer. 2015;15:424. https://doi.org/10.1186/s12885-015-1396-5.

7. Nathan SS, Healey JH, Mellano D, Hoang B, Lewis I, Morris CD, et al. Survival in patients operated on for pathologic fracture: implications for end-of-life orthopedic care. J Clin Oncol. 2005;23(25):6072–82. https://doi.org/10.1200/jco.2005.08.104.

8. Issack PS, Barker J, Baker M, Kotwal SY, Lane JM. Surgical management of metastatic disease of the proximal part of the femur. J Bone Joint Surg Am. 2014;96(24):2091–8. https://doi.org/10.2106/jbjs.n.00083.

9. Steensma M, Healey JH. Trends in the surgical treatment of pathologic proximal femur fractures among Musculoskeletal Tumor Society members. Clin Orthop. 2013;471(6):2000–6. https://doi.org/10.1007/s11999-012-2724-6.

10. Laitinen M, Parry M, Ratasvuori M, Wedin R, Albergo JI, Jeys L, et al. Survival and complications of skeletal reconstructions after surgical treatment of bony metastatic renal cell carcinoma. Eur J Surg Oncol. 2015;41(7):886–92. https://doi.org/10.1016/j.ejso.2015.04.008.

11. Lin PP, Mirza AN, Lewis VO, Cannon CP, Tu SM, Tannir NM, et al. Patient survival after surgery for osseous metastases from renal cell carcinoma. J Bone Joint Surg Am. 2007;89(8):1794–801. https://doi.org/10.2106/jbjs.f.00603.

12. Krygier JE, Lewis VO, Cannon CP, Satcher RL, Moon BS, Lin PP. Operative management of metastatic melanoma in bone may require en bloc resection of disease. Clin Orthop. 2014;472(10):3196–203. https://doi.org/10.1007/s11999-014-3761-0.

13. Sharma K, Marcus JR. Bevacizumab and wound-healing complications: mechanisms of action, clinical evidence, and management recommendations for the plastic surgeon. Ann Plast Surg. 2013;71(4):434–40. https://doi.org/10.1097/SAP.0b013e31824e5e57.

14. Marco RA, Sheth DS, Boland PJ, Wunder JS, Siegel JA, Healey JH. Functional and oncological outcome of acetabular reconstruction for the treatment of metastatic disease. J Bone Joint Surg Am. 2000;82(5):642–51.

15. Tsagozis P, Wedin R, Brosjo O, Bauer H. Reconstruction of metastatic acetabular defects using a modified Harrington procedure. Acta Orthop. 2015;86(6):690–4. https://doi.org/10.3109/17453674.2015.1077308.

16. Sim FH. Metastatic bone disease of the pelvis and femur. Instr Course Lect. 1992;41:317–27.

17. Steensma M, Boland PJ, Morris CD, Athanasian E, Healey JH. Endoprosthetic treatment is more durable for pathologic proximal femur fractures. Clin Orthop. 2012;470(3):920–6. https://doi.org/10.1007/s11999-011-2047-z.

18. Jacofsky DJ, Haidukewych GJ. Management of pathologic fractures of the proximal femur: state of the art. J Orthop Trauma. 2004;18(7):459–69.

19. Townsend PW, Smalley SR, Cozad SC, Rosenthal HG, Hassanein RE. Role of postoperative radiation therapy after stabilization of fractures caused by metastatic disease. Int J Radiat Oncol Biol Phys. 1995;31(1):43–9. https://doi.org/10.1016/0360-3016(94)e0310-g.

20. Patterson BM, Healey JH, Cornell CN, Sharrock NE. Cardiac arrest during hip arthroplasty with a cemented long-stem component. A report of seven cases. J Bone Joint Surg Am. 1991;73(2):271–7.

21. Xing Z, Moon BS, Satcher RL, Lin PP, Lewis VO. A long femoral stem is not always required in hip arthroplasty for patients with proximal femur metastases. Clin Orthop. 2013;471(5):1622–7. https://doi.org/10.1007/s11999-013-2790-4.

22. Moon B, Lin P, Satcher R, Lewis V. Simultaneous nailing of skeletal metastases: is the mortality really that high? Clin Orthop. 2011;469(8):2367–70. https://doi.org/10.1007/s11999-011-1814-1.

Rehabilitation of Patients with Bone Metastatic Disease

22

Sandra Miccinilli, Federica Bressi, Marco Bravi, and Silvia Sterzi

Abstract

Treatment of patients affected by bone metastases requires a multidisciplinary team of different specialists. Rehabilitation medicine works beside oncology, radiotherapy, orthopedics, and palliative care to reduce the impact of this pathology on patients' quality of life. Medical evidence shows that, even if rest prevents the occurrence of fractures in bone metastatic patients, rehabilitation seems to be effective in providing pain relief, preventing joint degeneration, increasing survival, and therefore reducing the occurrence of disuse syndrome in cancer patients. This condition, in fact, increases the risk of death and complications, such as muscle contractures, weakness and atrophy, osteoporosis, orthostatic hypotension, pressure sores, pneumonia, confusion and disorientation, and increased risk of thromboembolic disease. Rehabilitative interventions do not differ from rehabilitative treatments for patients affected by disabilities caused by other pathologies; however, they will depend on the subjects' general health conditions, on the site of the metastases, and on the involvement of other organs. In all cases, the ultimate goal for the patient will be the achievement of the highest possible functional status within the limits of the disease.

Keywords

Rehabilitation · Bone metastases · Cancer

22.1 Introduction

The increased survivorship of patients affected by cancer due to the development of more effective therapies has raised interest toward rehabilitation in this field. Rehabilitation improves the quality of life of patients affected by advanced cancer, aims to achieving the highest possible functional status within the condition of the disease, and is directed toward the limiting of the disability due to neoplasms and related therapies. Patients affected by advanced cancer need a multidisciplinary approach and several professional figures involved in relation to the stage of the disease and to the patients' specific issues. The identification of methods of intervention and of different roles of the various characters, and their integration in a team, can provide effective responses to the needs of patients. The clinical pathway of patients affected by cancer, in fact, is an exclusive model

S. Miccinilli · F. Bressi · M. Bravi · S. Sterzi (✉)
Department of Physical and Rehabilitation Medicine,
University Campus Bio-Medico of Rome,
Rome, Italy
e-mail: s.sterzi@unicampus.it

of interaction between neoplastic disease and various kinds of disabilities, often characterized by chronicity. Many patients, even in the case of being healed from tumor, often do not show complete recovery of functions. Rehabilitative treatments are variable and depend on cancer typology, location, aggressiveness and staging, on the patients' age, on their comorbidities, and on cultural, social, or family environment; therefore, these require a highly customized plan which needs to be frequently updated. Disabilities in cancer patients can be organ-specific (related to the localization of the primary tumor and to its surgical exeresis) or common to all kinds of tumors (due to iatrogenic causes or to the progression of the disease). The rehabilitation project is elaborated on the basis of the evaluation of the clinical and functional overall picture, by defining intervention strategies, objectives of autonomy, and quality of life, selecting and giving priority to the rehabilitation of patients at increased risk of functional damage, and limiting permanent damage and the resulting health and social consequences.

22.2 Cancer Rehabilitation

The different stages of the neoplastic disease are responsible for different gradients of clinical stability and autonomy. Rehabilitation can take place, therefore, in different care settings at the time of diagnosis, staging, treatment, recurrence, and palliative phase. In all phases of the therapeutic process, rehabilitative medicine is able to diversify the settings to ensure appropriate treatments. Flexibility of rehabilitation is necessary in this field, since cancer patients rarely present conditions of stability, and the changes in the clinical status impose continuous revision of the rehabilitative interventions in relation to the new

disabilities. The American Cancer Society distinguishes five stages of symptoms and functional disabilities according to the stage of cancer.

Stage IV and V are characterized by the presence of bone metastases. In these stages, we can also recognize other sub-phases, as described in Fig. 22.1. Each one is characterized by different disabilities, clinical evaluations, rehabilitative programs, and settings.

However, is rehabilitation always recommended in bone metastatic patients? Shibata et al. in 2016 [1], in a guideline for the diagnosis and treatment of bone metastases, analyze the medical evidence from meta-analyses, randomized controlled trials published from 2003 to 2013, and a guideline developed in Japan in 2014, according to the Medical Information Network Distribution Service Handbook for Clinical Practice Guideline Development. This analysis reveals that it is not strongly suggested that rehabilitation improves ADL and quality of life and that it prevents disuse syndrome in bone metastatic subjects. Conversely, rehabilitation seems to be effective in providing pain relief, preventing degeneration, and increasing survival [1]. In spite of these considerations, it is generally accepted, however, that even if bed rest prevents skeletal fractures, it also reduces autonomy and quality of life, resulting in disuse syndrome. This condition increases the risk of death and complications, such as muscle contractures, weakness and atrophy, osteoporosis, orthostatic hypotension, pressure sores, pneumonia, confusion and disorientation, and thromboembolic disease [1, 2]. If an accurate evaluation of risks and benefits assesses that no major contraindications to rehabilitation treatment are present, it might then be preferable to make the rehabilitation treatment to prevent hypomobility complications rather than forcing the patient to rest.

Phase	Disability	Evaluation	Rehabilitative programs	Setting	Activity limitation
Onset symptoms	✓ Pain ✓ Distrectual ipomobility ✓ Reduction of distrectual range of movement ✓ Fatigue	Clinical scales (VAS, brief pain inventory, brief fatigue Inventory, Barthel index, ECOG, EORTC, SF12), clinical evaluation (manual testing of strength, sensibility, and range of motion)	Pharmacologic therapy Physical therapy Occupational therapy Orthoses and aids prescription	DH Outpatient clinic Patients' domicile	ADL, IADL, self-care, familiar, social and job activities
Treatment (radiotherapy, surgery chemotherapy)	✓ Pain ✓ Distrectual Ipomobility ✓ Reduction of distrectual range of movement ✓ Respiratory failure ✓ Para- or tetra-paresis/plegia ✓ Neuropathies ✓ Post-actinic fibrosis ✓ Fatigue	Clinical scales (VAS, brief pain inventory, brief fatigue inventory, Barthel Index, ECOG, EORTC, SF12, borg, Ashworth, SCIM, Tinetti Scale, borg, 6MWT), clinical evaluation (manual testing of strength, sensibility, and range of motion)	Pharmacologic therapy Physical therapy Exercises for range of motion recovery Respiratory exercises Balance and coordination exercises Postural rehabilitation Occupational therapy Orthoses and aids prescription Education of the patient	Intensive post-acute rehabilitation DH Outpatient clinic Patients' domicile	ADL, IADL, self-care, familiar, social and job activities
Post-treatment	✓ Pain ✓ Distrectual Ipomobility ✓ Reduction of distrectual range of movement ✓ Respiratory failure ✓ Para- or tetra-paresis/plegia ✓ Neuropathies ✓ Post-actinic fibrosis ✓ Fatigue	Clinical scales (VAS, brief pain inventory, brief fatigue inventory, Barthel Index, ECOG, EORTC, SF12, Ashworth, SCIM, Tinetti, Borg, 6MWT, Barthel Index, ECOG, EORTC, SF12), clinical evaluation (manual testing of strength, sensibility, and range of motion), respiratory performance tests	Re-education to postural transfers Exercises for range of motion recovery Balance and coordination exercises Postural rehabilitation Orthoses and aids prescription Reconditioning exercises Education of the patient	DH Outpatient clinic Long-term care structures Patients' domicile	ADL, IADL, self-care, familiar, social and job activities
Terminal	✓ Pain ✓ Distrectual ipomobility ✓ Reduction of distrectual range of movement ✓ Respiratory failure ✓ Scare retractions ✓ Neuropathies ✓ Post actinic ✓ Fatigue ✓ Ipomobility	Clinical scales (VAS, brief pain inventory, brief fatigue inventory, Barthel, ECOG), clinical evaluation (manual testing of strength, sensibility, and range of motion)	Pharmacologic therapy Respiratory exercises Drainage Massotherapy Relaxation techniques Education to postural transfers Prevention of damages due to ipomobility	Hospice Patients' domicile	ADL, IADL, self-care, familiar, social and job activities

Fig. 22.1 Rehabilitative treatment in patients affected by disability due to neoplastic disease, Working Group on Rehabilitation, Italian Ministry of Health, Prof.ssa Silvia Sterzi, Campus Bio-Medico University of Rome

22.3 Rehabilitation in Bone Metastases

To draft a rehabilitative program, a correct clinical evaluation should be done. Bone metastatic patients assessment requires particular attention, since the manual testings could be detrimental. To prevent pathologic fractures, the examinator should elicit only active movements, which should be limited by the evocation of pain. Resistive exercise involving an affected area is generally contraindicated. The presence of rib metastases should be ascertained before starting physical examination of the thorax [2]. Rehabilitative programs should reduce hypomobility, improve deconditioning and osteopenia, prevent joint limitations, and increase autonomy by educating the patient to the usage of assistive devices. Bone metastases are usually distinguished into vertebral metastases and long bone metastases. This distinction is important since there are different rehabilitative issues depending on the site of the disease.

22.4 Vertebral Metastases

Bone metastases are mainly localized in the vertebral column [3]. Since this structure is the main support for our body, its integrity is of crucial importance. The principal concern with vertebral metastases is therefore the risk of fracture and the possible involvement of the spinal cord. Once the nature of the lesion and the possible involvement of the spinal cord are ascertained, a multidisciplinary evaluation of oncologists, radiotherapists, and orthopedics is needed to define which therapeutic treatment is more appropriate. According to the guidelines of Italian Association of Medical Oncology (AIOM) of 2015, radiation therapy is required in the following situations: when cancer is radiosensitive or moderately responsive to radiotherapy in patients with minimal or no neurologic deficits, when there is an epidural isolated compression, when pain is confined, when life expectancy is of less than 3 months, when the patient cannot undergo surgery, or, in the worst case, when the neurologic injury is no more reversible. Conversely, surgery aims to ensure the

local control of the disease consistent in remission of painful symptoms, prevention of deterioration of neurological function, and possible improvement and stabilization of the column. It is the only possible treatment in case of lesions resistant to radiotherapy or chemotherapy; otherwise, it can be used in association with radiotherapy treatments. Surgery of vertebral metastases can be classified as palliative therapy, adjuvant, or excisional and can be performed by anterior, posterior, or combined technique [4]. The guidelines of AIOM of 2015 also suggest the use of surgery in case of bone fragments causing neural compression, spinal deformities causing pain or neurologic compression, spinal instability, progressive neurologic deficit, no radiotherapy response, and unknown primary tumor. Rehabilitation treatment will be different depending on the presence of stable and unstable lesions and in case of involvement of the spinal cord. Common objectives of the rehabilitative program are pain control, prevention of secondary hypomobility damages, maintenance of articular range of movement of immobilized segments, practice of neuromuscular facilitation techniques, hypertone prevention or inhibition, optimization of residual functions and development of compensatory strategies, training for the management of sphincter functions, and training for the autonomous management of activities of daily living and for the management of aid and orthoses [5].

Clinical manifestation of vertebral bone metastases are common to those of other spine disorders (e.g., pain at rest, pain during movement, sensory-motor deficits, paraplegia, tetraplegia, cauda equina syndrome, sphincter disorders, spasticity, pressure sores, joint contractures, etc.). Neurologic deficits can present insidiously or acutely, according to the growth speed, location, and appearance of pathologic fractures. Low progression deficits are more frequent in lumbar-sacral tumors involving cauda equina, whereas thoracic tumors can cause sudden vertebral fractures with direct compression signs or medullary ischemia. Thoracic metastases are almost the 70% of all spine compressions causing paraplegia. As for frequency, 60% of patients present with thoracic metastases, 30% of patients present with lumbar-sacral metastases, and 10% with cervical metastases [6].

A correct initial assessment of neurological level and of completeness of the lesion and of consequent impairments is therefore needed. Administration of clinical scales, such as American Spinal Injury Association (ASIA) Impairment Scale, Spinal Cord Injury Measure (SCIM), Barthel Index (BI) for activities of daily independence, Rivermead Mobility Index (RMI), Walking Index for Spinal Cord Injury (WISCI), etc., helps clinicians with the definition of the main domains of intervention.

The rehabilitative treatment of patients affected by vertebral metastases will be the same adopted for vertebral fractures and for spinal cord injuries. Rehabilitation treatment of patients without spinal cord involvement will aim to pain relief, maintenance of muscle tropism and articular functions, education to the proper management of the spine, education to the proper transfer activities (e.g., from supine to sitting position, from sitting to standing position, from standing position to the toilet, etc.), ambulatory training when needed, education to the use of aids and orthoses, reinforcement of abdominal muscles and of the stabilizing muscles of the spine, and improvement of proprioception, coordination, and balance. Spinal cord involvement can lead to different clinical presentations: involvement of a single limb, paraplegia, tetraplegia, cauda equina syndrome, conus medullaris syndrome, with loss of movement, loss of sensitivity, loss of vasomotor control, loss of voluntary control of bladder and bowel, and loss of sexual functionality. Pain, pressure sores, deep vein thrombosis, pulmonary embolism, heterotopic ossification, spasticity, joint contractures, vasomotor, urological, and bowel and respiratory problems are the most common complications for these patients. Such variability requests rehabilitative programs which need to be tailored on each patient. Rehabilitation program is systematically reviewed on the basis of clinical conditions and disease phases.

Unstable lesions with no surgical treatment indication or in patients in bad clinical conditions who could not undergo surgery need spinal orthoses to be stabilized. Orthoses typology choice vary according to the grade of the instability, to the function of the orthoses (kinetic immobilization, immobilization and static support, immobilization and support associated with distraction) and to the vertebral level (cervical, dorsal, or lumbar). Cervical unstable lesions necessarily request orthoses for the elevated risk of spinal involvement (e.g., Halo Jacket, SOMI Brace, etc.) and can be integrated with an halo except in the case of concomitant skull metastases. The use of cervical-thoracic orthoses is recommended in case of more stable lesions (e.g., Philadelphia collar with sternal support or SOMI Brace without halo). Semirigid collars, such as Schanz Collar, are suggested, instead, in case of cervical contractures in patients with small stable lesions. As for dorsal and lumbar metastases C35 orthoses can be used in case of stable small lesions. Dorsal and lumbar unstable lesions, instead, require tailored plastic orthoses with distal iliac or acromial support (e.g., Cheneau/antigravity corset). In cases of elevated instability or in patients with multiple lesions, tailored plastic orthoses with both occipitocervical and iliac distal support are needed [5].

22.5 Long Bone Metastases

Long bone metastases are less frequent than vertebral metastases; however, there is an elevated risk of pathological fracture, and, in case this event occurs, patients can experience a sudden loss of function and disability. Treatment strategy for the management of metastatic limbs depends on biological and biomechanical characteristics of the lesions, which can be distinguished into four classes, described in Table 22.1.

Treatment of long bone metastases is usually surgical and varies from osteosynthesis to endoprostheses or tumor endoprostheses. It aims to relief pain and restore the patient lost function. The choice of surgery technique should consider patient's life expectancy, should save as much tissue as possible (within the limits of disease extent), should preserve limb function, and should influence recovery prognosis and rehabilitation programs. Recent studies show that modu-

Table 22.1 Differentiation in classes of bone metastases patients according to Capanna and Campanacci [7]

	Phase of cancer	Patient needs	Symptoms	Impact of symptoms on functions
I	Pre-treatment and evaluation	Information about treatment, options and impact of illness	Pain Anxiety Depression	Daily routines Sleep/Fatigue
II	Treatment	Information Support Rehabilitation interventions Help with daily routines Vocational, home, etc...	Pain Anxiety Loss of mobility Wound/skin care Speech/Swallowing	Daily routines Sleep/Stamina Self-care Cosmesis Communication
III	Post-treatment	Support, Rehabilitation intervention	Pain/Weakness Anxiety/Depression Loss of mobility Edema Fatigue/Stamina	Sleep/Fatigue ADL Vocational/Avocational Cosmesis
IV	Recurrence	Education Support Rehabilitation intervention	Pain/Weakness Anxiety/Depression Fatigue/Stamina Edema Anorexia Bone instability	Sleep/Fatigue Disability Disruptions of routines Cosmesis Vocational/Avocational
V	End of life	Education Support Palliative Rehabilitation	Pain Fatigue Anorexia	Dependence Immobility

lar tumor endoprosthesis, which requires tumor resection, is also associated with an increased survival, whereas osteosynthesis is associated with incomplete pain relief and with increased risk of local progression of tumor [8]. An impending fracture could also require a surgical treatment. There are definite limitations in the clinical ability to predict which lesions are at risk of fracture, whether the system used to identify them is based on the size or the percentage of erosion of the cortex. Criteria for definition of impending fractures are osteolytic lesion of the cortex >2.5 cm large; dysruption of cortex of ≥50% of the diameter; persistent pain or progression after radiotherapy or chemotherapy; >30 mm of axial cortex; and >50% of circumferential extension. It is generally accepted that wide resection and reconstruction are indicated in case of good prognosis, whereas rigid internal osteosynthesis and radiotherapy are suggested in case of poor prognosis. In particular prosthesis is indicated for femoral head or neck fractures and in solitary metastases with a good prognosis, whereas intramedullary nailing is locked for metadiaphyseal and diaphyseal fractures in patients with cancer in advanced stage.

Main concerns with prosthesis are immediate stability, good fixation, high mechanical strength, fast mobilization and loading, implant survival 10 years >80%, early mobilization, early load, early recovery of ADL and IADL, and maintenance of the best possible QoL [9].

Upper limb metastases mainly interest humerus, whereas pathologic fractures in the distal humerus are uncommon [10–13]. Humeral metastases can be distinguished into type I (proximal humerus), type II (humeral diaphysis), and type III (distal humerus). Prosthesis in humerus metastases is more functional than osteosynthesis and is indicated in lesion with large osteolysis, whereas reverse prosthesis is indicated in rotator cuff-deficient patient. Results are dependent from rotator cuff functionality, deltoid preservation, and patient's endurance, strength, and participation in rehabilitation. Type I metastases can be treated with cemented prosthesis which allow the attachment of rotator cuff tendons to the prosthetic head, whereas in type II metastases, a nail is introduced in the tumor cavity, which is filled with cement. Nail stability is reinforced either with interlocking screws or with a side plate. In case of intercalary resection, cement is used for bone filling. In order to cover the humeral diaphysis, the deltoid and brachialis muscles are sutured over the bone. Rehabilitative program in type I and type II metastases should consider the necessary initial immobilization of the arm in a sling for 3 weeks, during which the physiotherapist should work on the maintenance of the range of motion of the elbow, wrist, and fingers. After sling removal, gradual passive and active mobilization in flexion and abduction of the shoulder is started. In case of bone curettage only, arm mobilization should not be delayed after drainage tubes removal. Type III metastases, which involve humeral condyles, are generally treated with curettage, intramedullary rod, and cement reconstruction. Only in rare cases of massive destruction of the distal humerus, endoprosthetic reconstruction is performed. Passive and active mobilization of the elbow is started after drainage tubes removal [14–16].

Proximal femur metastases can be treated either with tumor removal by curettage and osteosynthesis (introduction of an intramedullary nail and cement filling or introduction of a side plate and a sliding screw) or with osteotomy below the lower border of the tumor and cemented tumor prosthesis placement. The abductor tendon is joined laterally to the prosthesis, whereas psoas muscle is attached medially. When a proximal femur resection is done, the gluteus medius muscle is detached and reflected from its insertion site at the greater trochanter muscle. Drainage tubes are left for 3–5 days. In case of tumor curettage, rehabilitation should include early mobilization of the hip joint for range of motion recovery and early ambulation with free weight-bearing. In case of endoprosthetic reconstruction, the extremity is kept in suspension for 5 days, and subsequently mobilization is started. Finally, in case of total hip replacement, the same precautions adopted for usual prostheses are adopted, even though an abduction brace and weight-bearing as tolerated can be continued for 6 weeks. Up to 3 months, in order to prevent hip prosthesis dislocation, it is also suggested to avoid maximum adduction and internal rotation movements and hip flexion to more than 80°. Patients are then required to respect specific daily rules, such as avoiding low seats, using WC aids, avoiding leg crossing, using aids for dressing, and undressing to limit forward bending.

Femoral diaphysis metastases are treated with curettage, introduction of an intramedullary nail, and cement. After drainage tube removal, patients can start rehabilitation programs, which should include passive and active mobilization of the knee joint and early ambulation with unrestricted weight-bearing and global muscular strengthening exercises, such as ankle rotations, bed-supported knee bends, buttock contractions, abduction exercise, quadriceps isometric contractions, straight leg raises, standing exercises, standing knee raises, standing hip abduction, standing hip extensions, walking, and stair climbing and descending.

Distal femur metastases are treated with cemented tumor prostheses. If tumor curettage had been done, rehabilitation should include early ambulation with unrestricted weight-bearing as well as passive and active range of motion of the knee joint. In the case of distal femur resection, the lower extremity is elevated for 3 days to prevent wound edema. Knee motion is restricted in an immobilizing brace for 2–3 weeks to allow healing of the surgical flaps and until the extensor mechanism is again functional. During that time, isometric exercises are carried out and weight-bearing is allowed [16–23].

References

1. Shibata H, Kato S, Sekine I, et al. Diagnosis and treatment of bone metastasis: comprehensive guideline of the Japanese Society of Medical Oncology, Japanese Orthopedic Association, Japanese Urological Association, and Japanese Society for Radiation Oncology. ESMO Open. 2016;1:e000037. https://doi.org/10.1136/esmoopen-2016-000037.
2. Bunting RW. Rehabilitation of cancer patients with skeletal metastases. Clin Orthop Relat Res. 1995;312:197–200.
3. Coleman RE. Metastatic bone disease: clinical features, pathophysiology and treatment strategies. Cancer Treat Rev. 2001;27:165–76.

4. Santini D. Linee Guida Trattamento Delle Metastasi Ossee AIOM. 2015. http://www.aiom.it/professionisti/documenti-scientifici/linee-guida/metastasi-ossee.

5. Scivoletto G, Lapenna LM, Di Donna V, Laurenza L, Sterzi S, Foti C, Molinari M. Neoplastic myelopathies and traumatic spinal cord lesions: an Italian comparison of functional and neurological outcomes. Spinal Cord. 2011;49:799–805. 2011 International Spinal Cord Society 1362-4393/11.

6. Galasko CSB, Norris HE, Crank S. Current concepts review spinal instability secondary to metastatic cancer. J Bone Joint Surg Am. 2000;82:570.

7. Capanna R, Piccioli A, Di Martino A, Italian Orthopaedic Society Bone Metastasis Study Group, et al. Management of long bone metastases: recommendations from the Italian Orthopaedic Society bone metastasis study group. Expert Rev Anticancer Ther. 2014;14(10):1127–34.

8. Henrichs MP, Krebs J, Gosheger G, et al. Modular tumor endoprostheses in surgical palliation of long-bone metastases: a reduction in tumor burden and a durable reconstruction. World J Surg Oncol. 2014;12:330. http://www.wjso.com/content/12/1/330.

9. Gosheger G, Gebert C, Ahrens H, et al. Endoprosthetic reconstruction in 250 patients with sarcoma. Clin Orthop Relat Res. 2006;450:164–71.

10. Bickels J, Kollender Y, Wittig JC, et al. Function after resection of humeral metastases. Analysis of 59 consecutive patients. Clin Orthop Relat Res. 2005;137:201–8.

11. Eckardt JJ, Kabo M, Kelly CM, et al. Endoprosthetic reconstructions for bone metastases. Clin Orthop Relat Res. 2003;415(suppl):S254–62.

12. Enneking WF, Dunham W, Gebhardt M, et al. A system for the classification of skeletal resections. Chir Organi Mov. 1990;75(suppl 1):217–40.

13. Gainor BJ, Buchert P. Fracture healing in metastatic bone disease. Clin Orthop Relat Res. 1983;178:297–302.

14. Bickels J, Malawer MM. Surgical management of metastatic bone disease: humeral lesions, part 4, oncology, section II shoulder girdle and upper extremities. In: Malawer MM, Wittig JC, Bickels J, editors. Operative techniques in orthopaedic surgical oncology. Philadelphia: Wolters Kluver and Lippincott Williams & Wilkins; 2012.

15. Flemming JE, Beals RK. Pathologic fractures of the humerus. Clin Orthop Relat Res. 1968;203:258–60.

16. Harrington KD, Sim FH, Enis JE, et al. Methylmethacrylate as an adjuvant in internal fixation of pathological fractures: experience with three hundred and seventy-five cases. J Bone Joint Surg Am. 1976;58A:1047–55.

17. Aaron AD. Treatment of metastatic adenocarcinoma of the pelvis and the extremities. J Bone Joint Surg Am. 1997;79A:917–32.

18. Bickels J, Meller I, Henshaw RM, et al. Reconstruction of hip joint stability after proximal and total femur resections. Clin Orthop Relat Res. 2000;375:218–30.

19. Bickels J, Wittig JC, Kollender Y, et al. Distal femur resection with endoprosthetic reconstruction: a long-term followup study. Clin Orthop Relat Res. 2002;400:225–35.

20. Capanna R, Morris HG, Campanacci D, et al. Modular uncemented prosthetic reconstruction after resection of tumours of the distal femur. J Bone Joint Surg Br. 1994;76B:178–86.

21. Dobbs HS, Scales JT, Wilson JN, et al. Endoprosthetic replacement of the proximal femur and acetabulum. J Bone Joint Surg Br. 1981;63B:219–24.

22. Harrington KD. Impending pathologic fractures from metastatic malignancy: evaluation and management. AAOS Instr Course Lect. 1986;35:357–81.

23. Kawai A, Muschler GF, Lane JM, et al. Prosthetic knee replacement after resection of a malignant tumor of the distal part of the femur: medium to long-term results. J Bone Joint Surg Am. 1998;80A:636–47.

Part IV

Minimally Invasive Tumor Treatment

Interventional Radiology, Thermoablation and Cryoablation

23

Mario Raguso, Salvatore Marsico,
Christine Ojango, and Salvatore Masala

Abstract

It is estimated that each year around 5% of all cancer patients develop metastases to the spine. In these patients, pain is the most cardinal symptom. The treatment of bone metastases is determined by a multidisciplinary team where the interventional radiologist is increasingly taking on a crucial role. Open surgery is not frequently used for treatment of bone metastases, owing to its morbidity and the often short life span of the patients. Surgical indications include a fracture with associated a neurologic compromise or high risk of developing pathologic fracture, which could result in neurological damage. Percutaneous cryoablation and thermoablation procedures are the therapeutic choices with a good efficacy in the treatment of painful metastatic lesions refractory to traditional therapies. These ablative methods can also be performed in combination with percutaneous cementoplasty to support and stabilisation for metastases in weight-bearing bones at risk for pathologic fracture.

23.1 Metastatic Bone Disease

The incidence of many cancers is increasing globally. Concurrently, the earlier diagnosis and modern treatments have attributed to the improved survival rates for many common forms of cancer and for all cancers combined [1, 2]. As the number of new cases and of long-term cancer survivors is growing, the incidence of metastatic bone disease (MBD) is increasing [3, 4]. The rise in occurrence of bone metastases is also accented by better diagnostic detection of distant malignant growths in various sites. Bone is the third most common target for the metastatic spread after the lung and liver, and prevalent primary malignancies to disseminate to bone are breast, prostate, thyroid, lung and kidney cancer [3, 5]. In autopsy studies, ca 70–80% of patients, dying with breast or prostate cancer, have evidence of MBD [3, 5]. The most commonly involved skeletal sites are the spine, pelvis (Fig. 23.1), femur and rib [3].

It is estimated that each year around 5% of all cancer patients develop metastases to the spine [6]. In these patients, pain is the most cardinal symptom and affects around 80% of patients with MBD [7]. In addition, patients with bone metastases are at risk to develop skeletal complications, termed as skeletal-related events (SRE). The SREs include debilitating bone pain requiring radiotherapy or surgery,

M. Raguso · S. Marsico · C. Ojango · S. Masala (✉)
Department of Diagnostic and Molecular Imaging,
Interventional Radiology and Radiation Therapy,
University of Rome "Tor Vergata", Rome, Italy
e-mail: salva.masala@tiscali.it

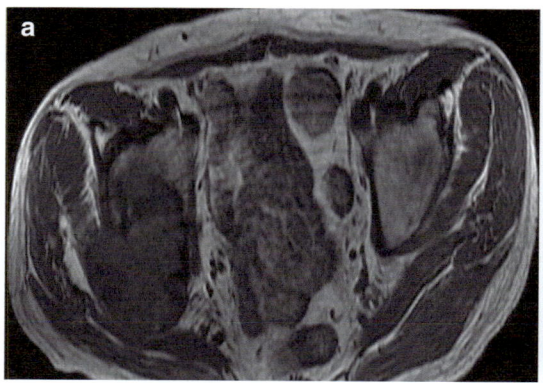
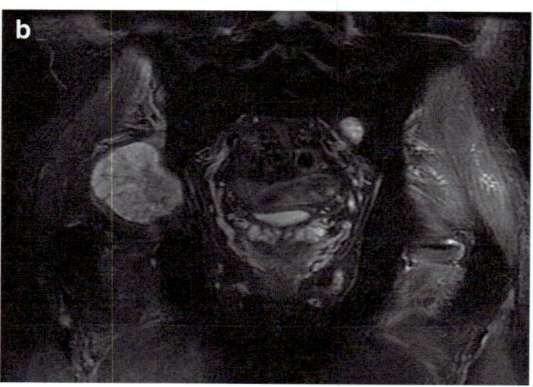

Fig. 23.1 A 60-year-old man affected by a large hip metastasis from lung cancer. Axial T1-weighted image (**a**) and coronal T2-SPIR-weighted image (**b**) show the pres- ence of a metastatic osteolytic lesion located in the right hip with infiltrative phenomena on surrounding muscle and subcutaneous tissues

pathological fracture, spinal cord compression or hypercalcaemia. In a large study, 20% of patients with skeletal metastases had a SRE concomitant with the diagnosis of bony metastases. The rate increased to 40–50% in the follow-up studies [3]. Pain and other SREs are common causes of morbidity in cancer patients with osseous metastases and affect negatively mobility. Reduced quality of life and mood changes with depression and anxiety are often present in this patient group [8].

The treatment methods for patients with MBD are critical to sufficiently control pain, to reduce tumour mass and to prevent SREs with the objective to improve quality of life and to maintain functional status of patients. The evaluation of every patient is interdisciplinary and includes various specialist, among others, oncologists, orthopaedic surgeons, interventional radiologists and palliative care specialists. The collaborative approach in choosing the optimal treatment or combined treatments should consider manifold factors, such as the histology of the primary tumour, the site and the extent of the metastatic spread and the general status of the patients. Analgesia with non-steroidal anti-inflammatory drugs or opioids is the first-line treatment in cancer patients with bone pain [8]. In addition, specific oncologic systemic or local therapies would be considered where appropriate. The systemic ones include chemo-,

hormonal and immunotherapies, radiopharmaceuticals and bisphosphonates. Chemotherapy is a systemic method that can deal even with small foci of metastases [9]. The treatment is effective in pain relief and also in reducing the burden of primary tumour and its related lesion [8]. However, pain in patients with MBD is often refractory to standard chemotherapy [10, 11]. Furthermore, it is not always well tolerated and associated with various side effects. The systemic radiopharmaceuticals are used to palliate pain in patients with diffuse painful bone metastases but are not suitable for patients with oligometastatic disease. Bisphosphonates are systemic bone-targeted agents that inhibit osteoclast activity. The agents are used as additional method alongside with other treatments to control bone pain and to prevent SREs [5]. Locally applied external beam radiation therapy stays the standard treatment for bone metastases [12]. Radiation therapy is effective in 60% of patients but requires several weeks to occur [12, 13]. Around 20–30% of patients do not experience pain relief after radiotherapy and 50% will suffer from recurrent pain [13]. Surgery is considered for patients with limited MBD, who present with pathological fracture or to resolve complications from the fracture. However, pain, from osseous metastases, is often undertreated, and patients experience moderate to severe pain and rely on the increasing doses of analgesics.

23.2 Image-Guided Thermal Ablation Techniques

The minimally invasive percutaneous procedures are the alternative choices of locally administered treatments. These include thermal or chemical ablation techniques, cementoplasty or percutaneous grafting. There are techniques which use the energy of heat to destroy a target tissue: i.e. thermal ablation procedures of radiofrequency, microwave, high-intensity focused ultrasound and laser ablation. In contrary, cryoablation technique damages the tissue with generated freezing temperatures of below −20 °C. Thermal ablation procedures are monitored by imaging. Ultrasound, computed tomography (CT) or magnetic resonance imaging (MRI) provides the possibility to choose the optimal route before the procedure, to monitor the placement of the cannula from the entry point to the selected site in real time or with small steps and to monitor the anatomical site during the procedure when necessary.

The main goal of the thermal ablation procedures is to reduce pain and to reduce the amount of analgesic opioid treatment. The procedures are considered in patients with refractory pain for conventional therapies. The indications for the procedures include pain intensity of more than 4/10 on visual analogue scale (VAS), localised pain in one or two places with the corresponding lesions seen on the imaging and life expectancy of more than 2 months [13]. Contraindications for the procedure include disseminated painful metastases, risk of fracture, prevalently osteoblastic metastases and a distance of less than 1 cm from a critical structure [7].

23.2.1 Radiofrequency Ablation

The energy of the radiofrequency (RF) current is the source for various interventional radiology procedures. The common aspect in these procedures is to generate and disperse heat and achieve the anomalous tissue coagulation in the specific site. Radiofrequency ablation (RFA) is the most widespread thermal ablation procedure for tumours in different sites (Fig. 23.2). It has become the gold standard as the curative treatment of benign bone tumour of osteoid osteoma. The use of RF for the malignant tumours is largely palliative, although the method may have effect to the local tumour growth [7].

Dupuy et al. were the first to report RFA method for the palliative treatment of painful bone metastases in 1998 [13]. Two large multicentre studies have shown the method to be effective and safe for the treatment of painful bone metastases [14, 15]. In the first multicentre study by Goetz et al., 43 patients were treated with RFA. From these, 41 patients (95%) experienced pain relief that was considered clinically significant. The reduction in worst pain, average pain, pain interference and significant improvement in pain relief was extending up to 24 weeks [14]. In the other multicentre study by Dupuy et al., 55 patients, who completed RFA, had on a 100-point scale an average increase of pain relief by around 26 points [15]. In addition, other scales of mood, pain intensity and pain severity showed significant improvement during follow-up studies [15]. Both of the multicentric studies reported a few significant adverse events related to the procedure. Other single site studies confirmed the efficacy and safety of the RFA treatment [9]. In addition to the positive effect on the pain scores, all of the conducted studies reported the decrease in the need for opioid analgesics [14, 15].

The aim of RFA is the destruction of cancer cells with the high temperature, with the final destruction or with the stop of the progression of the tumour mass. In single-electrode RFA systems, a closed-loop circuit is created with a RF generator, a large dispersive electrode (ground pad), the patient and a needle electrode in series [16]. The RFA procedure uses the alternating electrical current that oscillates in the radiofrequency band in the range of 400–500 kHz. The electrode has a non-insulated tip which leads the energy into the tissue, where the energy is dissipated as heat.

The current is lead into the site of the bone lesion through the inserted electrode [17]. The local ionic agitation and subsequent frictional heat are the final effect with a significant increase in temperature. Endosteal nerve endings are also

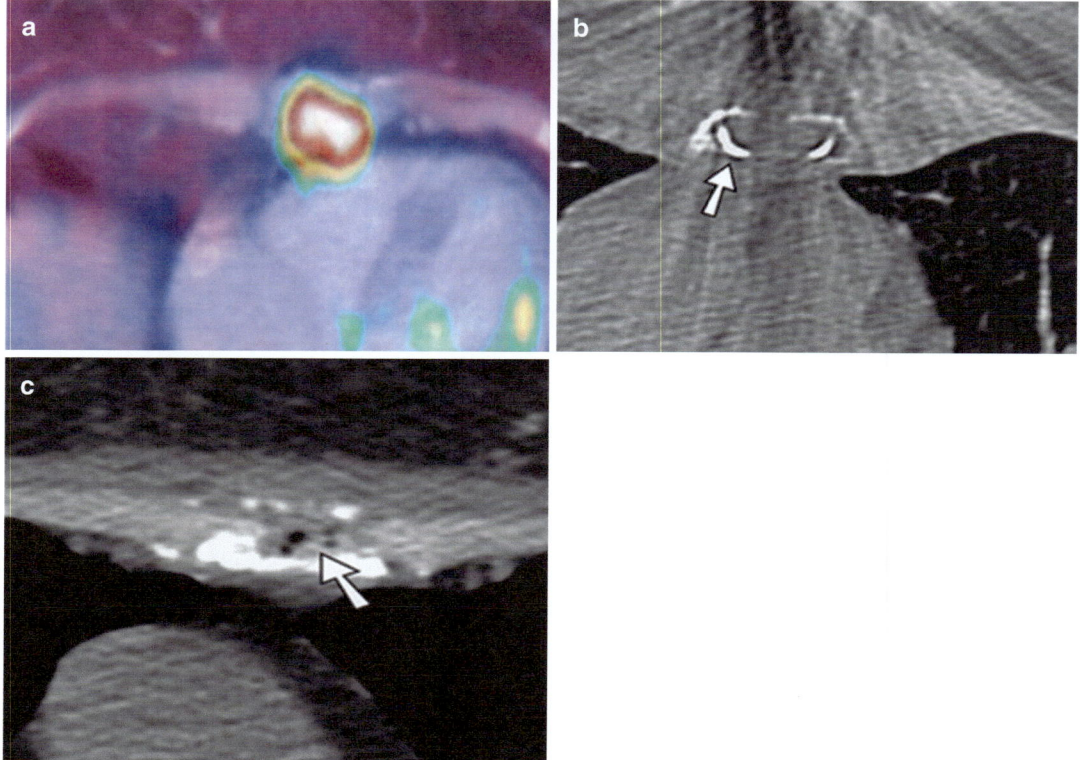

Fig. 23.2 A 50-year-old woman affected by a metastasis from breast cancer. (**a**, **b**) Axial PET and CT image shows a metastatic osteolytic lesion localised in the sternum. (**c**) CT axial image showing the results of radiofrequency treatment with air microbubbles in the context of the treated lesion

destroyed, with a reduction in production of chemicals involved in pain signalling, such as prostaglandins and bradykinin, substance P or histamine, released by the destroyed bone [13]. Cortical bone has heat insulating activity, which protects neighbouring structures [18].

Some studies proved the cells die, resulting in tissue necrosis, when the temperature exceeds 60 °C [19]. Authors then supposed the use of a 'higher-than-ideal temperatures', typically over 90–100 °C, for ablation of tissues with a greater distance from the RF source: a complete coverage of the tumour should be obtained by the ablation zone with an adequate margin, typically 1 cm otherwise the boundary of the treated cancer lesion [20].

There are many types of electrodes, which differ for the length and the thickness of the tip, and the choice depends on the characteristics of the lesion to be treated. The area of tissue coagulation necrosis is a sphere and its size increases linearly in function of the tip length [21]. There is a major ionic agitation in the molecules of the neighbour tissues to the electrode tip, therefore, a higher temperature increase [22]. A lot of systems include a single active electrode. Some companies produce bipolar electrodes: two serially non-insulated metallic surfaces at the tip electrode act as double poles [23, 24]. For larger tumours, RFA systems with multiple electrodes are preferred because of their faster and wider coagulation than single-electrode systems: multitine conventional or cooled electrode systems range from 3 to 12 active tips of variable size and cluster configurations, with a final ablation zone of 3–4 cm [25, 26].

RFA is performed under fluoroscopy or combined fluoroscopy/CT guidance, in local anaesthesia. With the patient in prone position and two rolls of soft material under the chest and the pelvis, a stiff cannula of a diameter between 11 and 13 gauge is introduced with uni-

lateral or bilateral trans-pedicular pathway (or inter-costovertebral for thoracic vertebrae or posterolateral for the lumbar levels) in the vertebral body (Fig. 23.3). A flexible working cannula

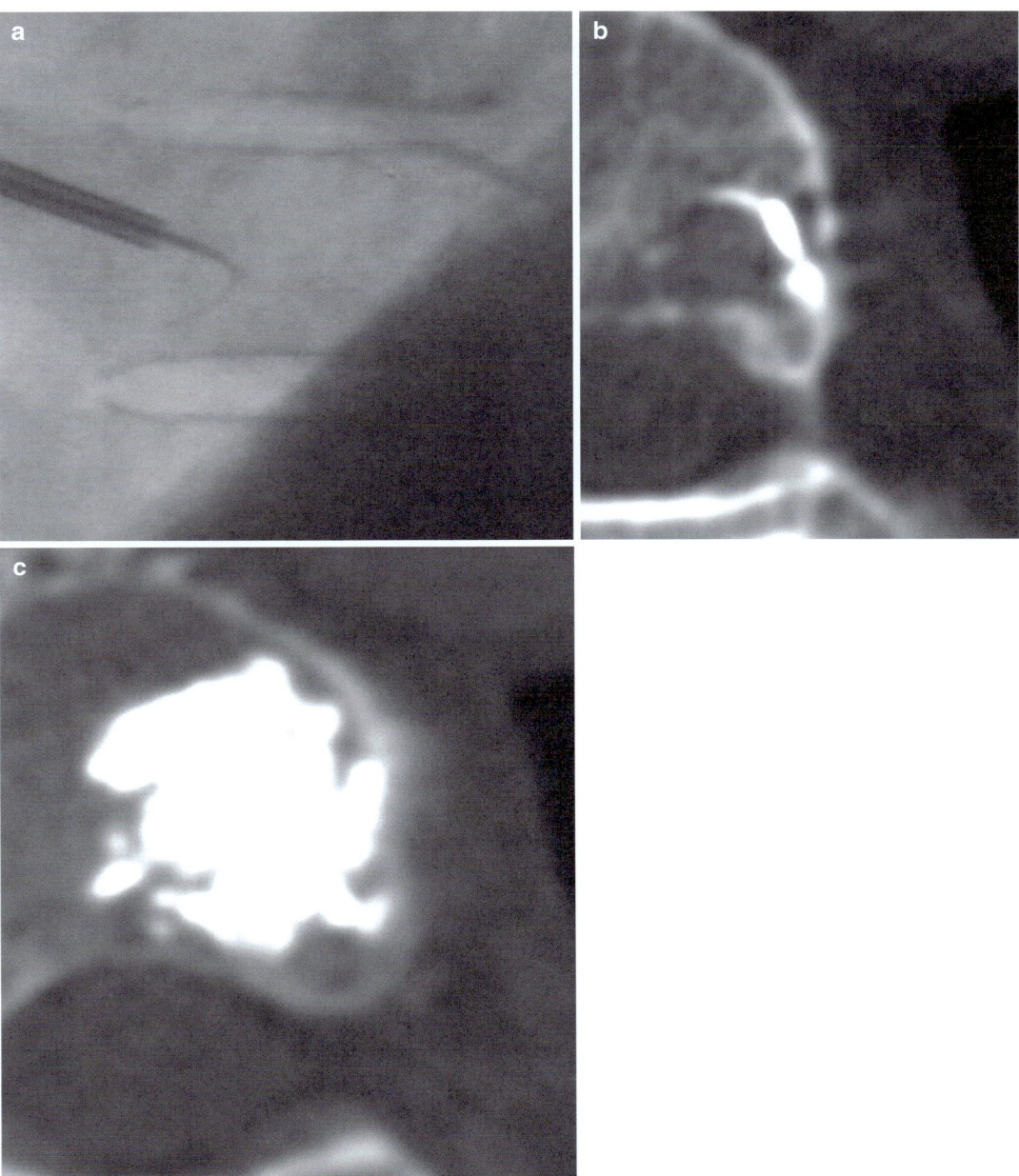

Fig. 23.3 A 66-year-old woman affected by a spinal metastases from breast cancer. (**a**) Placement under fluoroscopic guidance of the radiofrequency needle (white arrow) within the lesion. (**b**) Axial CT image showing the metastatic osteolytic lesion in a thoracic vertebral body. (**c**) CT axial image showing the results of the treatment after the stabilisation with PMMA augmentation

is introduced to allow the subsequent introduction of RF electrode that is then positioned with a coaxial technique in the target lesion.

There are contraindications to RFA: vertebral fractures with fragments within neural foramen, spread of tumour within the epidural space, local or systemic infection, coagulative disorders, asymptomatic fractures and tumour involvement of posterior arc [27]. The RFA induces temperature of over 45 °C; with this temperature, the heat sensitive nerve tissues may be damaged permanently. Damage to the nerve or vascular tissues is one of the most severe complications occurring [12]. Furthermore, the ablation margin of the targeted tissue cannot be visualised with ultrasound or CT, and significant increase of pain is reported immediately after the procedure [11].

Skin heat injuries and damages to neurovascular structure or other closer soft tissues should be prevented with thermal protection techniques: gas dissection (air or CO_2 in the soft tissues) or hydro-dissection with subcutaneous fluid injection as saline solution or the anaesthetic drugs, which have an insulating function [28]. Sterile gloves containing cooled fluid can be placed on the skin near to the entry site to prevent burns [28]. Some companies created temperature monitoring system as a thermocouple included in the RFA electrodes [28].

23.2.2 Cryoablation

Cryoablation (CA) is a thermal ablation technique with alternating rapid freezing and thawing cycles, with the aim to achieve tumour destruction. The freezing temperature is reached by rapidly conducting argon gas through the probe. The passage decompresses argon gas (Joule-Thomson effect) and leads within a few seconds to cooling with temperatures of below −100 °C. Thawing is achieved passively or by circulation of helium gas in the probe. During the procedure, the freezing temperature causes formation of ice crystals in the target site. Tissue destruction is complete at temperature from −20 to −40 °C. With very low temperature, direct cell destruction is obtained, while less icy temperature causes osmotic differences across the cell membranes, with resulting cellular dehydration and ischaemia [13].

Patients are treated under general anaesthesia or moderate sedation. There are two major producers of cryoprobes, Galil Medical (Yokneam, Israel) and Endocare, Inc. (HealthTronics/Endocare Incorporated, Irvine, California). Both industries produce an argon/helium pairing-based system and possess independent console to evaluate statistics of probes status and the different temperatures recorded. Galil Medical produces an MRI-compatible system. Following sterile preparation, one or more cryoprobes are straight inserted, introduced through the skin under CT or both CT and ultrasound guidance. Hydro-dissection is used to differentiate directly contiguous structures. This is a potential advantage over the RFA to visualise the ablation margins and adjacent critical structures. Cryoprobes localisation is monitored by CT imaging. Although, the ultrasound provides the real-time visualisation, its use is limited to the more superficial sites, including breast, thoracic or abdominal wall. CT is preferred for lung, bone, kidney and visceral structures. A series of freeze-thaw-freeze cycles are used for the treatment of metastasis with a goal of 10 min–8 min–10 min, respectively, for a single cycle (Fig. 23.4). The temperature at the outer edge of the iceball is around 0 °C [11]. However, the cell death reliably has been found around 3–5 mm from the edge. Non-contrast-enhanced CT is performed every 2–5 min of freezing cycles and displayed with good body window width and level settings (W 400 HU, L 40 HU) to show location and dimensions of the iceball. A limitation of CA is the long time-consuming procedure.

Percutaneous CA was used first for the curative treatment of lesions in the liver and consequently has been used for lesions in the kidney, lung, breast, bone and soft tissues [29]. In the first prospective study evaluating the efficacy and safety of CA procedure, 14 patients were treated with CA for the painful osseous metastases. During the follow-up evaluations up to 24 weeks, 12 patients of 14 had a drop of 3 points in the worst pain at some point during the follow-up [10]. In addition, the average pain intensities decreased at 1, 4, 6

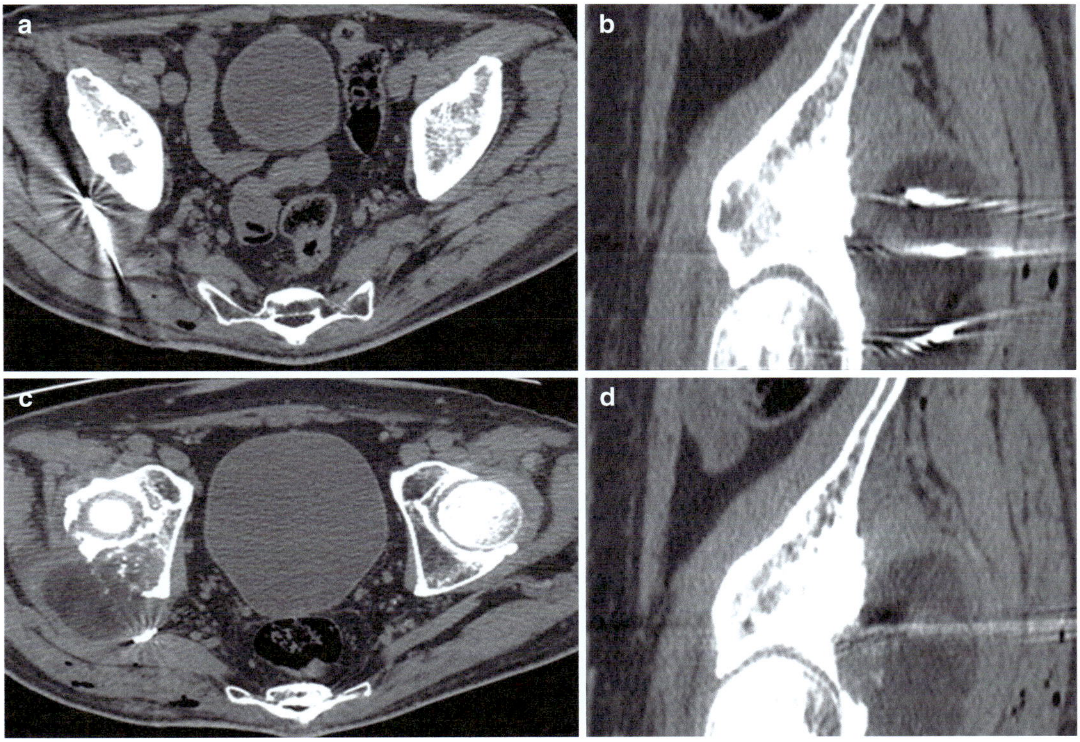

Fig. 23.4 A 60-year-old man affected by a large metastasis from lung cancer and hip pain. (**a**, **b**) Axial and sagittal CT images show the correct position of the cryoprobes in the centre of the lesion. (**c**, **d**) Axial and sagittal CT images show the iceball lesion formed in the metastatic target after the freezing cycles

and 8 weeks post-procedurally [10]. The multi-centre single-arm trial of the efficacy of cryoabla-tion by Callstrom et al. evaluated 61 cancer patients with MBD and reported highly significant reductions in pain scores [30]. In that study, 75% of patients achieved 90% or higher pain relief at some point in the follow-up period.

CA has been utilised in combination with radiotherapy for the treatment of solitary painful bone metastases. The combined approach had favourable impact on pain and quality of life scores compared with the radiotherapy treatment only [31]. The study by Zugaro et al. compared the outcomes of pain relief and quality of life in patients with painful osseous metastases treated with CA or RFA [32]. Pain relief has evaluated post-procedurally with complete and partial response. The study demonstrated that CA sig-nificantly improved complete or partial response with respect to baseline at 12 weeks following ablation. By contrast, only partial response sig-nificantly improved with respect to baseline fol-lowing RFA treatment [32].

23.3 Image-Guided Bone Augmentation Techniques

Vertebral cementoplasty (VP) is a well-established percutaneous technique to stabilise the spine with the injection of viscous material or cement into the weakened and pathological vertebral body. The VP was first performed in 1984 for the treat-ment of haemangioma in the cervical metamer and after a few years later was applied to treat porotic vertebral fractures [33]. The VP has been used to treat pain in various pathological pro-cesses involving the vertebrae, including Paget's disease, osteogenesis imperfecta, Langerhans cell histiocytosis and spinal pseudoarthrosis [34].

However, the main indications remain the painful osteoporotic and malignant vertebral compression fractures refractory to medical conservative treatment and aggressive vertebral haemangiomas. VP has been validated extensively and is an efficient pain management procedure in patients with spinal neoplasms who have classified as stable and possibly unstable [33]. Eighty-four to ninety-two percent of patients in these groups have shown rapid pain relief and the recorded safety data showed 4–9.2% of patients with asymptomatic paravertebral cement leakage [33]. The use of the radiofrequency ablation (RFA) before the cementoplasty appears to be useful to achieve tumour necrosis and stabilise the ablated lesions. The combined use of cryoablation and cementoplasty is thought to provide additional pain relief [35].

Polymethyl methacrylate (PMMA) is injected via the percutaneously inserted needles into the site of interest under imaging guidance. The optimal needle placement into the bone and accurate cement injection and distribution, including detection of cement leaks during the procedure, should be monitored sufficiently under fluoroscopy or CT guidance. The PMMA or cement flows into the cavities and spaces of bone and the viscous fluid hardens in 8–18 min [36]. The characteristic of the cement is that it is extremely stable but does not attach strongly to the bone. Therefore, it is considered as a treatment option for vertebral bodies or acetabulum, where the compression forces are present, but less so to treat meta-diaphysis of long-bone that are subjected to shear forces [36].

The main indication for the VP is the treatment of pain due to osteopenic or osteolytic lesions in the vertebral bodies that has not been sufficiently controlled with 3 weeks of conservative medical treatment. The baseline evaluation of patients before the VP treatment must be thorough to decide the probable site of pain in cases of involvement of multiple sites, to exclude the contraindications for the VP procedure or to evaluate the risk factors that are associated with complications. The contraindications for the VP procedure include the spinal cord compression, local or systemic infections, response to medical therapy, allergy to cement or diffuse bone metastases or uncorrectable coagulopathy [33, 34].

Over 70% of patients undergoing VP will have a visible leakage on CT scans into the soft tissues, perivertebral veins and intervertebral disks [36]. These leaks are usually asymptomatic. The complication of leakage into the spinal canal is also relatively well tolerated if the volume of the cement is small [36]. However, rarely the posterior cement overflow into the spinal canal and subsequent spinal cord compression may require urgent intervention. Less often complication is the leakage into the intervertebral foramen causing radiculopathy. Cement embolism is usually asymptomatic and has been estimated to be present 4.0–6.8% of cases [34]. As with all interventional procedures, sterile conditions and strict procedural protocol must be followed to minimise the risk of local infections [37].

Conclusions

The thermal ablation procedures are promising technique that could be part in the management plan for cancer patients with skeletal metastases. PMMA augmentation can be finally performed with good results in term of pain relief and bone stabilisation, by preventing pathologic fractures. However, especially for CA, the procedures are still relatively new, and more published data about the efficacy would be needed.

References

1. Jemal A, Siegel R, Ward E, Hao Y, Xu J, Thun MJ. Cancer statistics, 2008. CA Cancer J Clin. 2008;59(4):225–49.
2. Ferlay J, Autier P, Boniol M, Heanue M, Colombet M, Boyle P. Estimates of the cancer incidence and mortality in Europe in 2006. Ann Oncol. 2007;18(3):581–92.
3. Ashford RU, Randall RL. Bone metastases: epidemiology and societal effect. In: Randall RL, editor. Metastatic bone disease. New York: Springer; 2006. p. 793–810.
4. Schulman KL, Kohles J. Economic burden of metastatic bone disease. Cancer. 2007;109(11):2334–42.
5. Coleman RE. Clinical features of metastatic bone disease and risk of skeletal morbidity. Clin Cancer Res. 2006;12(20 Pt 2):6243s–9s.

6. Georgy BA. Metastatic spinal lesions: state-of-the-art treatment options and future trends. Am J Neuroradiol. 2008;29(9):1605–11.
7. Ringe KI, Panzica M, von Falck C. Thermoablation of bone tumors. Fortschr Röntgenstr. 2016;188(6):539–50.
8. Santiago FR, del Mar Castellano García M. Treatment of bone tumours by radiofrequency thermal ablation. Eur Oncol. 2008;4(2):92–9.
9. Thanos L, Mylona S, Galani P, et al. Radiofrequency ablation of osseous metastases for the palliation of pain. Skelet Radiol. 2008;37(3):189–94.
10. Callstrom MR, Atwell TD, Charboneau JW, et al. Painful metastases involving bone: percutaneous image-guided cryoablation--prospective trial interim analysis. Radiology. 2006;241(2):572–80.
11. Callstrom MR, Kurup AN. Percutaneous ablation for bone and soft tissue metastases-why cryoablation? Skelet Radiol. 2009;38(9):835–9.
12. Nicholas Kurup A, Callstrom MR. Ablation of musculoskeletal metastases: pain palliation, fracture risk reduction, and oligometastatic disease. Tech Vasc Interv Radiol. 2013;16(4):253–61.
13. Rosenthal D, Callstrom MR. Critical review and state of the art in interventional oncology: benign and metastatic disease involving bone. Radiology. 2012;262(3):765–80.
14. Goetz MP, Callstrom MR, Charboneau JW, et al. Percutaneous image-guided radiofrequency ablation of painful metastases involving bone: a multicenter study. J Clin Oncol. 2004;22(2):300–6.
15. Dupuy DE, Liu D, Hartfeil D, et al. Percutaneous radiofrequency ablation of painful osseous metastases: a multi-center American College of Radiology Imaging Network trial. Cancer. 2010;116(4):989–007.
16. Davis KW, Choi JJ, Blankenbaker DG. Radiofrequency ablation in the musculoskeletal system. Semin Roentgenol. 2004;39(1):129–44.
17. Curley SA. Radiofrequency ablation of malignant liver tumors. Ann Surg Oncol. 2003;10(4):338–47.
18. Dupuy DE, Hong R, Oliver B, et al. Radiofrequency ablation of spinal tumors: temperature distribution in the spinal canal. AJR Am J Roentgenol. 2000;175(5):1263–6.
19. Mertyna P, Dewhirst MW, Halpern E, et al. Radiofrequency ablation: the effect of distance and baseline temperature on thermal dose required for coagulation. Int J Hyperth. 2008;24(7):550–9.
20. Di Staso M, Zugaro L, Gravina GL, et al. A feasibility study of percutaneous radiofrequency ablation followed by radiotherapy in the management of painful osteolytic bone metastases. Eur Radiol. 2011;21(9):2004–10.
21. Frezza EE. Therapeutic management algorithm in cirrhotic and noncirrhotic patients in primary or secondary liver masses. Dig Dis Sci. 2004;49(5):866–71.
22. Haines DE, Verow AF. Observations on electrode-tissue interface temperature and effect on electrical impedance during radiofrequency ablation of ventricular myocardium. Circulation. 1990;82(3):1034–8.
23. Buy X, Basile A, Bierry G, et al. Saline-infused bipolar radiofrequency ablation of high-risk spinal and paraspinal neoplasms. AJR Am J Roentgenol. 2006;186(5 Suppl):S322–6.
24. Gazis AN, Beuing O, Franke J, et al. Bipolar radiofrequency ablation of spinal tumors: predictability, safety and outcome. Spine J. 2014;14(4):604–8.
25. Gulesserian T, Mahnken AH, Schernthaner R, et al. Comparison of expandable electrodes in percutaneous radiofrequency ablation of renal cell carcinoma. Eur J Radiol. 2006;59(2):133–9.
26. Pereira PL, Trübenbach J, Schenk M, et al. Radiofrequency ablation: in vivo comparison of four commercially available devices in pig livers. Radiology. 2004;232(2):482–90.
27. Masala S, Fiori R, Massari F, et al. Kyphoplasty and vertebroplasty: new equipment for vertebral fractures treatment. J Exp Clin Cancer Res. 2003;22(4 Suppl):75–9.
28. Tsoumakidou G, Buy X, Garnon J, et al. Percutaneous thermal ablation: how to protect the surrounding organs. Tech Vasc Interv Radiol. 2011;14(3):170–6.
29. Callstrom MR, Charboneau JW, Goetz MP, et al. Image-guided ablation of painful metastatic bone tumors: a new and effective approach to a difficult problem. Skelet Radiol. 2006;35(1):1–15.
30. Callstrom MR, Dupuy DE, Solomon SB, et al. Percutaneous image-guided cryoablation of painful metastases involving bone: multicenter trial. Cancer. 2013;119(5):1033–41.
31. Di Staso M, Gravina GL, Zugaro L, et al. Treatment of solitary painful osseous metastases with radiotherapy, cryoablation or combined therapy: propensity matching analysis in 175 patients. PLoS One. 2015;10(6):1–11.
32. Zugaro L, Di Staso M, Gravina GL, et al. Treatment of osteolytic solitary painful osseous metastases with radiofrequency ablation or cryoablation: a retrospective study by propensity analysis. Oncol Lett. 2016;11(3):1948–54.
33. Muto M, Guarnieri G, Giurazza F, Manfrè L. What's new in vertebral cementoplasty? Br J Radiol. 2016;89(1059):20150337. https://doi.org/10.1259/bjr.20150337.
34. Katsanos K, Sabharwal T, Adam A. Percutaneous cementoplasty. Semin Interv Radiol. 2010;27(2):137–47. https://doi.org/10.1055/s-0030-1253512.
35. Yilmaz S, Özdoğan M, Cevener M, et al. Use of cryoablation beyond the prostate. Insights Imaging. 2016;7(2):223–32. https://doi.org/10.1007/s13244-015-0460-7.
36. Laredo J-D, Chiras J, Kemel S, Taihi L, Hamze B. Vertebroplasty and interventional radiology procedures for bone metastases. Joint Bone Spine. 2017. https://doi.org/10.1016/j.jbspin.2017.05.005.
37. Masala S, Chiocchi M, Taglieri A, et al. Combined use of percutaneous cryoablation and vertebroplasty with 3D rotational angiograph in treatment of single vertebral metastasis: comparison with vertebroplasty. Neuroradiology. 2013;55(2):193–200.

Electrochemotherapy

24

Laura Campanacci and Flavio Fazioli

Abstract

Bone metastatic disease is a major cause of pain and decreased quality of life in patients with cancer. In addition to systemic therapy and pain control with narcotic analgesics, standard local treatments include palliation with radiation therapy, surgery, embolization or focused ultrasound treatment. However 20–30% of patients do not respond to conventional treatments, increasing the interest in alternative therapies.

Electrochemotherapy (ECT) – a combination of high-voltage electric pulses and of an anticancer drug – has demonstrated high effectiveness in the treatment of cutaneous and subcutaneous tumours and proved to be successfully used in the treatment of tumours regardless of its histological origin. Because of its demonstrated efficacy in the treatment of cutaneous and subcutaneous tumours, its application deserves to be extended to the treatment of internal tumours. To advance electrochemotherapy to treating internal solid tumours, new technological developments enabled treatment of internal tumours in daily clinical practice. Preclinical studies and clinical trial demonstrated the feasibility and efficacy of electrochemotherapy for the treatment of bone metastases.

ECT should be considered a new feasible tool in the treatment of bone metastases in place or in combination with standard local treatments; further developments are required to extend the use of this technique to spine metastases.

Keywords

Electroporation · Electrochemotherapy
Cancer treatment · Treatment planning

24.1 Introduction

Bone cancers greatly impact patients' quality of life due to associated symptoms such as pain, pathological fractures, spinal cord compression, hypercalcaemia and reduction of movement and performance status [1, 2].

The metastatic pain without mechanical failure of the skeletal segment is often effectively treated with analgesics, radiotherapy, hormone therapy, chemotherapy and bisphosphonates.

L. Campanacci (✉)
Oncological Orthopaedic Department,
Istituto Ortopedico Rizzoli, Bologna, Italy
e-mail: laura.campanacci@ior.it

F. Fazioli
Musculoskeletal Oncologic Surgery,
Istituto nazionate Tumori Fondazione Pascale,
Naples, Italy
e-mail: f.fazioli@istitutotumori.na.it

The surgical treatment is often necessary to prevent or stabilize pathological fractures or decompress the spinal cord in case of vertebral metastasis in order to preserve the function and allow a rapid patient mobilization. When surgery is not indicated, for example in the case of hardly accessible metastases, radiotherapy in divided doses is considered the treatment of choice with success rates of around 60% as regards the control of pain and to 25% for the control of local disease. Adjuvant radiation therapy, when possible, is also performed to complete the surgical treatment. Radiotherapy is more effective in some histological type metastases, mainly breast, prostate and lung, while its effectiveness in other types of metastases (as for metastases from kidney carcinomas) is lower. But radiotherapy cannot be repeated in the same anatomical area over 40–50 Gy, and there is a cumulative dose-dependent risk of collateral effects due to its toxicity to the surrounding healthy tissues.

Other local treatments may be selective arterial embolization, radiofrequency thermal ablation, focused ultrasound treatment and cryosurgery, with similar results or inferior to radiotherapy in terms of local progression or pain control.

Radiofrequency thermal ablation has been described to induce as well connective and vascular degeneration due to the heat dissipation, and when applied to the bone tissue, it leaves the trabecular structure brittle and not mechanically competent. Cryosurgery is particularly time consuming, requires multiple probes, and has a number of side effects [3–8].

Although the treatment of patients suffering from bone metastases has always been primarily aimed at palliation of pain, currently the local control of the disease is becoming an important goal, especially in a growing population of oligometastatic patients with a long life expectancy. The progression of neoplastic disease limited to one anatomical region can significantly impair the patient's quality of life with serious local complications.

When surgery finds no indication, for example, in difficult sites as pelvis and extended metastases, fractional dose radiotherapy is considered the treatment with success rates of about 60% for pain control and 25% for the control disease site [5]. Adjuvant radiotherapy, whenever possible, is also performed upon completion of the surgical treatment.

However, some bone metastases may not benefit from radiotherapy because they are not radiosensitive (e.g. kidney cancer metastases) or because they are located in districts already irradiated at the maximum dose allowed.

24.2 Electrochemotherapy

Electrochemotherapy is a local treatment for malignant tumours, which was first described by Mir in 1991 for cutaneous nodules of head and neck malignant tumours [9, 10].

Electrochemotherapy is based on electroporation associated to intravenous infusion of a chemotherapeutic drug to which the cellular membranes are usually poor or not permeant.

Electroporation is the local application of pulses of electric current to the tumour tissue: this opens the transmembrane canals of the cellular membranes, rendering the cell membranes permeable to otherwise impermeant or poorly permeant anticancer drugs, thereby facilitating a potent localized cytotoxic effect.

The permeabilization can be temporary (reversible electroporation) or permanent (irreversible electroporation) as a function of the electrical field magnitude and duration and the number of pulses. The appropriate electric pulses (short and intense square-wave electric pulses) have no apparent cytotoxic or systemic effects [11–16].

Among several clinically approved drugs that have been tested in preclinical studies, bleomycin and cisplatin have been demonstrated to be the most effective and suitable drugs for clinical use of electrochemotherapy.

After electroporation of the tumoral cells, to electroporation, the cytotoxicity of bleomycin increases of almost 8000-fold compared to its normal activity and that of cisplatin increases of 80-fold. In vivo application of electric pulses to the tumours significantly increases antitumour effectiveness of bleomycin given intravenously or cisplatin given intratumourally. The treatment results in complete responses of the tumours with drug doses that by themselves have minimal or no antitumour activity and induce no side effects [17].

The antitumoural activity of bleomycin depends on its capability to enter the cellular membrane and interact with the DNA; thus, with electroporation, the drug is forced to enter the cell, and its activity does not depend on the histology of the tumour. The real limit of its effectiveness is the possibility to completely induce electroporation in the entire tumoural mass.

24.3 Electrochemotherapy for Bone Metastases

In 2006 the European Standard Operating Procedures of Electrochemotherapy (ESOPE) has been published. It is a multicentre study which demonstrated the feasibility and safety of electrochemotherapy for the treatment of superficial tumours, with an objective response rate of 85% (74% complete response rate) in treated tumour lesions [18]. In 2013, a meta-analysis of the use of electrochemotherapy in the treatment of cutaneous metastasis confirmed that the cytotoxicity of bleomycin and cisplatin is vastly increased when electroporation pulses are delivered to tumours in the presence of sufficiently high extracellular concentration of chemotherapeutic drug [19].

24.4 Preclinical Studies

Following extensive clinical studies confirming the safety and efficacy of ECT, clinicians and researchers have developed new strategies to extend its use to the treatment of deep-seated tumours [20–24]. Before applying the ECT to the bone tissue, it was necessary to verify the effectiveness of the method in the presence of a mineralized matrix. In particular it was necessary to assess whether the electric fields inside a calcified matrix were equally effective in the permeabilization of the cell membranes. Fini et al.

published a preclinical study on the use of ECT on the bone [21, 22]. They first performed electroporation on healthy bone tissue with the aim of developing a reproducible technique to introduce electrodes into the target bone tissue in order to identify the electroporation protocols (applied voltage and numbers of pulses) sufficient to ablate all bone cells in the target area. Furthermore they investigated the biological activity in the electroporation area 30 days after complete cell ablation and finally tested the mechanical competence of the mineralized bone trabeculae after electroporation, demonstrating that electroporation did not alter bone mineral structure, regenerative activity and mechanical competence. In order to investigate not only the effectiveness but also the safety of the treatment in the vicinity of noble structures such as peripheral nerves or the spinal cord, the effect of the electric field applied directly at the level of the sciatic nerve of the rabbit and at the spinal cord of sheep through electrodes inserted through the vertebral pedicles was evaluated. Histological examination of the nervous structures showed that these had a transient oedema in the absence of irreversible structural alterations [23, 25].

24.5 Clinical Application

Based on these encouraging results, the technology was developed to permit the use of ECT for bone malignant tumours, and the first clinical trial was performed to demonstrate the feasibility and safety of the procedure in vivo. Bianchi et al. reported the results of ECT performed in 29 patients affected by bone metastases [26]. Primary endpoints of the study were the feasibility and safety of ECT when applied to metastases to the bone; secondary endpoints were patients' clinical and radiological outcome. The inclusion criteria were metastatic involvement of the appendicular skeleton from melanoma or carcinoma confirmed histologically, maximum length of metastases below 6 cm, the absence of local treatment in the previous 3 months and life expectancy greater than 3 months. The exclusion criteria were pathological fractures, visceral involvement, allergy to bleomycin, cumulative doses of bleomycin in excess of 250 mg/m², bleeding disorders, chronic renal failure, arrhythmias and pregnancy and breastfeeding.

Feasibility was assessed by evaluating the possibility of reliably inserting electrodes percutaneously in bone, according to a predefined geometry to ensure proper electroporation of cell membranes in the bone metastasis. All adverse events after treatment and at follow-up were recorded and evaluated according to Common Terminology Criteria for Adverse Events.

Tumour cell electroporation was performed using the Cliniporator-VG (Variable Geometry) (Igea, Modena, Italy), which has been designed to treat large volumes of tissue (up to several tens of cubic centimetres) and uses up to six independent electrodes that can be freely positioned to completely treat the tumour regardless of its shape and size [27–29]. This pulse generator delivers standard electric pulses of 100 μs of up to 3000 V in amplitude being able to provide up to 50 A of current. New needle-like electrodes were developed of 1.8 mm diameter with trocar tip to be inserted directly into the bone and bone metastasis by means of drilling machine. The electrodes are 20, 16 or 12 cm long with insulation except for the upper 3 or 4 cm. An external reference system was designed to keep the relative positioning of the electrodes (Fig. 24.1).

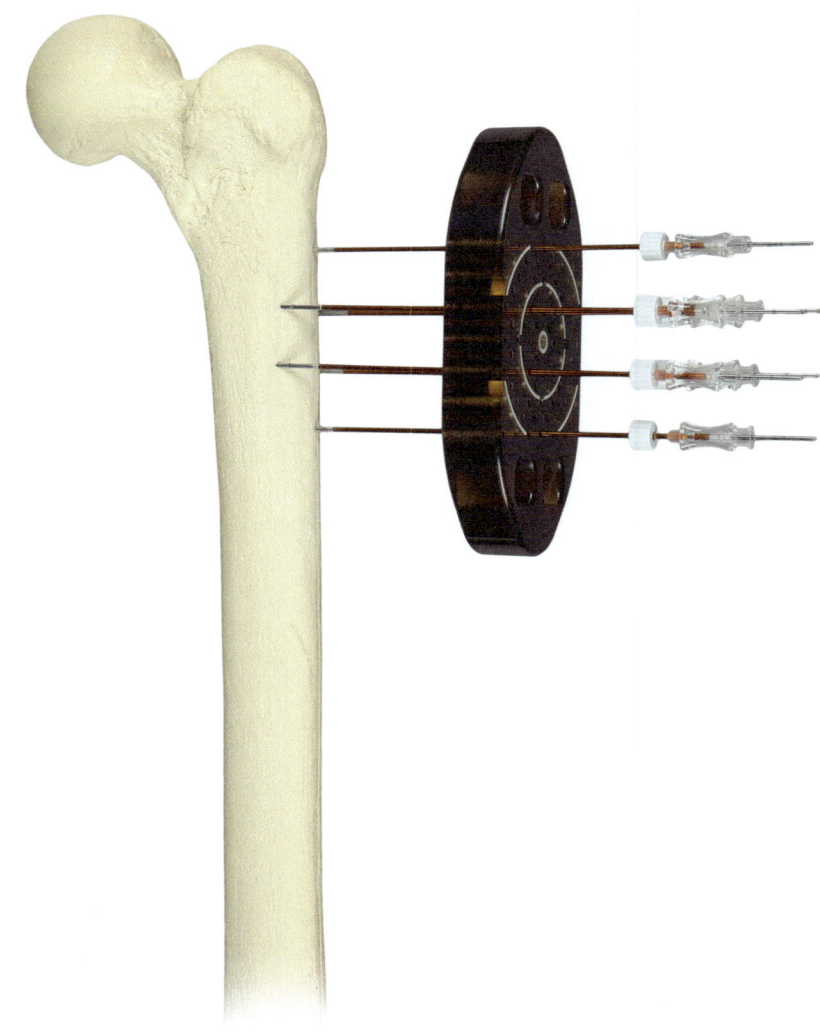

Fig. 24.1 Scheme of the ECT treatment in the bone: needle-like electrodes of 1.8 mm diameter with trocar tip are inserted directly into the bone lesion by means of drilling machine. The electrodes are 20, 16 or 12 cm long with insulation except for the upper 3 or 4 cm. An external reference system maintains the relative position of the electrodes

ECT procedure was performed according to the ESOPE study: eight pulses of 1000 V/cm are delivered between each couple of electrodes to homogeneously cover the lesion with local electric field (>350 V/cm) to induce cell membrane electroporation. Bleomycin, 15 mg/m^2 of body surface (Bleomycin Nippon Kayaku, Sanofi-Aventis, Milan, Italy), is administrated intravenously in bolus 8 min before applying the electric pulses. The time is required to allow the distribution of the drug in all the interstitial spaces at an effective concentration. The treatment has to be completed within 25 min from bleomycin injection.

The patients may be treated under general or peripheral anaesthesia. Usually when peripheral anaesthesia is performed, a deep sedation is associated during the electric current administration to the patient. The type of anaesthesia does not influence the ECT treatment outcome. ECT could be

performed in the proximity of vital structures considered there is no thermal denaturing effect; furthermore, applied electric pulses have showed no damaging effect on nerves and vessels [14, 15, 20].

Under radiological control (CT or image intensifier, depending on lesion accessibility), six to eight electrodes were inserted, depending on the volume and geometry of the metastases (Fig. 24.2). The treatment was repeated in some patients (43 ECT in 29 patients); in fact, after a significant clinical benefit after the first treatment, the procedure was repeated in order to further improve local control of the disease. One patient developed a pathological fracture at the target site after the second treatment and required internal fixation (Fig. 24.3).

Two major complications were observed. The first was an extensive ulceration of the skin of patient whose proximal tibia had previously

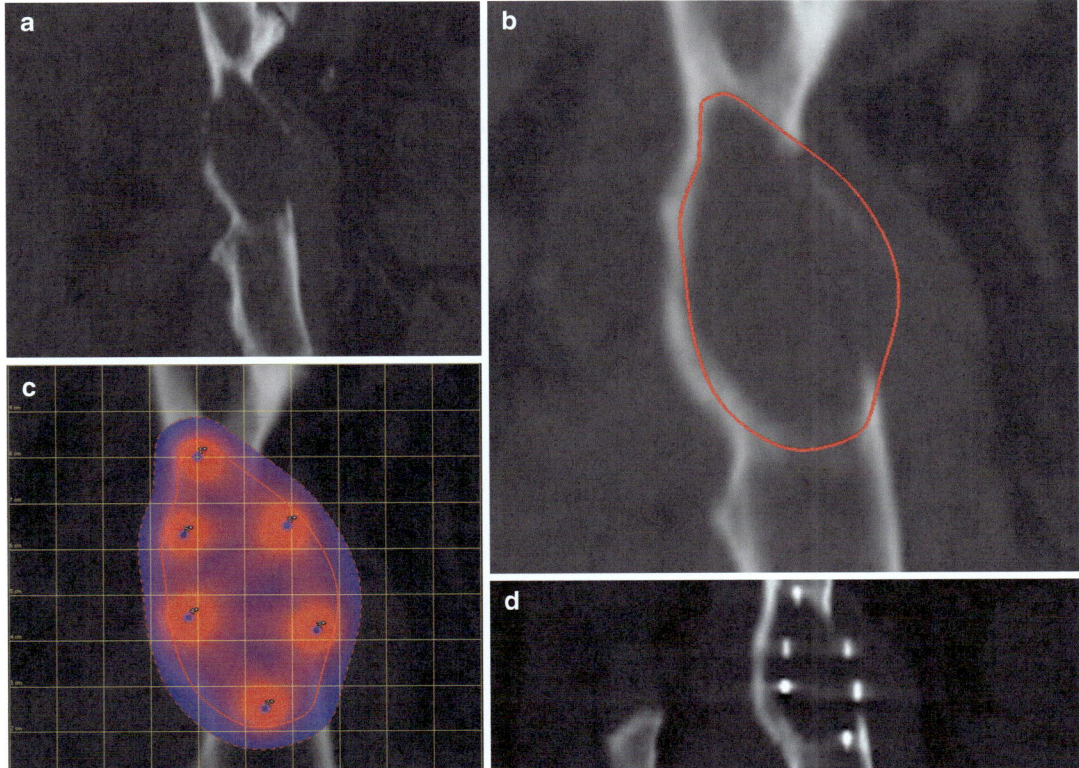

Fig. 24.2 (**a–d**) 68-year-old patient: (**a**) right peri-acetabular region bone metastasis, clear cell kidney carcinoma, radiation therapy already performed; pre-ECT planning with Pulsar® software: (**b**) the tumour area is drawn on the CT image, and (**c**) the software simulates the best positioning of the electrodes for optimal treatment. (**d**) CT-guided ECT needles positioning, coronal plane, reproducing the preoperative planning

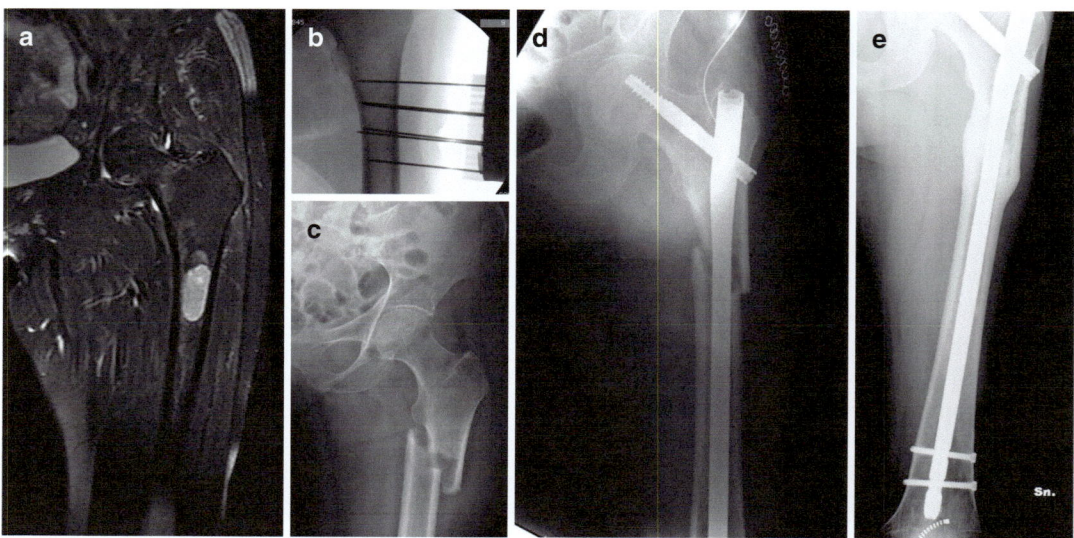

Fig. 24.3 (**a–e**) 65-year-old patient. (**a**) T2-weighted MRI of left femur painful bone metastasis, follicular thyroid carcinoma. (**b**) Fluoroscopy-guided ECT needle positioning. The patient was treated with two ECT settings: treatments one 3 months after the other. (**c**) A pathological fracture occurred 4 months after the second treatment, treated with reduction and intramedullary nail (**d**). (**e**) Radiograph performed 2 years later shows the complete healing of the fracture

been irradiated and that required thigh amputation. The second was the appearance of a neurogenic bladder after the third treatment with ECT in the sacral region, which was attributed to disease progression.

Pain relief was achieved in 84% of patients. Use of pain killers, quality of night's sleep and daily activities improved in 55–73% of patients. Local tumour control (stable disease) was achieved in most patients, with only 10% of the lesions showed progression at follow-up.

On CT, a progression of the disease was observed in only 10% of patients.

The results of the study showed that ECT was safe and effective in the treatment of painful bone metastases even when previous treatments have proved ineffective.

The spine ideally represents the main goal of treatment with ECT. In fact it is not only the seat skeletal more frequently affected by metastases, but in consideration of the contiguity with the spinal cord, it is technically complex to approach surgically. Moreover, it shows some limits to radiation treatment because of the limit dose of radiation to which the spinal cord may be exposed. Other minimally invasive treatments

such as microwave ablation or vertebroplasty are incomplete and poorly effective therapeutic strategies. The first aims at tumour ablation which is however often partial to the need to save the adjoining noble structures and compromises the mechanical competence of the vertebra. The second mechanically stabilizes the vertebral body by preventing or supporting a pathological fracture but is devoid of meaning oncology leaving room for local progression of neoplastic disease.

In the case of painful vertebral metastasis not candidates for radiation therapy (e.g. melanoma, renal cell carcinoma) or in the case where it has proved to be ineffective, in order to avoid a surgical vertebrectomy, complex and burdened with high morbidity, a mini-invasive approach through ECT may be indicated.

Gasbarrini et al. performed a minimally invasive treatment with ECT in a metastatic lesion from melanoma of the fifth lumbar vertebra [30] in order to avoid an en bloc resection of the involved vertebra. Through L5 hemilaminectomy, four electrodes were positioned in the vertebral body, and after the intravenous administration of a bolus of bleomycin, electrical impulses were conveyed. At 48-month follow-up, the patient was free of pain with FDG-PET negative for examination for tumour recurrence. Development of electrodes dedicated to the percutaneous treatment of spinal lesions is on study, because electrodes specifically developed for the treatment of bone lesions are unable to maintain the parallelism necessary for optimal electroporation.

Conclusions

Choosing the best therapeutic strategy for bone metastases is often difficult and depends on many factors which include patients' life expectancy and quality of life, clinical symptoms (pain, neurological symptoms), the risk of fracture and the risk/benefit ratio of surgery.

The ECT includes many benefits by combining the effectiveness in local control of the disease to the preservation of the mechanical competence of the skeletal segment. Furthermore, the selective cytotoxicity saves vascular and nerve structures that may be included in the volume of cancer treatment by allowing large margins when radical surgery is not feasible [14, 16, 23].

ECT has the advantage of avoiding surgical exposure, allowing to reach anatomical districts difficult to access through percutaneous approach.

A dedicated software (Pulsar®) allows to plan the placement of each individual electrode, so as to ensure complete coverage of the tumour volume with the electric field, minimizing the risk of disease recurrence. Furthermore, the electrical insulation of the electrode portion that crosses the skin and the subcutaneous tissue prevents the necrosis of the integuments in case of repeated treatments [26–29].

The ECT in the treatment of bone metastases is currently an effective treatment option with low morbidity for the patient, repeatable, and good cost/benefit ratio; in particular, its use is possible even when other strategies have failed.

Although palliation is the main objective in the treatment of patients suffering from bone metastases, currently oligometastatic patients with long life expectancy local control of disease deserve to be prosecuted. Local complications arising from local progression of neoplastic disease, such as pathological fractures, failure of osteosynthesis, neurological disorders, skin ulceration, etc., will have time to manifest itself in the long-surviving patients resulting in impaired quality of life and increased health and social costs.

ECT allows reduction of pain and local control of the disease. In case of impending fracture, ECT can be performed during the same surgical session of preventive osteosynthesis, with slight increase of the surgical time. In patients who are not candidates for surgery, ECT can be performed percutaneously, under CT or intensifier guidance, thus minimizing the risks and morbidity for the patient. In view of these advantages, it is currently included in the guidelines of the Italian Society of Orthopaedics and Traumatology (SIOT) for the treatment of non-resectable tumours of the sacrum [31].

The preclinical evidence and clinical experience support the use of ECT in the treatment of bone metastases. The selection of the candidate who can most benefit from treatment with ECT is multidisciplinary and must consider not only the characteristics of the patient but also the different available therapeutic possibilities, their limitations and their success rates.

It has recently been developed by the Registry on Electrochemotherapy in Bone (ReinBone) study, a national registry which collects all the cases of bone metastases treated by ECT. The increased knowledge that will result from the sharing of different clinical and surgical experiences will form the basis for improving the quality of care offered to cancer patients.

References

1. Coleman RE. Metastatic bone disease: clinical features, pathophysiology and treatment strategies. Cancer Treat Rev. 2001;27:165–76.
2. Jacofsky DJ, Frassica DA, Frassica FJ. Metastatic disease to bone. Hosp Physician. 2004;39:21–8.

3. Bickels J, Dadia S, Lidar Z. Surgical management of metastatic bone disease. J Bone Joint Surg Am. 2009;91(6):1503–16. (Review).
4. Callstrom MR, Charboneau JW, Goetz MP, et al. Image-guided ablation of painful metastatic bone tumors: a new and effective approach to a difficult problem. Skelet Radiol. 2006;35:1–15.
5. Culleton S, Kwok S, Chow E. Radiotherapy for pain. Clin Oncol. 2010;23:399–406.
6. Jeremic B, Shibamoto Y, Acimovic L, et al. A randomized trial of three single dose radiation therapy regimens in the treatment of metastatic bone pain. Int J Radiat Oncol Biol Phys. 1998;42:161–7.
7. Sze WM, Shelley M, Held I, Mason M. Palliation of metastatic bone pain: single fraction versus multifraction radiotherapy a systemic review of randomized trial. Clin Oncol (R Coll Radiol). 2003;15(6):345–52.
8. Yang L, Du S. Efficacy and safety of zoledronic acid and pamidronate disodium in the treatment of malignant skeletal metastasis: a meta-analysis. Medicine (Baltimore). 2015;94(42):e1822.
9. Mir LM, Belehradek M, Domenge C, et al. Electrochemotherapy, a new antitumor treatment: first clinical trial. C R Acad Sci III. 1991;313:613–8.
10. Mir L, Glass L, Sersa G, Teissie J, Domenge C, Miklavcic D, et al. Effective treatment of cutaneous and subcutaneous malignant tumours by electrochemotherapy. Br J Cancer. 1998;77:2336–42.
11. Belehradek M, Domenge C, Luboinski B, Orlowski S, Belehradek J, Mir LM. Electrochemotherapy, a new antitumor treatment. First clinical phase I-II trial. Cancer. 1993;72:3694–700.
12. Colombo GL, Di Matteo S, Mir LM. Cost-effectiveness analysis of electrochemotherapy with the Cliniporator™ vs other methods for the control and treatment of cutaneous and subcutaneous tumors. Ther Clin Risk Manag. 2008;4(2):541–8.
13. Kotnik T, Pucihar G, Miklavcic D. Induced transmembrane voltage and its correlation with electroporation-mediated molecular transport. J Membr Biol. 2010;236:3–13.
14. Li W, Fan Q, Ji Z, et al. The effects of irreversible electroporation (IRE) on nerves. PLoS One. 2011;6(4):e18831.
15. Mali B, Jarm T, Corovic S, et al. The effect of electroporation pulses on functioning of the heart. Med Biol Eng Comput. 2008;46:745–57.
16. Maor E, Ivorra A, Leor J, Rubinsky B. The effect of irreversible electroporation on blood vessels. Technol Cancer Res Treat. 2007;6(4):307–12.
17. Horiuchi A, Nikaido T, Mitsushita J, et al. Enhancement of antitumor effect of bleomycin by low-voltage in vivo electroporation: a study of human uterine leiomyosarcomas in nude mice. Int J Cancer. 2000;88(4):640–4.
18. Marty M, Sersa G, Garbay JR, et al. Electrochemotherapy - an easy, highly effective and safe treatment of cutaneous and subcutaneous metastases: results of ESOPE (European standard operating procedures of electrochemotherapy) study. EJC Suppl. 2006;4:3–13.
19. Mali B, Jarm T, Snoj M, Sersa G, Miklavcic D. Antitumor effectiveness of electrochemotherapy: a systematic review and meta-analysis. Eur J Surg Oncol. 2013;39(1):4–16.
20. Agerholm-Larsen B, Iversen HK, Ibsen P, Moller JM, Mahmood F, Jensen KS, et al. Preclinical validation of electrochemotherapy as an effective treatment for brain tumors. Cancer Res. 2011;71:3753–62.
21. Fini M, Tschon M, Ronchetti M, et al. Ablation of bone cells by electroporation. J Bone Joint Surg Br. 2010;92(11):1614–20.
22. Fini M, Salamanna F, Parrilli A, Martini L, Cadossi M, Maglio M, Borsari V. Electrochemotherapy is effective in the treatment of rat bone metastases. Clin Exp Metastasis. 2013;30(8):1033–45.
23. Tschon M, Salamanna F, Ronchetti M, Cavani F, Gasbarrini A, Boriani S, Fini M. Feasibility of electroporation in bone and in the surrounding clinically relevant structures: a preclinical investigation. Technol Cancer Res Treat. 2016;15(6):737–48.
24. Campana LG, Mocellin S, Basso M, et al. Bleomycin-based electrochemotherapy: clinical outcome from a single institution's experience with 52 patients. Ann Surg Oncol. 2009;16(1):191–9.
25. Sersa G, Jarm T, Kotnik T, et al. Vascular disrupting action of electroporation and electrochemotherapy with bleomycin in murine sarcoma. Br J Cancer. 2008;98(2):388–98.
26. Bianchi G, Campanacci L, Ronchetti M, Donati D. Electrochemotherapy in the treatment of bone metastases: a phase II trial. World J Surg. 2016;40(12):3088–94.
27. Miklavcic D, Beravs K, Semrov D, et al. The importance of electric field distribution for effective in vivo electroporation of tissues. Biophys J. 1998;74:2152–8.
28. Miklavcic D, Corovic S, Pucihar G, et al. Importance of tumour coverage by sufficiently high local electric field for effective electrochemotherapy. EJC Suppl. 2006;4:45–51.
29. Miklavcic D, Snoj M, Zupanic A, et al. Towards treatment planning and treatment of deep-seated solid tumors by electrochemotherapy. Biomed Eng Online. 2010;9:10.
30. Gasbarrini A, Campos WK, Campanacci L, Boriani S. Electrochemotherapy to metastatic spinal melanoma: a novel treatment of spinal metastasis? Spine. 2015;40(24):1340–6.
31. Gruppo di Studio SIOT sulle Metastasi Ossee, coordinator A. Piccioli. Linee guida: trattamento delle metastasi ossee nello scheletro appendicolare. GIOT. 2014;40:1–15.

MR-Guided Focused Ultrasound Treatment

25

Alessandro Napoli, Roberto Scipione,
Rocco Cannata, and Oreste Moreschini

Abstract

Magnetic resonance-guided focused ultrasound (MRgFUS) is an innovative noninvasive technique for pain management in skeletal metastases. This technology enables the performance of three-dimensional treatment planning with MR imaging and continuous real-time temperature monitoring of target zone with MR thermometric map, ensuring an accurate identification of the lesion and its margins and preventing surrounding healthy tissues from unwanted procedure-related damages. Acoustic energy application on the intact bone surface determines a rapid heating that induces critical thermal damage to the adjacent periosteum, with necrosis of local nerve endings and effective pain management. This procedure has also a potential role in effective local tumor control, allowing the complete ablation of target lesion, or the reduction of its size, and remineralization of trabecular bone. The whole MRgFUS protocol for ablation of bone metastases includes a pre-procedural imaging study, the choice for a strategy of simple palliation of pain or of local tumor control, the choice of the most appropriate anesthetic approach, the technical planning stage, the focal ablation treatment, the post-intervention management, and the clinical and imaging evaluation of treatment outcomes at different subsequent follow-ups.

Keywords

MRgFUS · Skeletal metastases · Pain management · High-intensity focused ultrasound · Ablative treatment

25.1 Introduction

Magnetic resonance-guided focused ultrasound (MRgFUS) has emerged as an innovative and promising technique that can treat a variety of solid benign and malignant lesions [1, 2]. The application of this procedure is under current investigation for pancreas, liver, prostate, and breast carcinomas and for soft-tissue sarcomas, while uterine fibroids represent the target with the most consolidated experience; this technique also represents a feasible option for bone lesions, such as osteoid osteoma and painful bone metastasis [3]. Another FDA and CE marked application of high interest is the treatment of functional neurological disorders (essential tremor or Parkinson).

A. Napoli · R. Scipione
Department of Radiological, Oncological and Anatomopathological Sciences - Radiology, "Sapienza" University of Rome, Rome, Italy

R. Cannata · O. Moreschini (✉)
Department of Anatomical Sciences, Histological, Forensic Medicine and Locomotive System, "Sapienza" University of Rome, Rome, Italy.
e-mail: oreste.moreschini@gmail.com

MRgFUS couples the use of focused ultrasound mechanical energy with MR scan. The first one induces a rise of target tissue temperature, resulting in a focal thermal ablation, while the second ensures an accurate three-dimensional visualization for treatment planning, thermal real-time monitoring, and immediate assessment of therapy.

Differently from other ablative procedures, such as cryoablation or radiofrequency, MRgFUS is completely noninvasive and does not require ionizing radiation, so it can be easily repeated in case of symptom recurrence or new tumor appearance. The treatment can be performed in an outpatient protocol.

The procedure is performed by an interventional radiologist, who has direct control over the areas to be ablated, while a dedicated software automatically determines the optimal treatment parameters.

25.2 MR-Guided Focused Ultrasound Technique: Basic Technical Principles

25.2.1 Interaction Between High-Intensity Focused Ultrasound and Biological Tissues

Acoustic energy of focused ultrasound systems (ExAblate, InSightec, Tirat Carmel, Israel) is generated by a piezoelectric transducer housed within the MR patient table. The transducer features a 208-element annular phased array (diameter, 120 mm; radius of curvature, 160 mm; focal distance, 60–200 mm; frequencies, 0.95–1.35 MHz; and energy range, 100–7200 J) and operates at frequency values between 200 kHz and 4 MHz, with an intensity that ranges between 100 and 10,000 W/cm^2 in the focal region, and with peak compression pressure of up to 70 MPa and peak rarefaction pressure of up to 20 MPa. At these energy levels, the focused ultrasound beams determine a heating of biological tissues inside the treated region. The increased cell temperature leads to coagulative

necrosis at a thermal range of 65–85 °C, depending on the tissue absorption coefficient [4].

In order to pursue an accurate control of the borders of the treated area, to maximize the efficacy of the focal ablation, and to guarantee an optimal synergy with MR temperature monitoring, focused ultrasound delivery is usually fractioned in sequential *sonications*, each of those is usually limited to focal volumes of 0.2–5 mm^3. A single sonication has duration of only a few seconds, and therefore, the potential detrimental effects of perfusion and blood flow on energy distribution are reduced. Thereby, multiple subsequent sonications are required to ensure the ablation of large volumes and to create homogeneous thermal damage and coagulative necrosis of the target lesion [5].

Another potential effect induced by focused ultrasound energy on biologic tissues is represented by cavitations, a nonthermal phenomenon due to microbubbles formation at high acoustic intensities within the treated area; when the size of the microbubbles exceeds a critical threshold, they may implode, producing micro-shock waves that can damage surrounding tissues. Cavitations can have unpredictable results; therefore, their application in clinical practice is usually avoided.

25.2.2 Role of MR Imaging Guidance

High-intensity focused ultrasound treatment is usually performed under imaging control with a 1.5T or 3T MR scanner that ensures the optimal US beam delivery. Specifically, the quantitative thermometry map is a technique based on phase-difference fast spoiled gradient-echo MR sequences that enables calculation of thermal dose and its distribution over anatomic MR structures, with particular attention to the regions in which it has reached cytotoxic levels. In other words, this technique provides a real-time mapping of the thermal dose on a preferred imaging plane during MRgFUS treatment, allowing for a closed-loop control of energy deposition, with temperature accuracy of 1 °C, spatial resolution of 1 mm, and temporal resolution of 3 s. In the specific clinical application of bone lesions, MR thermometry does not measure direct temperature variations in the bone (because of the absence of mobile protons in the cortical bone), so it is necessary to evaluate the tightly adjacent soft tissues that instead present a linear response to bone temperature increase.

Sapareto and Dewey equation [6] allows to establish the needed time for each employed temperature in order to obtain a critical treatment (defined as the 100% killing of target tissue cells). The treatment can be modulated according to the real-time MR feedback: US energy can be increased or decreased, if the measured temperature is insufficient or excessive, respectively; the possibility of modifying previously established sonication parameters represents one of the greatest strengths of MR control and provides an optimization of the treatment plan.

25.3 MRgFUS Application in Clinical Practice for Bone Lesions Ablation

Cortical bone is characterized by a particularly high ultrasound absorption rate, so that the wide majority of delivered energy is reflected by the interface between bone surface and adjacent soft tissue, while only a minimal fraction penetrates across the cortex [5]. Consequently, the first years of experience with MRgFUS application to the bone were limited to the palliation of pain from superficial lesions, while deep lesions inside the bone structure were considered as non-feasible targets.

As it was shown in subsequent works [7], the application of acoustic energy on the cortical bone intact surface determines a critical thermal damage to the adjacent periosteum, the highest innervated component of mature bone, and its ablation is an extremely effective approach for pain management.

Moreover, even if cortical bone is characterized by high acoustic absorption and low thermal conductivity that significantly limit the diffusion of US energy to the bone cortex surface in conventional protocols, innovative protocols with modulated parameters seem to reach a therapeutic effective heating threshold even at deeper levels within the bone [8]. In particular, the increase of acoustic energy levels, the increase of sonication duration, and the decrease of the frequency are potential modulations that can be used separately or in conjunction to facilitate penetration inside intact cortical bone. If cortical bone disruption is present, there is no absorption barrier, and the ultrasound beam can be delivered following standard protocols, thus potentially obtaining local tumor control.

25.4 Patient Selection

25.4.1 Clinical Indications

MRgFUS treatment can be considered as a reasonable option for the management of painful bone lesions from metastatic disease; this technique should address only patients with known history of malignancy, and the clinical condition should always be confirmed by imaging examinations [7]. MRgFUS is particularly recommended in those cases known as *radiation failures*: this category includes patients with no adequate clinical benefit after radiation administration, those who refuse additional radiation treatment, and those who can no longer receive radiation therapy because of safety issues.

25.4.2 Inclusion Criteria

- Accessible sites to MRgFUS treatment are posterior parts of the dorsal, lumbar, and sacral vertebra, ribs, sternum, pelvis, shoulders, or extremities (excluding the joints).
- The lesion must be identified on MR or CT images.
- The ultrasound beam path must reach the target lesion without crossing shielding or reflecting

anatomic structures, such as hollow viscera, nontargeted bone, or extensive scarring.

- The interface bone lesion should be deeper than 10 mm from the skin surface.

25.4.3 Exclusion Criteria

- General contraindications to MR (e.g., severe claustrophobia, permanent cardiac pacemaker, metallic implant likely to contribute significant artefact to images) and to gadolinium injection
- Concomitant acute or chronic medical conditions (e.g., cardiovascular, respiratory, neurologic, or infectious disorders) that may impair imaging acquisition, anesthesia, or technical intervention
- Affected bone at high risk of fracture, requiring surgical stabilization, or affected bone already surgically stabilized with metallic tools.
- Planned US beam path passing through extensive scarring or other reflecting structures (see inclusion criteria)
- Target lesion localization inside the skull, the vertebral body, at less than 1 cm from the skin surface, or at less than 1 cm from nerve bundles

25.5 MRgFUS Procedure Protocol

25.5.1 Pre-procedural Imaging Study

An optimal treatment planning requires an accurate preliminary lesion localization and characterization with imaging; both CT and MR scans should be acquired in order to guarantee the best quality of the study. Key parameters that must be considered during this process are tumor size, location, and extent, device accessibility to the tumor, and the presence of scarring, metal clips, or other reflecting structure along the planned ultrasound beam path.

Unenhanced CT is highly indicated to evaluate bone structures: it allows to study only the mineralized component of the lesions and to distinguish between osteoblastic and osteolytic metastases; the integrity or infiltration of adjacent cortical bone can also be investigated.

MR imaging exploits both T1- and T2-weighted morphologic sequences, with and without fat signal saturation. Additional functional studies are performed with diffusion-weighted imaging sequences (including calculation of apparent diffusion coefficient [ADC]) and three-dimensional dynamic contrast-enhanced T1-weighted sequences and are a fundamental starting point for the evaluation of treatment outcomes at follow-up.

Pre-procedural imaging is essential for the establishment of the optimal acoustic window and the ultrasound beam conformation, two technical issues that lead the whole MRgFUS procedure. Target volume must be accurately defined, because tumor margins must be correctly identified and included inside it. Air and nontarget bone structures must be avoided by the energy path, as they shield the propagation of ultrasound and obscure targets beyond them, generating potential reflection phenomena along their interfaces. Rib metastases are a feasible target only if there is enough bone thickness interposed between the lesion and the lung that blocks the undesirable heating of lung tissue, as a safety measure.

25.5.2 Choice of Anesthetic Approach

Case-specific factors, such as target lesion localization, clinical presentation, and anamnesis (age, allergies, renal function, current pharmacologic therapy, cardiovascular and respiratory risk factors, infections), guide the choice of anesthetics. In our experience, the use of local anesthetics is not a first choice due to the poor pain control during treatment that can be highly painful at high energy dose.

General anesthetics are usually reserved to procedures targeting upper trunk lesions (proximal humerus, scapula, sternum, and clavicle); on the contrary, lesions involving the limbs can be managed by ultrasound-guided peripheral nerve blocks, and lesions located in the lower trunk, spine, or proximal femur, through a spinal block.

25.5.3 Planning Phase

The planning phase is conducted just before the actual treatment, with the patient already on the table inside the MR unit. Patient positioning is an important step of planning procedure and aims to center target lesion directly over the focused ultrasound transducer; an MR acquisition is obtained afterward to confirm the optimal position.

Subsequent steps include calibration, loading, segmentation, planning, and verification.

- During the *calibration* step, the operator chooses the most appropriate initial position and orientation of the ultrasound transducer, consistently with previous patient positioning.
- In the *loading* step, MR scans are collected, and these images represent the base for subsequent planning stages.
- In the *segmentation* step, the interventional radiologist manually defines the region of treatment, the skin surface, the bone cortex, and the areas surrounding the target lesion; particular attention is needed for the so-called limited energy density regions, sensitive structures close to target region that may determine energy dispersion and unwanted thermal damage: these critical areas must be carefully identified and highlighted in order to avoid side effects during the treatment phase. During the segmentation step, the treatment volume may be limited to the superficial periosteum, or it can involve also the deeper tumor tissue to attempt a complete ablation of the lesion. During this step, the operator establishes on MR images fiducial anatomic

markers, useful for detection and compensation of physiologic or accidental motion of the patient during the treatment.

- In the *planning* step, starting from previous RM images, the dedicated software automatically calculates the optimal treatment plan that aims to cover the target with the minimal number of needed sonications, preventing unwanted damages to sensible adjacent tissue. Each established parameter can be modified by the operator at any moment: the sonication locations, the number of sonications, the energy levels, the sonication duration, the cooling duration, or the spot sizes.
- In the *verification* step, a low-energy sonication test, below ablation threshold, is performed to confirm the beam path into the target area. The direction of generated ultrasound can be modified to reach the optimal result.

25.5.4 Ablative Treatment

Once that all the steps of planning phase are completed and show favorable outcomes, the actual treatment phase can be started; at this point, target lesions receive full-energy sonications. Sonications are considered completely therapeutic beyond a threshold of 65 °C for both periosteum and target tissue. Intact cortical bone usually requires a lower level of ultrasound energy (1500–3000 J) to produce periosteal damage. When cortical erosion is present, the treatment can be limited to the surrounding vital periosteum. In addition, the soft-tissue component of the tumor can be ablated by using higher acoustic energies (2500–6500 J).

During ablation phase, real-time MR thermometric map is used to evaluate the temperature rise of neoplastic and healthy tissues and ensures a careful real-time monitoring of the delivered thermal dose into the desired tumor location that is monitored throughout the therapy.

25.5.5 Post-intervention Management

Posttreatment management is usually based on the anesthetic strategy: patients receiving local anesthetics or a spinal block follow an outpatient protocol, while patients under general anesthesia require 24-h hospitalization. During post-procedural management, it is important to evaluate the skin surface to identify skin burns, to monitor vital signs (oxygen saturation, ECG), and to administrate pain drug if necessary.

Nonsignificant or minor side effects of MRgFUS normally resolve without sequelae within 10–14 days after the procedure: pain in the area of treatment, first/second degree skin burns less than 2 cm in diameter or bruising in the treated area, and transient fever. Significant or major side effects may require medical treatment, may have sequelae, and their time of resolution is not defined: necrosis of tissue outside the targeted volume because of heat conduction from heated bone, bowel perforation, skin burns with ulceration, and complications of anesthetics (cardiac, pulmonary complications, drug reactions).

25.5.6 Assessment of Treatment Success

Treatment success is defined with both clinical evaluation of pain resolution and imaging studies to assess tumor control.

25.5.6.1 Clinical Evaluation
For the clinical evaluation, data are collected at 1, 3, 7, and 14 days after procedure and then at 30-day intervals for 1 year. Clinical data include an evaluation of a visual analog pain scale (VAS), changes in the drug schedule, and improvements in quality of life.

The VAS is a 0–10 pain scale, where 0 describes a complete absence of pain, and 10 is the worst possible pain. A complete response is defined as a VAS of 0 without an increase in medication, while a partial response is defined as a drop of two points in the VAS from the baseline conditions, with no increase in pain medication, or a reduction of 25% in pain medication without an increase in VAS score.

A change in the drug schedule is defined by a decrease in the analgesics or opiates intake.

The improvement in quality of life (as measured by the Brief Pain Inventory Quality of Life questionnaire) assesses changes in the impact of pain on key domains of daily living, such as physical activity, work, mood, ambulation, and sleep.

25.5.6.2 Imaging Evaluation
Real-time assessment of thermal damage with MR thermometry during treatment is completed by other MR studies after therapy, including immediately afterward and at 1-, 3-, 6-, and 12-month follow-up.

After treatment, diffusion-weighted imaging sequences and three-dimensional dynamic contrast-enhanced T1-weighted sequences are used to estimate the potential increase in ADC values and potential NPV of the lesions; NPV is defined as the ratio between the non-perfused posttreatment lesion volume and the whole pretreatment lesion volume and provides information about the ablated volume in both the periosteum and metastases. A complete overlap of the NPV with the original perfused lesion volume is considered as a successful ablation of both the periosteal component and metastasis. If the lesion was not completely accessible for ablation, the NPV should at least overlap with the periosteal component to achieve pain relief. ADC variations are not sensible for bone metastases, even after a complete ablation, especially at first follow-ups: ADC should always be combined with contrast-enhanced imaging to obtain a more reliable assessment of effective tissue ablation.

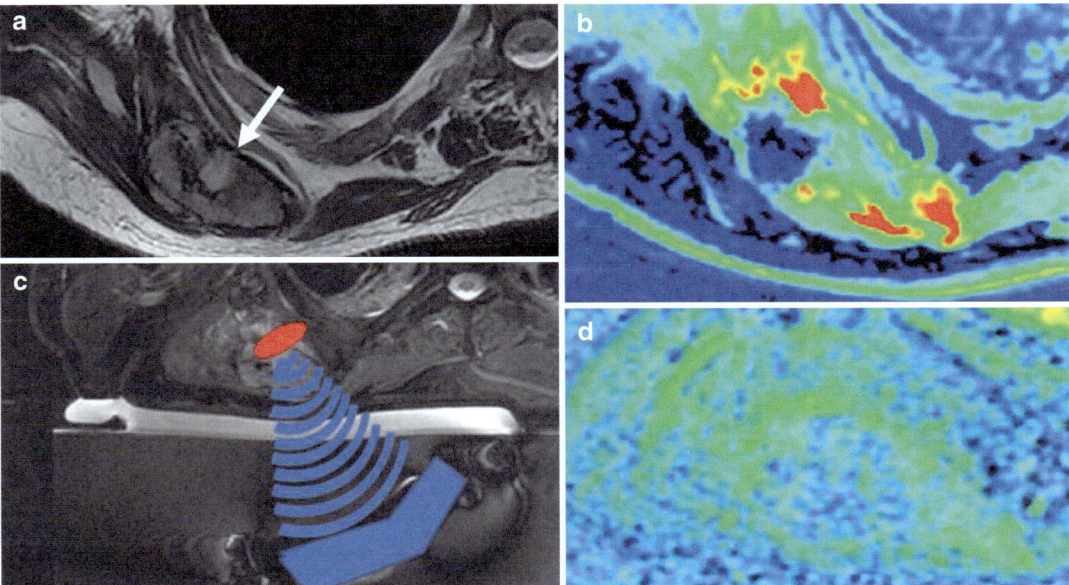

Fig. 25.1 74-year-old man affected by melanoma with multiple bone metastases previously treated with EBRT. Patient-reported high-intensity pain and disability (VAS = 8) on his right shoulder and right arm, due to the lesion located on the right scapula (**a**, axial T2-weighted MR image showing solid mass (*white arrow*) replacing the scapula bone); MRI perfusion sequence of the metastasis was also obtained (**b**) showing highly perfused peripheral zone of the metastasis with necrotic core. The lesion was then treated with single MRgFUS procedure (**c**) treatment lasted for 1 h and 20 min, requiring 26 sonications and average energy deposition of 2450 J. Three days after treatment, the patient discontinued medication for pain management (VAS = 0): the metastasis was successfully ablated at MRI perfusion control (**d**)

At 1, 3, 6, and 12 months after treatment, both MR imaging and CT examinations are used to assess treatment effects in the target zone and to evaluate potential tumor necrosis or recurrence. CT scan is used to demonstrate potential signs of de novo mineralization in the treated area as a further indicator of treatment success, while MR imaging evaluation follows the same criteria and sequences used for the aftertreatment control.

Figures 25.1 and 25.2 present two exemplificative cases of patients with bone metastasis treated with MRgFUS and provide specific imaging results together with clinical outcomes.

Fig. 25.2 36-year-old woman with breast cancer and multiple bone metastases that had exhausted the allowed X-ray maximum dose for EBRT; the patient presented high pain level (VAS = 10) at the right hip with dramatic impact on the quality of life, due to the lesion located on the right pelvic bone, just above the acetabulum roof. Images on the left column (**a**) show baseline condition detected on the pretreatment CT scan, while the right column (**b**) illustrates the corresponding images on 2-month CT follow-up; the first image of each column is taken from a frontal section, while the other two are axial views on different levels. The comparison of tomographic images highlights the effective impact of MRgFUS ablation. The large osteolytic lesion, located in a weight-bearing zone, demonstrated partial de novo mineralization as effect of the single MRgFUS treatment. The beneficial effect detected on imaging matches with a noticeable clinical improvement (VAS = 0 at 2 months)

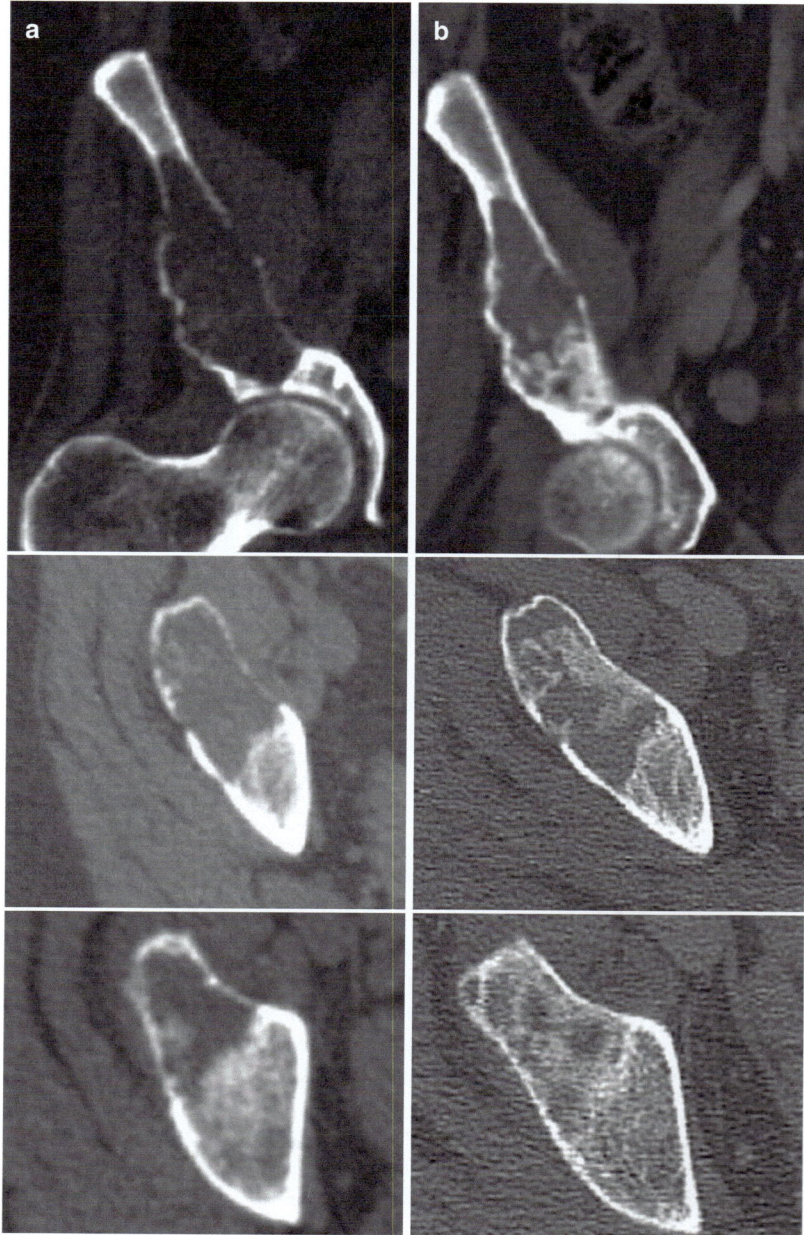

Conclusions

MR imaging-guided focused ultrasound ablation is an extremely promising alternative therapy for pain palliation and tumor control in patients suffering from bone metastases. The major advantages of the technique include its noninvasive nature; the ability to perform three-dimensional MR imaging visualization for precise treatment planning; continuous temperature mapping of treated tissue with MR thermometry, which enables real-time monitoring of thermal damage in the target zone; and immediate posttreatment assessment of therapy. Furthermore, MRgFUS treatment can be performed to patients regardless of concomitant chemotherapy regimen, limiting—wherever possible—radiation exposure and related toxic effects.

References

1. Napoli A, Anzidei M, Ciolina F, Marotta E, Marincola BC, Brachetti G, et al. MR-guided high-intensity focused ultrasound: current status of an emerging technology. Cardiovasc Intervent Radiol. 2013;36(5):1190–203.
2. Dick E, Gedroyc W. ExAblate® magnetic resonance-guided focused ultrasound system in multiple body applications. Expert Rev Med Devices. 2010;7(5):589–97.
3. Napoli A, Anzidei M, Marincola BC, Brachetti G, Noce V, Boni F, et al. MR imaging–guided focused ultrasound for treatment of bone metastasis. Radiographics. 2013;33(6):1555–68.
4. Simon CJ, Dupuy DE, Mayo-Smith WW. Microwave ablation: principles and applications 1. Radiographics. 2005;25(suppl_1):S69–83.
5. Jolesz FA, Hynynen K. Magnetic resonance image-guided focused ultrasound surgery. Cancer J (Sudbury, Mass). 2001;8:S100–12.
6. Sapareto SA, Dewey WC. Thermal dose determination in cancer therapy. Int J Radiat Oncol Biol Phys. 1984;10(6):787–800.
7. Catane R, Beck A, Inbar Y, Rabin T, Shabshin N, Hengst S, et al. MR-guided focused ultrasound surgery (MRgFUS) for the palliation of pain in patients with bone metastases—preliminary clinical experience. Ann Oncol. 2007;18(1):163–7.
8. Chen W, Zhu H, Zhang L, Li K, Su H, Jin C, et al. Primary bone malignancy: effective treatment with high-intensity focused ultrasound ablation 1. Radiology. 2010;255(3):967–78.

Part V

Future Directions

What Is New in Management of Bone Metastases

26

Costantino Errani and Davide Maria Donati

Abstract

Metastatic tumors are the most common malignancy of the bone. Traditional management techniques involve a combination of pharmacotherapy, radiotherapy, and surgical procedures. Novel medical treatments combined with less invasive surgical procedures can offer an effective palliative option in patients with limited life expectancy. Denosumab, a monoclonal antibody targeting receptor activator of nuclear factor kappa-B ligand (RANKL), was found to be a promising new therapeutic strategy for patients with bone metastases by restricting bone destruction. However, the scientific community should be aware of the possible association of denosumab treatment with occurrence of new malignancies.

Advancements in surgical techniques have led to the development of the concept of less invasive surgical procedures with the aim of achieving the same clinical results with less morbidity related to the surgical approach. Less invasive procedures include the following: endoscopic surgery, computer-assisted surgery, and minimally invasive percutaneous surgery. Benefits of less invasive techniques include decreased blood loss, less postoperative pain, and shortened recovery time. Less invasive procedures also allow earlier initiation of postoperative adjuvant treatments. Considering the limited expectancy of most patients with bone metastases, the main goal of novel medical and surgical treatments is to improve the quality of life of patients with bone metastases reducing the adverse effects related to the traditional medical or surgical treatments.

Keywords

Bone metastases · Novel therapies · Denosumab · Endoscopic surgery · Computer-assisted surgery · Minimally invasive percutaneous surgery

26.1 Introduction

The prevalence of metastatic bone disease in the United State is high (280,000 per year) [1] and is expected to increase as patients with cancer live longer [2]. The bone is the third most common site of metastatic disease after the lung and liver. Postmortem analysis shows that around 70% of all patients with breast and prostate cancer have skeletal metastases, and between 35 and 42% of

C. Errani (✉) · D. M. Donati
Orthopaedic Service, Istituto Ortopedico Rizzoli,
Bologna, Italy
e-mail: costantino.errani@ior.it

patients with lung, thyroid, and renal cancer [3]. The economic costs of treating metastatic bone disease in the United States per year are an estimated $12.6 billion, which is 17% of the total annual cost of cancer treatments [4].

Although malignant primary bone tumors are usually managed by orthopedic surgeons with expertise in oncology, patients with metastatic disease of the bone may be treated by general orthopedic surgeons at community hospitals [2].

Metastatic bone lesions have more similarities than differences. For the most part, surgical intervention is similar across the spectrum. Predicting survival in patients with bone metastasis often helps in directing care [5].

Over the last few decades, advances in medical and surgical treatment have been proposed regarding the management of metastatic bone disease. Immediate pain relief and improvement of the functional status is particularly important for patients with a short life expectancy [6]. If surgical or medical treatment is necessary, we have to consider the expected life span of the patient. Shorter life expectancies may require less invasive procedures that do not need prolonged rehabilitation [7]. New medical and surgical treatments should have the purpose of reducing trauma compared to conventional approaches.

26.2   New Medical Treatment

Bone metastases lead to local bone destruction and skeletal complications. Osteoclast inhibitors, such as bisphosphonates, have been used as the standard treatment for solid cancer or myeloma with bone metastases [8]. Bisphosphonates have been one of the key pharmaceutical treatments in patients with bone metastases. Within the class of bisphosphonates, zoledronic acid has been shown to effectively decrease the risk of pathologic fracture and other skeletal-related events, including hypercalcemia [9]. Some studies have shown that denosumab, a new monoclonal antibody, may delay and prevent skeletal-related events in metastatic bone disease more effectively than zoledronic acid [10]. However, other authors found similar results between denosumab and zoledronic acid in the treatment of bone metastases [9]. Denosumab is a new human monoclonal antibody that binds to the receptor activator of nuclear factor-k B ligand (RANKL). By binding to RANKL, denosumab inhibits the interaction between receptor activator of nuclear factor-k B (RANK) and RANKL, which in turn decreases osteoclast activity, decreases bone resorption, and increases bone mass [9]. Henry et al. reported a randomized double-blind study of denosumab versus zoledronic acid in the treatment of patients with bone metastases. Denosumab was found to be as effective as zoledronic acid in preventing or delaying skeletal-related events, including pathologic fractures [9]. A meta-analysis of six randomized controlled trials involving 13,733 patients confirmed only slightly superior effectiveness of denosumab compared to zoledronic acid in decreasing the rate of skeletal-related events. However, occurrences of adverse events such as hypocalcemia, renal adverse events, and new primary malignancy were significantly different between denosumab and zoledronic acid. Only the occurrence of osteonecrosis of the jaw showed no significant difference between the denosumab and zoledronic acid. Chen and Pu recently performed a meta-analysis of randomized controlled trials showing the safety of denosumab versus zoledronic acid in patients with bone metastases. They found that a new primary malignancy occurred significantly more frequently in patients treated with denosumab than with zoledronic acid [10]. Expression of RANKL plays an important role in B- and T-cell differentiation, and its inhibition could eventually increase the risk of new malignancies due to immunosuppression [11]. Zheng et al. [8] compared three randomized controlled trials with a total of 5544 patients with advanced solid tumors and bone metastases; there were 2776 patients treated with denosumab, and 2768 patients treated with zoledronic acid. This meta-analysis showed that denosumab was superior to zoledronic acid in delaying time to skeletal-related events. However, no significant difference was found in overall survival improvement between denosumab and zoledronic acid [8].

These data do not support denosumab as a potential novel treatment option for the management of bone metastases in advanced solid tumors, showing that the long-term safety of denosumab has not yet been assessed, and long-term treatment surveillance is still ongoing [11].

26.3   New Surgical Treatments

New surgical approaches for the management of patients with bone metastases include the following: endoscopic surgery, computer-assisted surgery, and minimally invasive percutaneous surgery (Table 26.1).

26.3.1 Endoscopic Surgery

Only few previous reports have shown the use of minimally invasive approaches using an endoscopic technique for the treatment of primary bone tumors [12, 13]. Minimally invasive tech-

niques using an arthroscope seem to be a method for accessing lesions in difficult locations, such as juxta-articular or spinal tumors. In fact, direct endoscopic visualization allows safer and less destructive excision. This minimal surgical approach could minimize morbidity and facilitate rapid functional recovery without compromising oncological principles [12].

Endoscopic surgery seems to have selective indications for the treatment of bone metastases in the thoracic spine, as an alternative to classic open anterior approaches [14]. The indications for spinal endoscopy are lesions of the anterior column caused by metastatic bone disease. The main advantage of endoscopy is that the upper thoracic spine (T2–T4) and the thoracolumbar junction (T11–L2) can be approached with no disinsertion of the scapula or minimal disinsertion of the diaphragm, enabling complex reconstructions without additional trauma [14]. The endoscopic surgery seems also be a useful adjunct to surgery in completing lateral approaches to the craniovertebral junction [15]. Severe pulmonary restriction and the impossibility of performing selective intubation are the most important contraindications for this procedure [14].

A cervical approach does not allow for good spinal cord decompression at levels T1, T2, or T3 because of the instability of seeing the posterior vertebral ligament and the difficulty of performing an osteosynthesis is not easy due to the obliquity of access [16]. Le Huec et al. reported an endoscopic approach to the cervicothoracic junction in two patients with spinal metastases. A strut graft was fixed anteriorly after decompression of the spinal cord. The use of the endoscope was the key to providing a good view of the spine without an extensile exposure [16]. The operating time for the two patients was 2 h 15 min and 3 h, and the blood loss was 300 and 400 cc, respectively [16].

The video-assisted technique could be a promising less invasive surgical procedure. The indications still seem limited, but in selected cases, this method could minimize the surgical approach and optimize visualization.

Table 26.1 Indications and limits of recently developed technologies in bone metastasis surgery

Procedure	Indications	Limits
Endoscopic surgery	• Bone metastases of cranio-vertebral junction • Bone metastases of upper thoracic spine (T2–T4) • Bone metastases of thoracolumbar junction	• Pachypleuritis • Pneumonectomy on the contralateral side of the approach • Severe pulmonary restriction • Selective intubation not possible
Computer-assisted surgery	• Pelvic bone metastases • Sacral bone metastases	• Bone metastases with extra-osseous soft tissue mass
Minimally invasive percutaneous stabilization	• Spinal bone metastases	• Patients with potentially long survival (>24 months) • Need for neural decompression

26.3.2 Computer-Assisted Surgery

In literature to date, computer-navigated surgery has been used to assist with the resection of primary musculoskeletal tumors [17]. The use of computer navigation systems seems to be promising in difficult tumor resections from regions with complex local anatomy, such as the pelvis or sacrum [17].

Young et al. reported 18 resections for sarcoma using computer-assisted surgery. The mean intraoperative registration error was 0.9 mm (0.2–1.6). All patients underwent a wide excision. Surgery was carried out under computer navigation as planned in 16 of the 18 patients. In one patient, the authors were unable to resect the tumor with computer navigation due to the patient's high body mass index (BMI). In the second patient, while planning the plane of acetabular osteotomy for an extra-articular resection of the proximal femur, the authors incorrectly used a mobile bone segment (the femoral head) during preoperative planning when marking the levels and planes of the acetabular osteotomy. Therefore, the authors concluded that a high BMI could increase the error during intraoperative registration by making fixed bony landmarks difficult to find [17].

Wong and Kumta evaluated the accuracy of computer-assisted tumor surgery in 21 malignant tumors. The diagnosis was primary bone sarcoma in 18 and solitary metastatic carcinoma in 3. These three solitary metastatic carcinomas were located in the pelvis, the right acetabulum, the left acetabulum, and the left ischial tuberosity, respectively. A histological examination of all resected specimens showed a clear tumor margin. The resulting bone resection matched the planned one with a difference of <2 mm. Four patients affected by chordoma developed local recurrence, and three were located at the sacral region. The authors postulated that all four patients had local recurrence because they all had large soft tissue extra-osseous tumor extension. In fact, navigation by itself could only assist and guide the bone resection at surgery. Moreover, surgeons still have to adopt a conventional technique in soft tissue resection [18].

The indication of computer-assisted surgery includes bone metastases of the pelvis or sacrum; limits are tumors with extra-osseous soft tissue mass.

26.3.3 Minimally Invasive Percutaneous Surgery

The incidence of spinal metastases is increasing due to early detection and advances in medical treatment of the primary tumor [19]. Recent studies have demonstrated better quality of life in patients with spinal metastases who were treated with surgery compared to radiotherapy [20]. Open surgical procedures are associated with significant risk and morbidities, such as higher risk of infection, postoperative pain, and longer hospitalization [21, 22]. With the development of minimally invasive stabilization of spinal metastases using percutaneous screws, the morbidity associated with open surgery can be avoided [23].

Several authors reported that a minimally invasive approach aims to reduce the amount of muscle dissection required, therefore reducing postoperative pain and duration of hospital stay [23–25].

Kwan et al. reported 50 cases of spinal metastases with pathological fractures treated by minimally invasive spinal stabilization using fluoroscopic-guided percutaneous screws. Thirty-seven patients (74%) required minimally invasive decompression in addition to percutaneous stabilization. The mean number of vertebral levels with pathological fractures was 1.8. The average number of instrumented vertebrae was 7.8 with the longest instrumentation spanning across 15 levels. The average operation time was 3.1 h (range, 1–7 h). The average blood loss was 1.4 L [23].

There was significant pain reduction 2 weeks and 3 months after surgery compared to preoperative pain (both $p < 0.001$). For patients with neurological deficit, 70% displayed improvement of one Frankel grade, and 5% had an improvement of two Frankel grades. There were no surgical complications. However, there was one case of implant failure diagnosed with renal cell carcinoma; this case had a breakage of both rods at the thoracolumbar junction 27 months after the index surgery [23]. The reason for the failure was attributed to the long survival of the patient.

Versteeg et al. performed a minimally invasive spinal stabilization in 101 patients with unstable spinal metastases between 2009 and 2014. The median operating time was 122 min with a median blood loss of 100 mL. Eighty-eight patients (87%) ambulated within the first 3 days after surgery. A complication rate of 18% was reported, suggesting that minimally invasive spinal stabilization may lead to fewer complications compared to open surgical procedures [26].

The limitation of minimally invasive percutaneous spinal stabilization is that this technique does not allow for any fusion of the diseased bone segment. Therefore, patients with potentially long survival (over 24 months) could present the risk of implant failure. In such cases, minimally invasive fusion in addition to minimally invasive percutaneous spinal stabilization could be safely performed [27].

Minimally invasive percutaneous stabilization of spinal metastases seems to be a promising surgical procedure. Using this technique, spinal stabilization and direct neural decompression could be achieved with minimal morbidity for patients with limited life expectancy [25].

The indication of minimally invasive percutaneous stabilization of the spine includes all spinal bone metastases in patients with a life expectancy shorter than 24 months.

Conclusions

Cancer survival has increased annually. Improvements in oncologic management have also increased the survival of patients with a metastatic disease [6]. Skeletal metastases influence the quality of life of patients with a metastatic disease. The indication for surgery depends on pain or impending or pathological fractures and differs between nations [7]. In the United States, up to 71% of patients have been treated due to impending fracture compared with only 18% in Nordic countries [6]. Decisions regarding potential surgery for metastatic disease require reliable data about the patient's survival and quality of life [28].

Patients with metastatic disease are often treated at community centers [2]. Therefore, general orthopedic surgeons need to be familiar with the treatment of these patients. As the treatment of metastatic disease is multidisciplinary, it is imperative that orthopedic surgeons are involved at an early stage with impending fractures and not only following pathological fractures. Immediate pain relief and improvement of the functional status is particularly important for patients with a short life expectancy [6].

The orthopedic surgeon who treats patients with metastatic bone disease needs to be familiar with the biological behavior of metastatic bone lesions that may not heal reliably [2]. Potential advantages of less invasive procedures consist of a decreased need for blood transfusion, a decreased need for analgesics, a shorter hospital stay, an early functional recovery, and an early initiation of postoperative adjuvant therapies [26].

References

1. Cheung FH. The practicing orthopedic surgeon's guide to managing long bone metastases. Orthop Clin North Am. 2014;45:109–19. https://doi.org/10.1016/j.ocl.2013.09.003.
2. Weber KL, Randall RL, Grossman S, Parvizi J. Management of lower-extremity bone metastasis. J Bone Joint Surg Am. 2006;88(Suppl 4):11–9. https://doi.org/10.2106/JBJS.F.00635.
3. Coleman RE. Clinical features of metastatic bone disease and risk of skeletal morbidity. Clin Cancer Res. 2006;12:6243s–9s. https://doi.org/10.1158/1078-0432.CCR-06-0931.
4. Schulman KL, Kohles J. Economic burden of metastatic bone disease in the U.S. Cancer. 2007;109:2334–42. https://doi.org/10.1002/cncr.22678.
5. Errani C, Mavrogenis AF, Cevolani L, et al. Treatment for long bone metastases based on a systematic literature review. Eur J Orthop Surg Traumatol. 2017;27:205–11. https://doi.org/10.1007/s00590-016-1857-9.
6. Ratasvuori M, Wedin R, Hansen BH, et al. Prognostic role of en-bloc resection and late onset of bone metastasis in patients with bone-seeking carcinomas of the kidney, breast, lung, and prostate: SSG study

on 672 operated skeletal metastases. J Surg Oncol. 2014;110:360–5. https://doi.org/10.1002/jso.23654.

7. Forsberg JA, Eberhardt J, Boland PJ, et al. Estimating survival in patients with operable skeletal metastases: an application of a Bayesian belief network. PLoS One. 2011;6:e19956. https://doi.org/10.1371/journal.pone.0019956.

8. Zheng GZ, Chang B, Lin FX, et al. Meta-analysis comparing denosumab and zoledronic acid for treatment of bone metastases in patients with advanced solid tumours. Eur J Cancer Care. 2016. https://doi.org/10.1111/ecc.12541.

9. Henry DH, Costa L, Goldwasser F, et al. Randomized, double-blind study of denosumab versus zoledronic acid in the treatment of bone metastases in patients with advanced cancer (excluding breast and prostate cancer) or multiple myeloma. J Clin Oncol. 2011;29:1125–32. https://doi.org/10.1200/JCO.2010.31.3304.

10. Chen F, Pu F. Safety of denosumab versus zoledronic acid in patients with bone metastases: a meta-analysis of randomized controlled trials. Oncol Res Treat. 2016;39:453–9. https://doi.org/10.1159/000447372.

11. Criscitiello C, Viale G, Gelao L, et al. Crosstalk between bone niche and immune system: osteoimmunology signaling as a potential target for cancer treatment. Cancer Treat Rev. 2015;41:61–8. https://doi.org/10.1016/j.ctrv.2014.12.001.

12. Errani C, Traina F, Chehrassan M, et al. Minimally invasive technique for curettage of chondroblastoma using endoscopic technique. Eur Rev Med Pharmacol Sci. 2014;18:3394–8.

13. Campos WK, Gasbarrini A, Boriani S. Case report: curetting osteoid osteoma of the spine using combined video-assisted thoracoscopic surgery and navigation. Clin Orthop. 2013;471:680–5. https://doi.org/10.1007/s11999-012-2725-5.

14. Rosenthal D. Endoscopic approaches to the thoracic spine. Eur Spine J. 2000;9(Suppl 1):S8–16.

15. Martins C, Cardoso AC, Alencastro LF, et al. Endoscopic-assisted lateral transatlantal approach to craniovertebral junction. World Neurosurg. 2010;74:351–8. https://doi.org/10.1016/j.wneu.2010.05.037.

16. Le Huec JC, Lesprit E, Guibaud JP, et al. Minimally invasive endoscopic approach to the cervicothoracic junction for vertebral metastases: report of two cases. Eur Spine J. 2001;10:421–6.

17. Young PS, Bell SW, Mahendra A. The evolving role of computer-assisted navigation in musculoskeletal oncology. Bone Joint J. 2015;97-B:258–64. https://doi.org/10.1302/0301-620X.97B2.34461.

18. Wong KC, Kumta SM. Computer-assisted tumor surgery in malignant bone tumors. Clin Orthop. 2013;471:750–61. https://doi.org/10.1007/s11999-012-2557-3.

19. Loblaw DA, Perry J, Chambers A, Laperriere NJ. Systematic review of the diagnosis and management of malignant extradural spinal cord compression: the Cancer Care Ontario Practice Guidelines Initiative's Neuro-Oncology Disease Site Group. J Clin Oncol. 2005;23:2028–37. https://doi.org/10.1200/JCO.2005.00.067.

20. Lee C-H, Kwon J-W, Lee J, et al. Direct decompressive surgery followed by radiotherapy versus radiotherapy alone for metastatic epidural spinal cord compression: a meta-analysis. Spine. 2014;39:E587–92. https://doi.org/10.1097/BRS.0000000000000258.

21. Kim D-Y, Lee S-H, Chung SK, Lee H-Y. Comparison of multifidus muscle atrophy and trunk extension muscle strength: percutaneous versus open pedicle screw fixation. Spine. 2005;30:123–9.

22. Veeravagu A, Patil CG, Lad SP, Boakye M. Risk factors for postoperative spinal wound infections after spinal decompression and fusion surgeries. Spine. 2009;34:1869–72. https://doi.org/10.1097/BRS.0b013e3181adc989.

23. Kwan MK, Lee CK, Chan CYW. Minimally invasive spinal stabilization using fluoroscopic-guided percutaneous screws as a form of palliative surgery in patients with spinal metastasis. Asian Spine J. 2016;10:99–110. https://doi.org/10.4184/asj.2016.10.1.99.

24. Rao PJ, Thayaparan GK, Fairhall JM, Mobbs RJ. Minimally invasive percutaneous fixation techniques for metastatic spinal disease. Orthop Surg. 2014;6:187–95. https://doi.org/10.1111/os.12114.

25. Zairi F, Arikat A, Allaoui M, et al. Minimally invasive decompression and stabilization for the management of thoracolumbar spine metastasis. J Neurosurg Spine. 2012;17:19–23. https://doi.org/10.3171/2012.4.SPINE111108.

26. Versteeg AL, Verlaan J-J, de Baat P, et al. Complications after percutaneous pedicle screw fixation for the treatment of unstable spinal metastases. Ann Surg Oncol. 2016;23:2343–9. https://doi.org/10.1245/s10434-016-5156-9.

27. Shim CS, Lee S-H, Jung B, et al. Fluoroscopically assisted percutaneous translaminar facet screw fixation following anterior lumbar interbody fusion: technical report. Spine. 2005;30:838–43.

28. Nathan SS, Healey JH, Mellano D, et al. Survival in patients operated on for pathologic fracture: implications for end-of-life orthopedic care. J Clin Oncol. 2005;23:6072–82. https://doi.org/10.1200/JCO.2005.08.104.

Treatment of Bone Metastases: Future Directions

27

Guido Scoccianti and Rodolfo Capanna

Abstract

Four main future directions in the treatment of bone metastases can likely be envisaged: fewer tumors in general population, fewer bone metastases in patients affected by tumors, less invasive therapies, and in selected cases highly invasive surgery also in metastatic patients who have been often banished to palliative treatment so far. Development and improvements of current techniques and introduction of new technological achievements are expected to improve actual therapeutic regimens. Nanotechnologies and a combination of diagnosis and treatment in the same time (theranostics) are likely to deeply change our approach to bone metastatic disease and, we hope, its results. New and less invasive surgical procedures are going to progressively decrease the surgical burden on most of the metastatic patients who will still need surgery, but at the same time, a growing number of these patients will undergo highly invasive surgery, due to the application of the criteria of primary tumor surgery also to metastatic patients, thanks to the improved survival. The future of the treatment of bone metastases will surely be a varied and variegated future, ranging from the use of extremely small devices, like nanoprobes, to the use of megaprostheses, and maybe also combinations of them. The clinician will have to be ready to manage a continuously growing range of therapeutic options and to have the capability to choose the right one for the specific patient.

Keywords

Bone metastases · Orthopedic oncology Mini-invasive surgery · Nanomedicine Future treatments

27.1 Introduction

Predicting the future is always a hard job and that's particularly true when dealing with an ever-evolving matter like medicine.

Innovations in the future treatment of bone metastases are likely to include some procedures which are already at their start today or which can already be envisaged on the basis of our actual knowledge and practice but also (at least, we hope so) completely new treatments following upcoming new theoretical and technical achievements. It's therefore very difficult to write a chapter about

G. Scoccianti (✉)
Department of Orthopaedic Oncology and Reconstructive Surgery, Careggi University Hospital, Florence, Italy
e-mail: scocciantig@aou-careggi.toscana.it

R. Capanna
Department of Orthopaedics and Traumatology, Translational Research and Innovative Techniques, University of Pisa, Pisa, Italy

future treatments, and maybe we can only focus on the main directions which have to be addressed in the forthcoming years to take us to the future of our practice on bone metastatic disease.

The most important directions, which we have to move to, are four:

1. Fewer tumors in our population
2. Fewer bone metastases in patients affected by tumors
3. Less invasive therapies
4. In selected cases, highly invasive surgery also in metastatic patients (who have been often banished to palliative treatment so far)

In this paper, we mostly address the third and fourth of the abovementioned directions, which are the ones which directly involve the surgical care of metastatic patients.

27.1.1 Direction 1: Fewer Tumors in Our Population

Lowering tumor rate in our population is the first and most important target. Addressing this issue is out of the aim and possibility of this chapter. Key factors to move in this direction will be a better understanding of tumor pathogenesis and spreading, together with an improved knowledge about tumor risk factors and causative agents. Consequent actions will have to be adopted about environment (pollution, climate, etc.), diet, and habits.

27.1.2 Direction 2: Less Bone Metastases Occurring in Patients Affected by Tumor

Bone metastatic disease is a heavy complication for patients affected by oncological diseases.

Spreading of the tumor to the bone causes to the patient pain, functional impairment, and the need of additional medical and surgical therapies. For many patients affected by tumor bone metastases constitute the first and worst cause of symptoms.

On this basis, reducing the rate of bone metastatic disease in a patient after the diagnosis of cancer is of outstanding importance.

Several pathways should be followed to obtain this result.

First, an earlier diagnosis of cancer can help us to prevent tumor progression with a treatment applied earlier and against tumors at their initial stage. More efficient, less invasive, and also cheaper screening methods of the population should be developed, involving a wider number of tumors in comparison with the few screening programs activated at the moment.

Not only an earlier but also a better diagnosis will be hopefully made available in the forthcoming decades. A better understanding of tumor characteristics of every single case could help us in choosing the best therapeutic approach case by case, with a tailor-made treatment choice. Identification of new methods of tumor tracing and follow-up diagnostics could anticipate metastases detection and treatment.

Improvements in medical treatment of oncological diseases could reduce the number of patients developing metastatic disease, making the prognosis of cancer patients better and lowering the burden of treatments necessary for oncological patients. Some aspects of the modalities for these improvements will be discussed in the following section.

27.1.3 Direction 3: Less Invasive Therapies

When bone metastatic disease has occurred, treatment must be undertaken. The metastatic cancer patient is a frail patient, affected by a widespread oncological disease with its direct and indirect (paraneoplastic) consequences and also affected by the effects of chemotherapy regimens on bone marrow, liver, kidney, and immunological system. Moreover, the life expectancy is still generally short. In this setting, treatments least invasive as possible are usually advocated, also to lessen the possibility of occurrence of postsurgical complications which can negatively affect the chances of undergoing further systemic treatment for the primary oncological disease.

A better understanding of cancer biology can lead to the introduction in the near future of more efficient and more selective medical therapies with the development of targeted therapeutic strategies designed to attack a single or a few targets governing the survival and proliferation of cancer cells. New therapies should address the survival strategies of tumor cells in order to kill cancer cells while sparing normal cells. Cancer cells have distinctive patterns of development, growing, and spreading, the so-called hallmarks of cancer [1, 2], which can be used as specific pathways to be targeted to succeed in inhibiting tumor growth. Therapeutic targeting of the hallmarks of cancer could and should be the keystone of development of more selective therapies [3]. These targets can involve genetic aberrations including mutations (single-base substitutions), amplifications, translocations (e.g., gene fusion), deletions, and insertions/deletions [4].

How can we get there? Definition of specific single or few targets governing the proliferation of genetically distinct populations of cancer cells can make it possible to find out selective and more efficient drugs. This is what is already ongoing and is generally called "targeted therapy," but it's nowadays still at its beginning, and major advancements are expected in the near future or, at least, we hope so. A better molecular understanding of cancer pathways can lead us to the production of new molecular weapons to fight tumors, optimizing not only drug mechanism of action but also drug delivering and on-site activation, thus obtaining increased drug efficacy and safety.

Another key factor in this evolution of our treatments can be molecular imaging. Imaging specific molecular patterns in vivo can in fact make us able to choose the best treatment and to monitor its effect in the patient. Direct monitoring of the response to treatment can let us modify our therapeutical choices and treat any patient with a tailor-made plan.

A personalized cancer therapy thus relies on a targeted therapy and on innovations in imaging technology. The introduction of nanoprobe technology and the possibility that nanomedicine offers for selective tracking and hitting of specific molecular targets has recently open the doors to enormous advancements in our capabilities of fighting cancer.

27.1.3.1 Theranostics and Nanomedicine

A combination of diagnostics and treatment in the same action can reduce treatment starting time and, most important, improve efficacy of treatment by a guided delivery of the drug. Furthermore, diagnostics monitoring can help to confirm or modify treatment schedule on the basis of its results.

This kind of approach has gained more and more interest in the latest years, and it's now known as "theranostics." This term describes any material that combines the modalities of therapy and diagnostic imaging into a single unit, and it's now used to describe image-guided therapy or therapeutic agents which concomitantly possess imaging capabilities. Theranostics includes diagnostic tests to identify patients most likely to be helped by a therapeutic procedure, targeted therapy, and in vivo imaging to tailor and monitor treatment.

For example, ErbB2 in breast cancer can be directly visualized, improving the MRI image with an ErbB2-specific antibody-conjugated MRI nanoprobe (molecular imaging); at the same time, therapeutic agents can be delivered to the tumor together with the ErbB2-specific nanoprobe, and the response to treatment can be monitored, thus completing the theranostics approach [3].

Nanoprobes can be conjugated with aptamers or antibodies to target specific molecules with the aim of both a diagnostic and therapeutic improvement, and they can be loaded with drugs or other agents with antitumoral activity. Furthermore, nanoprobes have an inherent tendency to a preferential delivery to tumor sites due to the EPR effect because of the leaky neovasculature of tumors and the absence of lymphatic drainage [5].

Treatment of bone metastases can greatly benefit from these ongoing technological developments.

A drug can be covalently bonded to an osteotropic moiety like bisphosphonates and thus targeted to the bone [6], or it can be added to a nanoprobe, using its tendency to target tumor environment. Using both strategies can furtherly enhance the efficacy of our treatment, and with this aim, bone-seeking osteotropic drug delivery systems (ODDS) were introduced in recent years, adding to the surface of a nanoprobe a targeting molecule (bisphosphonates) and loading the nanoprobe with an antitumoral drug [7–10]. This can offer several advantages, like protection of the drug from biodegradation in the bloodstream, higher drug delivery doses, and longer circulation times.

To selectively deliver drugs to bone metastases, we can use different targets, including bone (bisphosphonates), tumor cells (antibodies, aptamers), and tumor environment (nanocarriers exploiting EPR effect due to leaky tumor neovasculature; nanoprobes which can respond to specific characteristics of tumor environment like acidic condition).

Nanocarriers can deliver to the tumor not only drugs (cytotoxic or antiangiogenetic) but also radiopharmaceuticals, gene therapy vectors (DNA or RNA), hyperthermia, and photodynamic therapy.

Thermoablation with a temperature higher than 50 °C causes tumor destruction by direct cell necrosis, but normal tissue is involved by the necrosis as well. Hyperthermia with a temperature of 41–45 °C induces damages to intracellular proteins and consequently to cellular function; tumor cells are generally significantly more prone to this kind of damage, while normal tissue is minimally affected. Thus, delivery of a hyperthermic treatment at the site of the tumor can produce important damages to the neoplastic cells with only minor effects on normal tissues. Magnetic nanoparticles and gold nanoparticles are promising hyperthermia-inducing agents. Magnetic nanoparticles produce heat via energy loss pathways when an external alternating electromagnetic field is applied. If we deliver these nanoparticles to the tumors, we can then activate the heat production through application of an external electromagnetic field. First, clinical applications of this technique were recently reported in prostate and brain cancer [11, 12]; utilization in bone metastases could be available in the future.

Local heat can also be produced by nanoparticles able to absorb near-infrared light like gold nanoparticles, and their action can also be augmented by adding chemotherapeutics to the gold nanoparticle with a combined effect of hyperthermia and chemotherapy [13, 14].

Photodynamic therapy could be another treatment option. In this kind of treatment, photosensitizer molecules are activated by light, and, when this happens, they generate reactive oxygen species (ROS), which can kill cancer cells by damage to DNA, RNA, and proteins. The use of photosensitizer able to absorb near-infrared light permits to penetrate more deeply in the tissues. Some clinical experiences were reported in literature for different kinds of cancer [15–18].

27.1.3.2 Radiotherapy and Nuclear Medicine

Radiation therapy has always had a primary role in bone metastases treatment, and it's going to maintain it. In the last decades, huge technological advancements were made, improving both efficacy and delivery to the target of the radiation treatment. Nowadays, we can use several different radiation modalities, from the traditional (and still most used and widespread) photons to electrons, protons, neutrons, Π-mesons (pions), heavy-charged nuclei (carbon, helium, neon), and antiprotons.

If most bone metastases can be effectively treated with photons, the use of charged particles (hadrontherapy) in selected cases can increase efficacy and allow better sparing of the surrounding tissues. The limited availability and the cost of these treatments are actually limiting their use, but an increase in the number of centers with hadrontherapy facilities could make these treatments more widely available in the future.

In the last decades, great improvements have been obtained not only in efficacy but also in delivery modalities, leading to the development of techniques like intensity-modulated radiation therapy (IMRT), stereotactic radiotherapy (Gamma Knife, Cyberknife), and image-guided and electronic brachytherapy. These techniques allow us to perform a more precise and effective (higher dose) radiation treatment on the target with a better sparing of surrounding tissues. This possibility has led also to the development of new concepts on treatment of the metastatic patients like stereotactic body radiotherapy in oligometastatic disease [19, 20]. If we assume that at the beginning of metastatic disease a patient can present with only a few metastases before widespread dissemination of the disease and that in this phase we can still eradicate the disease [21], the role of radiotherapy in the management of metastatic disease can be no more limited only to palliation but could also constitute an attempt to really change disease progression, delivering radical ablative doses of radiation instead of subradical palliative doses. Such a treatment can nowadays be performed, targeting also several sites, because of the reduction of collateral effects and damages to the healthy tissues determined by the introduction of the abovementioned new techniques.

Developments in nuclear medicine techniques are also leading to important opportunities for a better control of bone metastatic disease. Different bone-seeking radiopharmaceuticals have been introduced to selectively deliver treatment to the bone, from beta-emitter strontium-89 to gamma-emitter samarium-153 and, more recently, alpha-emitter radium-223. Radium-223 dichloride is a bone-seeking calcium mimetic that selectively binds to areas of increased bone turnover (osteoblastic or sclerotic bone metastases), emitting short-range alpha particles which induce DNA damages with a consequent cytotoxic effect; the short range of these particles permits substantial sparing of nontarget tissue. Interesting results were reported in treatment of osteoblastic metastatic disease with radium-223, particularly in prostate cancer [22–24].

Combining of radiopharmaceuticals and bisphosphonates is also possible to selectively deliver the radiopharmaceutical to the bone [25]. Nanomedicine will further improve this delivery because of the higher doses of radiopharmaceutical which can be taken to the target by a nanoprobe, and development of similar delivery systems is ongoing [26].

27.1.3.3 Minimally Invasive Surgery

Minimally invasive surgery to treat bone metastases has greatly developed in the last years. Now we can percutaneously ablate a tumor with several different techniques. Radiofrequency ablation was the first technique to find a widespread use, but treatment of bone metastases can be performed also with cryotreatment by argon-helios cryoprobes, microwaves, and laser. Moreover, a transcutaneous treatment (without any incision) can be delivered with the expanding technology of MRI-guided high-intensity focused ultrasounds (HIFU). All these techniques are based on a thermal (with heat or cold) ablation of the tumor. A different strategy has led to the development of electrochemotherapy, recently expanded also to the bone [27], which is based on a percutaneous electric shock to the target area, which makes the tissue hundreds of times more vulnerable to the effects of chemotherapeutics systemically delivered.

All these techniques are showing interesting results in selected indications, but few consistent series were reported up to now and with usually short follow-up [28–34]. Specific description of percutaneous treatments of bone tumors and its results can be found in previous chapters, and it's not the matter of this paper. A recent review on different ablation techniques can be found in a paper of Kurup and Callstrom [35].

Minimally invasive treatment of bone metastases is surely destined to gain a more and more widespread use in the near future.

At the moment, there are some questions which remain open and unanswered:

– When choosing a percutaneous ablation treatment versus a radiation treatment?
– Which is the best technique?
– Are there specific characteristics which can lead us to a case-by-case patient-tailored choice of the ablation technique?

We hope that in the next years, we will have enough data to get these answers.

As far as we can now evaluate, among ablation treatments cryoablation and HIFU appear particularly promising. Cryoablation has in fact some advantages in comparison to radiofrequency ablation, particularly the possibility to visualize on CT images the treated area as an "ice ball" (Fig. 27.1), the chance to use multiple probes simultaneously to increase the treatment area and to better adapt it to the geometry of the target, a better toleration of the procedure by the patient due to a reduced postoperative pain, a reduced risk of damage to nearby critical structures due to visualization of the ablation margin on CT, and the possibility of tissue displacement with catheter-guided balloon [33, 36]; also a reduced damage to joint cartilage in iuxtarticular sites can be presumed.

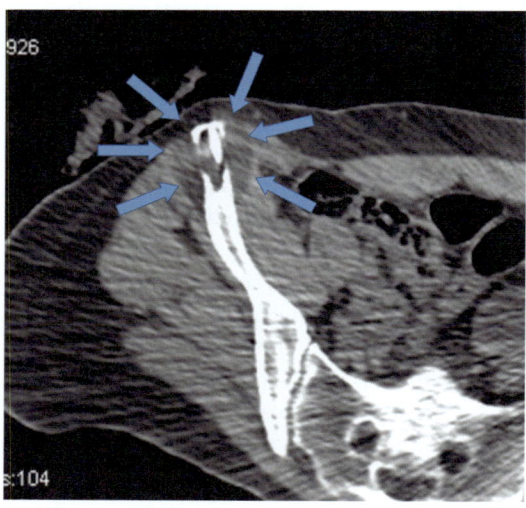

Fig. 27.1 CT visualization of the area of treatment ("ice ball") during cryoablation of a metastasis of the iliac wing from renal cell carcinoma

HIFU technique has the advantage of being a completely "closed" procedure with ultrasound delivered transcutaneously and not percutaneously and with the possibility to obtain a delivery which is well conformed to the geometry of the target [37, 38]. The MRI guide of the procedure permits to treat also the bone, but at the moment its diffusion is limited due to the high costs. A more widespread use of this technique is likely to occur in the forthcoming years.

Also, electrochemotherapy is a promising technique, particularly for its much higher effect on tumor cells than on healthy tissue and the possibility, at least theoretically, of a better sparing of normal bone in comparison to other ablative procedures, but further experience is needed to define its results and indications. In electrochemotherapy, an active drug is administered systemically and a local sensitizing treatment is performed. Also, the opposite can be hypothesized: for example, the systemic administration of a photosensitizer compound, and then a local percutaneous treatment with laser was recently proposed [39].

27.1.3.4 Improving Open Surgery

Surgical treatment of bone metastases presents peculiar aspects in diagnosis, treatment, and follow-up, which differentiate this field of orthope-dic surgery from trauma surgery or primary tumors surgery.

Following improvements in cancer patient survival during last decades, surgical treatment of bone metastases is not any more a minor issue, limited to procedures intended to offer a palliative treatment in pathological fractures, but it is becoming a major task in orthopedic surgery, particularly in centers devoted to oncological surgery but also in the general orthopedic units.

In this setting, new and specifically designed devices have been developed in recent years, and an increased attention should be expected for this kind of surgery in the future.

New Intramedullary Devices

In other chapters of this book, some of the recent most outstanding innovations are described, like carbon fiber nails and plates, which permit a better delivery of postoperative radiation treatment and allow a more effective follow-up with imaging diagnostics [40], or intramedullary implants with minimal invasiveness, which can conform to the intramedullary cavity, thanks to a combination of balloons, light-activated monomers, and flexible catheters [41].

These are important improvements for our surgical practice, and others are likely to follow in the near future, due to the increased interest in this field of orthopedic surgery.

Improving Excision of Metastatic Tissue

If in many cases a closed nailing can still be the treatment of choices in metastatic patients, a growing number of patients today can and should be better treated with excision of the tumor to avoid local oncological progression in patients who can present nowadays a long survival.

Excision of the tumor can be accomplished either with intralesional or wide procedures, according to tumor site and extension, to residual bone stability and prognosis of the patient, and to the expected response of the metastatic tumor to the adjuvant therapies.

Patients most fit for an excision procedure are the patients affected by one or a few bone metastases, in accordance to the definition of oligometastatic patient above reported when dealing with radiation treatment strategies, but also patients affected by plurimetastatic disease can need extended and even wide procedures due to the local condition of the bone. This is particularly true when dealing with metastases from tumors usually poor responding to radiation treatment, like renal cell carcinoma, where surgery is often the mainstay of treatment also for metastatic disease.

Improvements in curettage procedure can be expected in the near future, both in the identification and use of adjuvant local treatments for the residual bone walls and in the effectiveness of the procedure of excision itself.

For example, delivery of cryotreatment in the residual cavity after curettage, which has a long history with the use of liquid nitrogen, has recently become safer and more conforming to the different anatomical sites with the introduction of argon probes systems. This is going to expand the use of this technique, which seems to be at the moment the more effective for its capacity to act more deeply on the bone than the other commonly used adjuvant treatments.

Filling with cement with addition of chemotherapeutics or bisphosphonates can be another useful step to enhance our treatment effect on the residual bone after curettage, and further innovations are likely to appear in the future in this field.

We can expect also technological improvements to help us in the future to increase the precision itself and completeness of our curettage procedures. Fluorescence-guided surgery is a promising technique for in-the-field detection of tumor cells. First in-human results were reported in different fields of oncological surgery, mostly using fluorescence for lymph node mapping but also using specific tumor receptors to track tumor cells in glioma [42–44], pancreatic cancer [45], and ovarian cancer [46]. A similar technique could be quite helpful also in bone metastatic disease, using specific tumor receptors as targets. At the best of our knowledge, no in-human experience on bone metastases were reported so far, but some experimental works are already moving in this direction, for example, in experimental bone metastases from prostate cancer, demonstrating a better result after excision using fluorescence-guided surgery [47, 48]. Application of these techniques is rapidly growing in oncological surgery, and also bone metastases surgery could benefit of it in the forthcoming years.

27.1.4 Direction 4: Highly Invasive Surgery Also in Metastatic Patients

Also in surgery of bone metastases, minimally invasive or less invasive procedures are not always the procedures which best fit the patient requirements. Bone metastatic patients have been often banished to palliative treatment so far, but due to the improvements in medical treatments and prolonged survival, another direction of future treatment of bone metastases will be a growing application to the metastatic patient of procedures usually dedicated to primary bone tumors.

Revision surgery in bone metastases has become a not rare occurrence, due to a local progression of disease or a mechanical failure of the reconstruction in patients who present long survival (Fig. 27.2). It's therefore important to select the patients with better prognosis and to apply also to these patients the concepts of surgical treatment of primary bone tumors.

Resection and reconstruction with megaprostheses in metastatic patient is therefore likely to become a more and more frequent surgery in the near future.

Also in difficult locations, like the spine and pelvis, surgical treatment is going to increase its indications and applications, with major surgery applied also to secondary disease, when needed.

Improvements in anesthesiologic perioperative support to the patients make today possible to perform highly invasive procedures also in these patients. Dedicated medical teams are advised for this kind of surgery. In these settings, and in a frail patient like the metastatic patient, every effort to reduce the surgical burden on the patient is to be attempted. To reduce perioperative blood loss, preoperative selective arterial embolization will continue to be a fundamental aid for the surgeon. Another aid which can be used and maybe will increase its application in the near future is the application of intraoperative cryotreatment to reduce blood loss. The introduction of argon cryoprobes has made possible to freeze a tumor and to curette it with a minimum bleeding, also in highly vascularized tumors like many bone metastases (Fig. 27.3).

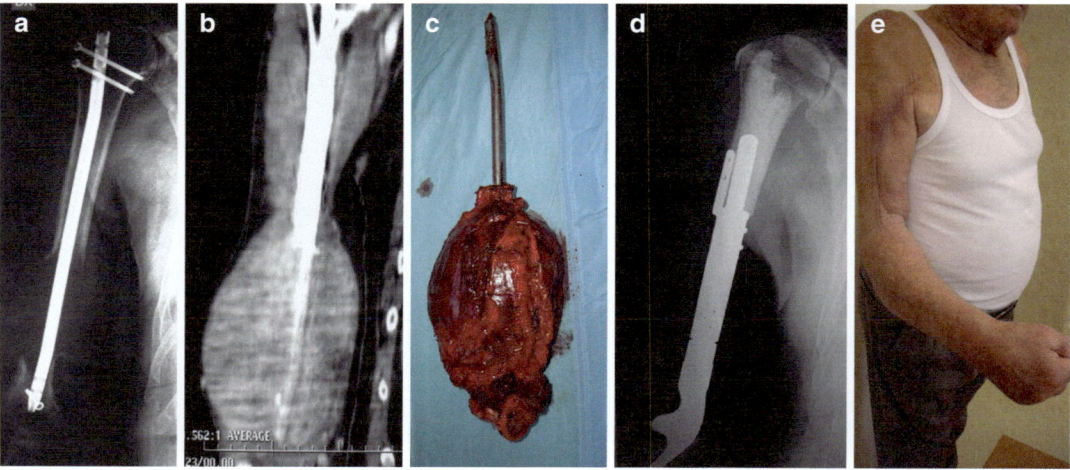

Fig. 27.2 Metastasis of the distal humerus from hepatic carcinoma with local progression after intramedullary nailing. (**a**, **b**) Preoperative X-ray and CT view. (**c**) Resected specimen. (**d**) Postoperative X-ray view after reconstruction with elbow megaprosthesis. (**e**) Postoperative elbow flexion

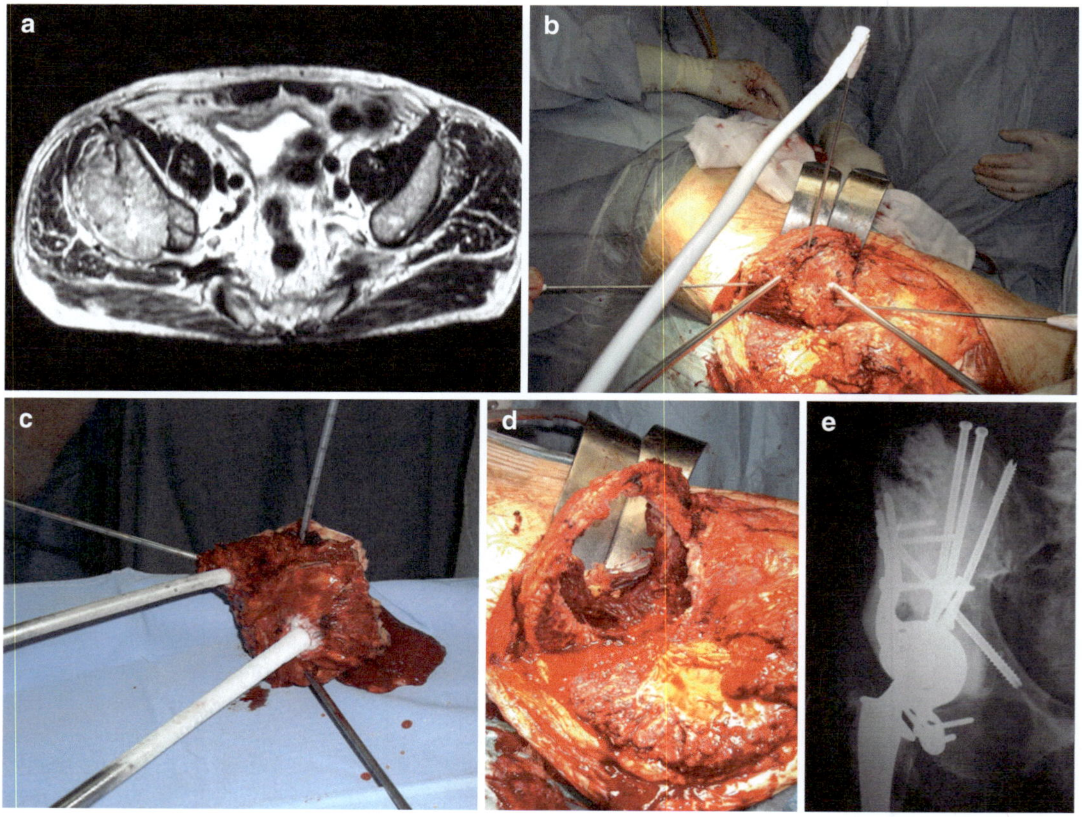

Fig. 27.3 Metastasis of the periacetabular region from renal cell carcinoma. (**a**) Preoperative MRI axial view. (**b, c**) Intraoperative views during freezing of the tumor to decrease bleeding while curetting the metastatic disease. (**d**) Intraoperative view after curettage. (**e**) Postoperative X-ray view after reconstruction with cement and hip arthroplasty

Conclusions

There are not conclusions when talking about future directions. We can say that the future of the treatment of bone metastases will surely be varied and variegated, ranging from the use of extremely small devices, like nanoprobes, to the use of megaprostheses, and maybe also combinations of them. The clinicians will have to be ready to manage a continuously growing range of therapeutic options and to have the capability to choose the right one for the specific patient.

They will have to be always ready to change their practices and to adopt new ideas and techniques, without forgetting the experience of the past. A multidisciplinary approach is and will be mandatory in this field.

References

1. Hanahan D, Weinberg RA. The hallmarks of cancer. Cell. 2000;100:57–70.
2. Hanahan D, Weinberg RA. Hallmarks of cancer: the next generation. Cell. 2011;144:646–74.
3. Lim EK, Kim T, Paik S, Haam S, Huh YM, Lee K. Nanomaterials for theranostics: recent advances and future challenges. Chem Rev. 2015;115:327–94.
4. Vogelstein B, Papadopoulos N, Velculescu VE, Zhou S, Diaz LA, Kinzler KW, et al. Cancer genome landscapes. Science. 2013;339:1546–58.
5. Iyer AK, Khaled G, Fang J, Maeda H. Exploiting the enhanced permeability and retention effect for tumor targeting. Drug Discov Today. 2006;11:812–8.
6. Hirsjärvi S, Passirani C, Benoit JP. Passive and active tumor targeting with nanocarriers. Curr Drug Discov Technol. 2011;8:188–96.
7. Bonzi G, Salmaso S, Scomparin A, Eldar-Boock A, Satch-Fainaro R, Caliceti P. Novel pullulan bioconjugate for selective breast cancer bone metastases treatment. Bioconjug Chem. 2015;26:489–501.
8. Chen H, Li G, Chi H, Wang D, Tu C, Pan L, Zhu L, Qiu F, Guo F, Zhu X. Alendronate-conjugated amphiphilic hyperbranched polymer based on Boltorn H40 and poly(ethylene glycol) for bone-targeted drug delivery. Bioconjug Chem. 2012;23:1915–24.
9. Miller K, Erez R, Segal E, Shabat D, Satchi-Fainaro R. Targeting bone metastases with a bispecific anticancer and antiangiogenic polymer-alendronate-taxane conjugate. Angew Chem. 2009;48:2949–54.
10. Pignatello R, Sarpietro MG, Castelli F. Synthesis and biological evaluation of a new polymeric conjugate and nanocarrier with osteotropic properties. J Funct Biomater. 2012;3:79–99.
11. Krishnan S, Diagaradjane P, Cho S. Nanoparticle-mediated thermal therapy: evolving strategies for prostate cancer therapy. Int J Hyperth. 2010;26:775–89.
12. Maier-Hauff K, Ulrich F, Nestler D, Niehoff H, Wust P, Thiesen B, et al. Efficacy and safety of intratumoral thermotherapy using magnetic iron-oxide nanoparticles combined with external beam radiotherapy on patients with recurrent glioblastoma multiforme. J Neuro-Oncol. 2011;103:317–24.
13. Agarwal A, Mackey MA, El-Sayed MA, Bellamkonda RV. Remote triggered release of doxorubicin in tumors by synergistic application of thermosensitive liposomes and gold nanorods. ACS Nano. 2011;5:4919–26.
14. Park JH, von Maltzahn G, Ong LL, Centrone A, Hatton TA, Ruoslahti E, et al. Cooperative nanoparticles for tumor detection and photothermally triggered drug delivery. Adv Mater. 2010;22:880–5.
15. Green B, Cobb ARM, Hopper C. Photodynamic therapy in the management of lesions of the head and neck. Br J Oral Maxillofac Surg. 2013;51:283–7.
16. Nahashima A, Nagayasu T. Current status of photodynamic therapy in digestive tract carcinoma in Japan. Int J Mol Sci. 2015;16:3430–40.
17. Simone CB, Cengel KA. Photodynamic therapy for lung cancer and malignant pleural mesothelioma. Semin Oncol. 2014;41:820–30.
18. Yano T, Muto M, Yoshimura K, Niimi M, Ezoe Y, Yoda Y, et al. Phase I study of photodynamic therapy using talaporfin sodium and diode laser for local failure after chemoradiotherpay for esophageal cancer. Radiat Oncol. 2012;7:113.
19. Dagan R, Lo SS, Redmond KJ, Poon I, Foote MC, Lohr F, et al. A multi-national report on stereotactic body radiotherapy for oligometastases: patient selection and follow-up. Acta Oncol. 2016;55:633–7.
20. Tree AC, Khoo VS, Eeles RA, Ahmed M, Dearnaley DP, Hawkins MA, et al. Stereotactic body radiotherapy for oligometastases. Lancet Oncol. 2013;14:e28–37.
21. Hellman S, Weichselbaum RR. Oligometastases. J Clin Oncol. 1995;13:8–10.
22. El-Amm J, Aragon-Ching JB. Targeting bone metastases in metastatic castration-resistant prostate cancer. Clin Med Insights Oncol. 2016;10:11–9.
23. Kairemo K, Joensuu T. Radium-223-dichloride in castration resistant metastatic prostate cancer-preliminary results of the response evaluation using F-18-fluoride PET/CT. Diagnostics. 2015;5:413–27.
24. Parker C, Nilsson S, Heinrich D, Helle SI, O'Sullivan JM, Fosså SD, et al. Alpha emitter radium-223 and survival in metastatic prostate cancer. N Engl J Med. 2013;369:213–23.
25. Yuan J, Liu C, Liu X, Wang Y, Kuai D, Zhang G, et al. Efficacy and safety of 177Lu-EDTMP in bone metastatic pain palliation in breast cancer and hormone refractory prostate cancer: a phase II study. Clin Nucl Med. 2013;38:88–92.
26. Song L, Falzone N, Vallis KA. EGF-coated gold nanoparticles provide an efficient nano-scale delivery system for the molecular radiotherapy of EGFR-positive cancer. Int J Radiat Biol. 2016;21:1–8.

27. Miklavčič D, Serša G, Brecelj E, Gehl J, Soden D, Bianchi G, et al. Electrochemotherapy: technological advancements for efficient electroporation-based treatment of internal tumors. Med Biol Eng Comput. 2012;50:1213–25.

28. Callstrom MR, Dupuy DE, Solomon SB, Beres RA, Littrup PJ, Davis KW, et al. Percutaneous image-guided cryoablation of painful metastases involving bone: multicenter trial. Cancer. 2013;119:1033–41.

29. Damian E, Dupuy DE, Liu D, Hartfeil D, Hanna L, Blume JD, et al. Percutaneous radiofrequency ablation of painful osseous metastases: a multicenter American College of Radiology Imaging Network trial. Cancer. 2010;116:989–97.

30. Deschamps F, Farouil G, Ternes N, Gaudin A, Hakime A, Tselikas L, et al. Thermal ablation techniques: a curative treatment of bone metastases in selected patients? Eur Radiol. 2014;24:1971–80.

31. Goetz MP, Callstrom MR, Charboneau JW, Farrell MA, Maus TP, Welch TJ, et al. Percutaneous image-guided radiofrequency ablation of painful metastases involving bone: a multicenter study. J Clin Oncol. 2004;22:300–6.

32. McMenomy BP, Kurup AN, Johnson GB, Carter RE, McWilliams RR, Markovic SN, et al. Percutaneous cryoablation of musculoskeletal oligometastatic disease for complete remission. J Vasc Interv Radiol. 2013;24:207–13.

33. Thacker PG, Callstrom MR, Curry TB, Mandrekar JN, Atwell TD, Goetz MP, et al. Palliation of painful metastatic disease involving bone with imaging-guided treatment: comparison of patients' immediate response to radiofrequency ablation and cryoablation. AJR Am J Roentgenol. 2011;197:510–5.

34. Thanos L, Mylona S, Galani P, Tzavoulis D, Kalioras V, Tanteles S, et al. Radiofrequency ablation of osseous metastases for the palliation of pain. Skelet Radiol. 2008;37:189–94.

35. Kurup AN, Callstrom MR. Ablation of musculoskeletal metastases: pain palliation, fracture risk reduction, and oligometastatic disease. Tech Vasc Interv Radiol. 2013;16:253–61.

36. Callstrom MR, Kurup AN. Percutaneous ablation for bone and soft tissue metastases—why cryoablation? Skelet Radiol. 2009;38:835–9.

37. Liberman B, Gianfelice D, Inbar Y, Beck A, Rabin T, Shabshin N, et al. Pain palliation in patients with bone metastases using MR-guided focused ultrasound surgery: a multicenter study. Ann Surg Oncol. 2009;16:140–6.

38. Tempany CM, McDannold NJ, Hynynen K, Jolesz FA. Focused ultrasound surgery in oncology: overview and principles. Radiology. 2011;259:39–56.

39. Lo VC, Akens MK, Moore S, Yee AJ, Wilson BC, Whyne CM. Beyond radiation therapy: photodynamic therapy maintains structural integrity of irradiated healthy and metastatically involved vertebrae in a pre-clinical in vivo model. Breast Cancer Res Treat. 2012;135:391–401.

40. Zimel MN, Hwang S, Riedel ER, Healey JH. Carbon fiber intramedullary nails reduce artifact in postoperative advanced imaging. Skelet Radiol. 2015;44:1317–25.

41. Vegt P, Muir JM, Block JE. The photodynamic bone stabilization system: a minimally invasive, percutaneous intramedullary polymeric osteosynthesis for simple and complex long bone fractures. Med Devices (Auckl). 2014;7:453–61.

42. Hadjipanayis CG, Widhalm G, Stummer W. What is the surgical benefit of utilizing 5-aminolevulinic acid for fluorescence-guided surgery of malignant gliomas? Neurosurgery. 2015;77:663–73.

43. Stummer W, Pichlmeier U, Meinel T, Wiestler OD, Zanella F, Reulen HJ, et al. Fluorescence-guided surgery with 5-aminolevulinic acid for resection of malignant glioma: a randomised controlled multicentre phase III trial. Lancet Oncol. 2006;7:392–401.

44. Zhao S, Wu J, Wang C, Liu H, Dong X, Shi C, et al. Intraoperative fluorescence-guided resection of high-grade malignant gliomas using 5-aminolevulinic acid-induced porphyrins: a systematic review and meta-analysis of prospective studies. PLoS One. 2013;8:e63682.

45. McElroy M, Kaushal S, Luiken GA, Talamini MA, Moossa AR, Hoffman RM, et al. Imaging of primary and metastatic pancreatic cancer using a fluorophore conjugated anti-CA19-9 antibody for surgical navigation. World J Surg. 2008;32:1057.

46. Van Dam GM, Themelis G, Crane LM, Harlaar NJ, Pleijhuis RG, Kelder W, et al. Intraoperative tumor-specific fluorescence imaging in ovarian cancer by folate receptor-α targeting: first in-human results. Nat Med. 2011;17:1315–9.

47. Miwa S, Matsumoto Y, Hiroshima Y, Yano S, Uehara F, Yamamoto M, et al. Fluorescence-guided surgery of prostate cancer bone metastasis. J Surg Res. 2014;192:124–33.

48. Miwa S, De Magalhães N, Toneri M, Zhang Y, Cao W, Bouvet M, et al. Fluorescence-guided surgery of human prostate cancer experimental bone metastasis in nude mice using anti-CEA DyLight 650 for tumor illumination. J Orthop Res. 2016;34:559–65.

MIX
Papier aus verantwortungsvollen Quellen
Paper from responsible sources
FSC® C105338

If you have any concerns about our products,
you can contact us on
ProductSafety@springernature.com

In case Publisher is established outside the EU,
the EU authorized representative is:
Springer Nature Customer Service Center GmbH
Europaplatz 3, 69115 Heidelberg, Germany

Printed by Libri Plureos GmbH
in Hamburg, Germany